An Introduction to Orthodontics

An Introduction to Orthodontics

FIFTH EDITION

Simon J. Littlewood

MDSc, BDS, FDS (Orth) RCPS (Glasg), M. Orth RCS (Edin), FDSRCS (Eng)
Consultant Orthodontist, St Luke's Hospital, Bradford, UK
Honorary Senior Clinical Lecturer, Leeds Dental Institute, Leeds, UK

Laura Mitchell MBE

MDS, BDS, FDSRCPS (Glasg), FDSRCS (Eng), FGDP (UK),
D. Orth RCS (Eng), M. Orth RCS (Eng)
Retired. Previously, Consultant Orthodontist, St Luke's Hospital, Bradford, UK
Honorary Senior Clinical Lecturer, Leeds Dental Institute, Leeds, UK

With contributions from

Benjamin R. K. Lewis

BDS, MFDS RCS (Eng), MClinDent, M. Orth. RCS (Eng), FDS (Orth) RCS (Eng)
Consultant Orthodontist, Wrexham Maelor Hospital & Glan Clwyd Hospital, Rhyl, UK
Honorary Clinical Lecturer, University of Liverpool, UK

Sophy K. Barber

BDS, MSc, M. Orth RCS (Edin), PG Cert. Health Res.
Post-CCST Registrar in Orthodontics, Leeds Dental Institute and St Luke's Hospital,
Bradford, UK

Fiona R. Jenkins

MDSc, BDS, MFDS RCS (Eng), FDS (Orth) RCS (Eng), M. Orth RCS (Eng)
Consultant Orthodontist, St Luke's Hospital, Bradford, UK
Honorary Senior Clinical Lecturer, Leeds Dental Institute, Leeds, UK

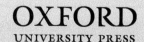

OXFORD
UNIVERSITY PRESS

OXFORD
UNIVERSITY PRESS

Great Clarendon Street, Oxford, OX2 6DP,
United Kingdom

Oxford University Press is a department of the University of Oxford.
It furthers the University's objective of excellence in research, scholarship,
and education by publishing worldwide. Oxford is a registered trade mark of
Oxford University Press in the UK and in certain other countries

Second edition 2001
Third edition 2007
Fourth edition 2013

Published in the United States of America by Oxford University Press
198 Madison Avenue, New York, NY 10016, United States of America

British Library Cataloguing in Publication Data

Data available

Library of Congress Control Number: 2018954270

ISBN 978–0–19–880866–4

Printed in Great Britain by
Bell & Bain Ltd., Glasgow

Oxford University Press makes no representation, express or implied, that the
drug dosages in this book are correct. Readers must therefore always check
the product information and clinical procedures with the most up-to-date
published product information and data sheets provided by the manufacturers
and the most recent codes of conduct and safety regulations. The authors and
the publishers do not accept responsibility or legal liability for any errors in the
text or for the misuse or misapplication of material in this work. Except where
otherwise stated, drug dosages and recommendations are for the non-pregnant
adult who is not breast-feeding

Links to third party websites are provided by Oxford in good faith and
for information only. Oxford disclaims any responsibility for the materials
contained in any third party website referenced in this work.

Preface for fifth edition

Orthodontics is both an art and a science, and, like most great works of art, at its best orthodontics can appear both deceptively simple and wonderfully aesthetic. The reality is of course that behind that apparent simplicity, there is real complexity that takes years to master. Gaining expertise in any subject requires sound foundations on which to build on, and we hope that this introduction to orthodontics provides these foundations.

In this new, significantly updated edition, we have tried to stay true to the ethos of the previous editions, providing key basic science and clinical information that is based on the best current evidence. We hope it will be useful to anyone involved in the treatment of orthodontic patients: undergraduate dental students, postgraduate students specializing in orthodontics, dentists with an interest in orthodontics, orthodontic therapists and orthodontic nurses, and perhaps even those more experienced orthodontists who would welcome a succinct evidence-based, sensible, and contemporary update on the subject of orthodontics.

We hope you enjoy it!

Simon J. Littlewood and Laura Mitchell

Acknowledgements

We would like to thank everyone who has assisted in completing this book, in particular our new contributing authors, Benjamin R. K. Lewis, Sophy K. Barber, and Fiona R. Jenkins. It has been a pleasure to work with these talented orthodontists on this project. We would also like to thank all those authors who have contributed to previous versions. Individual credits to clinicians who have provided figures for this edition are provided in the respective legends throughout the book. We would also like to sincerely thank all those patients who have provided consent to show their photos.

Working with busy authors is not always easy, so we would like to thank all those clinical and support staff who work with us on a daily basis.

For all those inspiring clinicians, teachers, and colleagues who have shared with us their knowledge, ideas, and experience throughout our careers, thank you.

We would also like to thank the staff of Oxford University Press for their help, patience, and expertise in guiding us through the publishing process.

And finally, to our respective families—Emma and Jack Littlewood, and David Mitchell—this book is dedicated to you.

Simon J. Littlewood and Laura Mitchell

Online Resources

 Further reading and references (including Cochrane Reviews) can also be found at:

www.oup.com/uk/orthodontics5e.

Where possible, these are presented as active links which direct you to the electronic version of the work, to help facilitate onward study. If you are a subscriber to that work (either individually or through an institution), and depending on your level of access, you may be able to peruse an abstract or the full article if available.

Brief contents

Detailed contents

1

The rationale for orthodontic treatment

S. K. Barber

Chapter contents

1.1 Orthodontics

Orthodontics is the branch of dentistry concerned with facial growth, development of the dentition and occlusion, and the diagnosis, interception, and treatment of occlusal anomalies.

1.2 Malocclusion

'Ideal occlusion' is the term given to a dentition where the teeth are in the optimum anatomical position, both within the mandibular and maxillary arches (intramaxillary) and between the arches when the teeth are in occlusion (intermaxillary). Malocclusion is the term used to describe dental anomalies and occlusal traits that represent a deviation from the ideal occlusion. In reality, it is rare to have a truly perfect occlusion and malocclusion is a spectrum, reflecting variation around the norm.

The prevalence of malocclusion and particular occlusal anomalies depends on the population studied (e.g. age and racial characteristics), the criteria used for assessment, and the methods used by the examiners (e.g. whether radiographs were employed). In the UK, it is estimated 9% of 12-year-olds and 18% of 15-year-olds are undergoing orthodontic treatment, with a further 37% of 12-year-olds and 20% of 15-year-olds requiring treatment (Table 1.1). This suggests the overall prevalence of moderate–severe malocclusion is around 40–50% in adolescents (Table 1.1).

Table 1.1 England, Wales, and Northern Ireland Child Dental Health Survey 2013

	Age band	
	12 years	**15 years**
Children undergoing orthodontic treatment at the time of the survey	9%	18%
Children not undergoing treatment but in need of treatment (IOTN dental health component)	37%	20%

Source data from Child Dental Health Survey 2013, England, Wales and Northern Ireland, 2015, Health and Social Care Information Centre.

1.3 Rationale for orthodontic treatment

Malocclusion may cause concerns related to dental health and/or oral-health-related quality of life issues arising from appearance, function, and the psychosocial impact of the teeth. The need for treatment depends on the impact of the malocclusion and whether treatment is likely to provide a demonstrable benefit to the patient. To judge treatment need, potential benefits of treatment are balanced against the risk of possible complications and side-effects in a risk–benefit analysis (Table 1.2).

1.3.1 Need for orthodontic treatment

Health and well-being benefits are the most appropriate determinant of treatment need. Orthodontic indices have been developed to help objective and systematic evaluation of the potential risk to dental health posed by the malocclusion and the possible benefits of orthodontic treatment (see Section 2.3). While indices were largely developed to measure treatment need, due to high treatment demand in many

Table 1.2 Risk–benefit analysis for orthodontics

Benefits of treatment	versus	Risks
Improved dental health Improved oral-health-related quality of life (OHRQoL) Improved aesthetics Improved function		Worsening of dental health Failure to achieve aims of treatment Relapse

countries, indices are also used to manage demand and support prioritization through some form of rationing. For example, in the UK acceptance for NHS orthodontic treatment is predominantly based on need for treatment determined by the Index of Orthodontic Treatment Need (IOTN) (see Section 2.3.3). Similarly, in Sweden treatment priority is estimated using a Priority Index developed by the Swedish Orthodontic

Board and the Medical Board, which aims to identify and treat the malocclusions judged to be most severe.

Unmet treatment need varies within and across countries, depending on individuals' desire for treatment and organizational factors, such as availability of treatment, access to services, and cost of treatment. In the UK, the unmet orthodontic treatment need for children from deprived households is higher than average; 40% for 12-year-olds and 32% for 15-year-olds. Similar patterns of inequality in access to treatment are seen in other countries.

1.3.2 Demand for orthodontic treatment

It can readily be appreciated that demand for treatment does not necessarily reflect objective treatment need. Some patients are very aware of minor deviations, such as mild rotations of the upper incisors, whilst others refuse treatment for malocclusions that are considered to be severe.

Research shows awareness of malocclusion and willingness to undergo orthodontic treatment is greater in females and those from higher socio-economic backgrounds. Demand is also higher in areas with a smaller population to orthodontist ratio, presumably due to increased awareness and acceptance of orthodontic appliances.

The demand for treatment is increasing, particularly among adults who are attracted by the increasing availability of less visible appliances, such as ceramic brackets and lingual fixed appliances (see Section 20.6) and orthodontic aligners (see Chapter 21). Orthodontic treatment has a useful adjunctive role to restorative work and as people are keeping their teeth for longer, this is contributing to more requests for interdisciplinary care (see Section 20.5). Increasing dental awareness and the desire for straight teeth, combined with the acceptability of orthodontic appliances and awareness of different types of orthodontic treatment means many adults who did not have treatment during adolescence are now seeking treatment.

1.4 Potential benefits to dental health

To determine whether orthodontic treatment is likely to carry a dental health benefit, it is necessary to consider first whether the malocclusion is likely to cause problems to dental health and secondly, whether orthodontic treatment is likely to address the problem.

There are specific occlusal anomalies where evidence suggests orthodontic treatment may provide a dental health benefit (Box 1.1). For other dental conditions, such as caries, plaque-induced periodontal disease, and temporomandibular joint dysfunction syndrome (TMD), there is currently insufficient evidence to suggest orthodontic treatment is beneficial. These conditions are complex and multifactorial in origin and as such, direct causal relationship with malocclusion is difficult to measure effectively.

1.4.1 Localized periodontal problems

Certain occlusal anomalies may predispose individuals to periodontal problems, particularly where the gingival biotype is thin, and in these cases orthodontic intervention may have a long-term health benefit. These include:

Box 1.1 **Occlusal anomalies where evidence suggests orthodontic correction would provide long-term dental health benefit**

Localized periodontal problems

- Crowding causing tooth/teeth to be pushed out of the bony trough, resulting in recession
- Periodontal damage related to tramatic overbites
- Anterior crossbites with evidence of compromised buccal periodontal support on affected lower incisors
- Increased overjet with increased risk of dental trauma
- Unerupted impacted teeth with risk of pathology
- Crossbites associated with mandibular displacement

- Crowding where one or more teeth are pushed buccally or lingually out of the alveolar bony trough, resulting in reduced periodontal support and localized gingival recession.
- Class III malocclusion where lower incisors in crossbite are pushed labially (Fig. 1.1).
- Traumatic overbites, which occur when teeth bite onto the gingiva, can lead to gingival inflammation and loss of periodontal support over time and this is accelerated by suboptimal plaque control.

1.4.2 Dental trauma

There is evidence that increased overjet is associated with trauma to the upper incisors. Two systematic reviews have found that the risk of injury is more than doubled in individuals with an overjet greater than 3 mm and the risk of injury appears to increase with overjet size and lip incompetence. Surprisingly, overjet is a greater contributory factor in girls than boys despite traumatic injuries being more common in boys. Orthodontic intervention may be indicated where assessment and history indicate the young person is at increased risk of dental trauma (see Section 9.2.2). Mouthguards are also important in reducing the risk of dental trauma, particularly for those participating in contact sports (see Section 8.9).

1.4.3 Tooth impaction

Tooth impaction occurs when normal tooth eruption is impeded by another tooth, bone, soft tissues, or other pathology. Supernumerary teeth can cause impaction and if judged to be impeding normal dental development, orthodontic input may be required (see Section 3.3.6).

Ectopic teeth are teeth that have formed, or subsequently moved, into the wrong position; often ectopic teeth become impacted. Unerupted impacted teeth may cause localized pathology, most commonly resorption of adjacent roots or cystic change. This is most frequently seen in relation to ectopic maxillary canine teeth, which can resorb roots of the incisors and premolars (Fig. 1.2). Orthodontic management of impacted teeth may be indicated to reduce the risk of pathology (see Section 14.8).

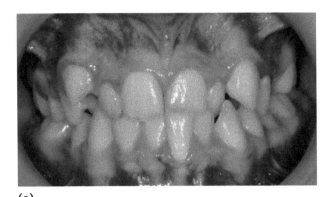

(a)

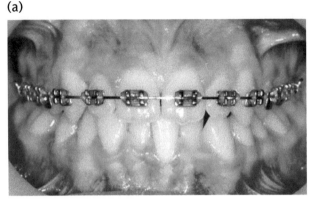

(b)

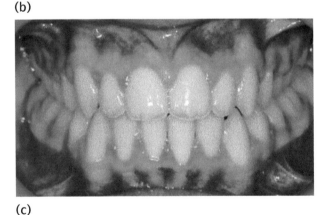

(c)

1.4.4 Caries

Caries experience is directly influenced by oral hygiene, fluoride exposure, and diet; however, research has failed to demonstrate a significant association between malocclusion and caries. Caries reduction is therefore rarely an appropriate justification for orthodontic treatment and placement of orthodontic appliances in an individual with uncontrolled caries risk factors is likely to cause significant harm.

In caries-susceptible children, for example those with special needs, malalignment may reduce the capacity for natural tooth cleansing and potentially increase the risk of caries. In these cases, an orthodontic opinion may be sought regarding methods for reducing food stagnation, such as extraction or simple alignment to alleviate localized crowding.

1.4.5 Plaque-induced periodontal disease

The association between malocclusion and plaque-induced periodontal disease is weak, with research indicating that individual motivation has more impact than tooth alignment on effective tooth brushing. In people with consistently poor plaque control, inadequate oral hygiene is more critical than tooth malalignment in the propagation of periodontal disease. Although patients report increased dental awareness and positive habits around diet and oral hygiene patients following orthodontic treatment, poor plaque control is a contraindication for orthodontic treatment. It is essential that oral hygiene is satisfactory and any periodontal disease is controlled prior to considering orthodontic treatment to prevent worsening of dental health.

Fig. 1.1 (a) A 12-year-old male presented with gingival recession on the left mandibular central incisor resulting from an anterior crossbite pushing the tooth labially. (b) Orthodontic treatment was indicated to prevent further damage to the periodontal tissues. Initially upper arch alignment was provided to correct the anterior crossbite. A small improvement was noted in the gingival recession. (c) Comprehensive treatment was provided and following treatment, the gingival condition of the left mandibular central incisor is similar to the other mandibular incisors.

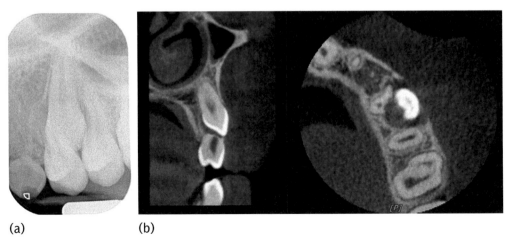

(a)   (b)

Fig. 1.2 (a) Periapical radiograph from a 14-year-old female patient who presented with resorption of the left maxillary first premolar caused by a transposed and ectopic canine. (b) Cone-beam computed tomography shows the extent of the root resorption of the first premolar more clearly.

For people with reduced dexterity or restricted access for cleaning, it is possible that irregular teeth may hinder effective brushing. In these cases, orthodontic alignment may aid plaque control but appliance treatment must be approached carefully to minimize the risk of periodontal damage during treatment.

1.4.6 Temporomandibular joint dysfunction syndrome

The aetiology and management of TMD has caused considerable controversy in all branches of dentistry. TMD comprises a group of related disorders with multifactorial aetiology including psychological, hormonal, genetic, traumatic, and occlusal factors. Research suggests that depression, stress, and sleep disorders are major factors in the aetiology of TMD and that parafunctional activity, for example bruxism, can contribute to muscle pain and spasm. Some authors maintain that minor occlusal imperfections can lead to abnormal paths of closure and/or bruxism, which then result in the development of TMD; however if this were the case, a much higher prevalence of TMD would be expected to reflect the level of malocclusion in the population.

The role of orthodontics in TMD has been extensively debated, with some authors claiming that orthodontic treatment can cause TMD, while others advocate appliance therapy to manage TMD. After considerable discussion in the literature, the consensus view is that orthodontic treatment, either alone or in combination with extractions, cannot be reliably shown to either 'cause' or 'cure' TMD.

The alleged success of a wide assortment of treatment modalities for TMD highlights both the multifactorial aetiology and the self-limiting nature of the condition. Given this, conservative and reversible approaches are advised to manage TMD in the first instance. It is advisable to carry out a TMD screen for all potential orthodontic patients, including questions about symptoms, examination of the temporomandibular joint and associated muscles, and a record of the range of opening and movement (see Section 5.4.6). Where signs or symptoms of TMD are found it is wise to refer the patient for a comprehensive assessment and specialist management before embarking on orthodontic treatment.

1.5 Potential benefits for oral health-related quality of life

The other key area where orthodontics may be beneficial is in improving oral health-related quality of life (OHRQoL). Research focussing on the effect of malocclusion suggests OHRQoL can be negatively affected by issues relating to dental appearance, masticatory function, speech, and psychosocial well-being.

1.5.1 Appearance

Dissatisfaction with dental appearance is often the principal reason people seek orthodontic treatment and, in most cases, treatment is able to deliver a positive change. Although improved dental appearance may be cited as the main goal of treatment by patients, it is likely that the perceived benefit is not a change in appearance per se, but the anticipated psychosocial benefit associated with improved appearance.

1.5.2 Masticatory function

Patients with significant inter-arch discrepancy including anterior open bites (AOB) and markedly increased or reverse overjet often report difficulty with eating, particularly when incising food (Fig. 1.3). This may manifest as avoidance of certain foods, such as sandwiches or apples, or embarrassment when eating in public. Patients with severe hypodontia may also experience problems with eating due to fewer teeth to bite on and concerns about dislodging mobile primary teeth and prosthetic teeth (see Chapter 21). Limited masticatory function rarely results in a complete inability to eat, but it can contribute to significant quality of life issues and this may be a driver for orthodontic treatment.

1.5.3 Speech

Speech is a complex neuromuscular process involving respiration, phonation, articulation, and resonance. Articulation is the formation of different sounds through variable contact of the tongue with surrounding structures, including the palate, lips, alveolar ridge, and dentition. It is unlikely that orthodontic treatment will significantly change speech in most cases, as speech patterns are formed early in life before the permanent dentition is present and the teeth are only one component in the complex system. However, where patients cannot attain contact between the incisors anteriorly, this may contribute to the production of a lisp (interdental sigmatism). In these cases correcting the incisor relationship and reducing interdental spacing may reduce lisping and improve confidence to talk in public.

1.5.4 Psychosocial well-being

Extensive research has been undertaken to examine the effect of malocclusion on psychosocial well-being in terms of self-perception, quality of life, and social interactions. Malocclusion has been linked to reduced self-confidence and self-esteem, with more severe malocclusion and dentofacial deformities causing higher levels of oral impacts. However, other research suggests visible malocclusion has no discernible negative effect on long-term social and psychological well-being. A possible explanation for this is that self-esteem is a mediator in the response to malocclusion, rather than a consequence of malocclusion. Furthermore, self-reported impact of malocclusion may not always reflect objective measurement of the severity of occlusal deviations; this has been attributed to an individual's resilience, ability to cope, as well as social and cultural factors.

Dental appearance can evoke social judgements that affect peer relations and childhood emotional and social development. People with an attractive dentofacial appearance have been judged to be friendlier, more interesting and intelligent, more successful, and more socially competent. On the other hand, deviation from the norm can cause stigmatization and a high correlation has been found between victimization, malocclusion, and quality of life. The incidence of peer victimization in adolescent orthodontic patients with untreated malocclusion has been estimated to be around 12% in the UK. The extent of malocclusion may not be proportionate to the psychosocial impact, for example, more severe forms of facial deformity can elicit stronger reactions such as pity or revulsion, while milder malocclusions can lead to ridicule and teasing.

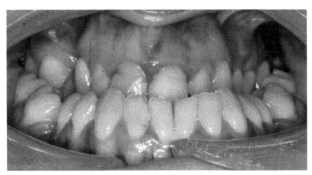

(a)

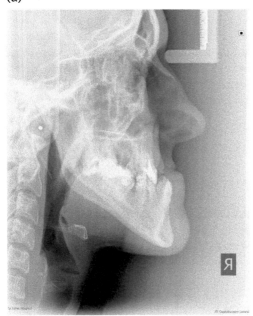

(b)

Fig. 1.3 A significant skeletal discrepancy can impact on masticatory function. This 28-year-old female patient reported that her Class III incisor relationship and bilateral buccal crossbite made incising and chewing food difficult.

Table 1.3 Potential risks of orthodontic treatment

Problem	Avoidance/Management of risk
Intra-oral damage	
Root resorption	Avoid treatment in patients with resorbed, blunted, or pipette-shaped roots In teeth judged to be at risk, roots should be monitored radiographically and treatment terminated if root resorption is evident
Loss of periodontal support	Maintain high level of oral hygiene Avoid moving teeth out of alveolar bone
Demineralization	Diet control, high level of oral hygiene, regular fluoride exposure Abandon treatment
Enamel damage	Avoid potentially abrasive components e.g. ceramic brackets where there is a risk of occlusal contact Use of appropriate instruments and burs to remove appliances and adhesives
Soft tissue damage	Avoid traumatic components Orthodontic wax or silicone to protect against ulceration Manage allergic reaction promptly
Loss of vitality	If history of previous trauma to incisors, counsel patient
Extra-oral damage	
Worsening facial profile	Careful treatment planning and appropriate mechanics
Soft tissue damage	Use of appropriate safety measures with headgear Manage allergy promptly
Ineffective treatment	
Relapse	Avoidance of unstable tooth positions at end of treatment Long-term retention
Failure to achieve treatment objectives	Thorough assessment and accurate diagnosis Effective treatment planning Appropriate use of appliances and mechanics

1.6 Potential risks of orthodontic treatment

Like any other branch of medicine or dentistry, orthodontic treatment is not without potential risks. These risks need to be explained to patients during the decision-making process and where possible, steps taken to manage the risk (Table 1.3). Patients should be made aware of their role in treatment and any self-care or behaviour required to achieve success, such as modifications to diet, oral hygiene practice, or use of a sports guard for participation in contact sports.

1.6.1 Root resorption

It is now accepted that some root resorption is inevitable as a consequence of tooth movement, but there are factors that increase the risk of more severe root resorption (Box 1.2).

Box 1.2 **Recognized risk factors for root resorption during orthodontic treatment**

- Shortened roots with evidence of previous root resorption
- Pipette-shaped or blunted roots
- Teeth which have suffered a previous episode of trauma
- Patient habits (e.g. nail biting)
- Iatrogenic—use of excessive forces, intrusion, and prolonged treatment time

On average, during the course of a conventional 2-year fixed-appliance treatment, around 1 mm of root length will be lost and this amount is not usually clinically significant. However, this average finding masks a wide range of individual variation, as some patients appear to be more susceptible and undergo more marked root resorption. Evidence would suggest a genetic basis in these cases. In teeth with periodontal attachment loss or already shortened roots, the impact of root resorption will be higher (Fig. 1.4).

1.6.2 Loss of periodontal support

An increase in gingival inflammation is commonly seen following the placement of fixed appliances as a result of reduced access for cleaning and if oral hygiene is consistently poor, gingival hyperplasia may develop (Fig. 1.5). This normally reduces or resolves following removal of the appliance, but some apical migration of periodontal attachment and alveolar bony support is usual during a 2-year course of orthodontic treatment. In most patients this is minimal but in individuals who are susceptible to periodontal disease, more marked loss may occur. Removable appliances may also be associated with gingival inflammation, particularly of the palatal tissues, in the presence of poor oral hygiene.

Orthodontic movement of teeth outside the envelope of alveolar bone can result in loss of buccal or less commonly lingual bone, increasing the risk of bony dehiscence and gingival recession. The risk is higher in patients with a narrow alveolus, thin gingival biotype, or existing crowding where teeth have been pushed outside the alveolar bone (Fig. 1.6).

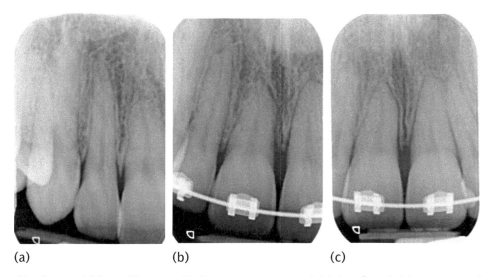

(a) (b) (c)

Fig. 1.4 (a) A patient with a shortened right maxillary central incisor root pre-treatment. A risk–benefit analysis is necessary to determine whether the risk of further resorption is justified by the potential benefit of treatment. (b) A monitoring periapical radiograph of the right central and lateral incisor 6 months into treatment shows little further resoprtion of the central incisor root; however, some resoprtion of the apical tip of the lateral incisor root was noted. (c) A further radiograph of the incisors 6 months later confirmed there was no significant progress in the root shortening.

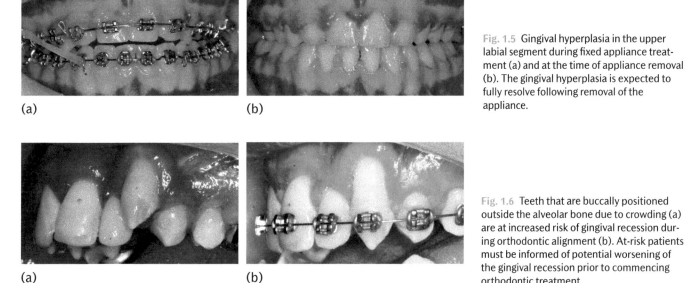

(a) (b)

Fig. 1.5 Gingival hyperplasia in the upper labial segment during fixed appliance treatment (a) and at the time of appliance removal (b). The gingival hyperplasia is expected to fully resolve following removal of the appliance.

(a) (b)

Fig. 1.6 Teeth that are buccally positioned outside the alveolar bone due to crowding (a) are at increased risk of gingival recession during orthodontic alignment (b). At-risk patients must be informed of potential worsening of the gingival recession prior to commencing orthodontic treatment.

1.6.3 Demineralization

Demineralized white lesions are an early, reversible stage in the development of dental caries, which occur when a cariogenic plaque accumulates in association with a high-sugar diet. If white spot lesions are not managed early and effectively they can cause permanent damage and even progress to frank caries. The presence of a fixed appliance predisposes to plaque accumulation, as tooth cleaning around the components of the appliance is more difficult. Demineralization during treatment with fixed appliances is a real risk, with a reported prevalence of between 2% and 96% (see Section 18.7). Although there is evidence to show that the lesions regress following removal of the appliance, patients may still be left with permanent 'scarring' of the enamel (Fig. 1.7).

1.6.4 Enamel damage

Enamel damage can occur as a result of trauma or wear from the orthodontic appliances. Band seaters, band removers, and bracket removal can cause fracture of enamel, or even whole cusps in heavily restored teeth. During removal of adhesives, the debonding burs can cause enamel damage, particularly if used in a high-speed handpiece. Certain components of orthodontic appliances can cause wear to opposing tooth enamel if there is heavily occlusal contact during function. This is a particular concern if ceramic brackets are used in the lower arch in cases with a deep overbite or where buccal crossbites are present.

1.6.5 Intra-oral soft tissue damage

Ulceration can occur during treatment as a result of direct trauma from both fixed and removable appliances, although it is more commonly seen in association with fixed components as an uncomfortable removable appliance is usually removed. Lesions generally heal within a few days without lasting effect.

Intra-oral allergic reactions to orthodontic components are rare but have been reported in relation to nickel, latex, and acrylate.

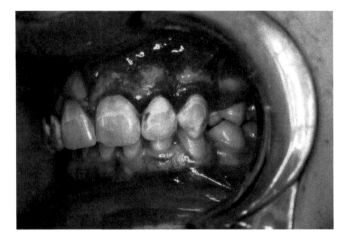

Fig. 1.7 Demineralization on the buccal surfaces of the incisor and canine teeth during fixed appliance treatment. After repeated attempts to control risk factors, treatment was abandoned to prevent further enamel damage.

Management depends on the location and severity of the allergic reaction and the scope for modifying treatment.

1.6.6 Pulpal injury

Excessive apical root movement can lead to a reduction in blood supply to the pulp and even pulpal death. Teeth which have undergone a previous episode of trauma appear to be particularly susceptible, probably because the pulpal tissues are already compromised. Any teeth that have previously suffered trauma or that are judged to be at risk of pulpal injury require thorough examination prior to orthodontic treatment, and any orthodontic treatment should be delivered with light force and careful monitoring.

1.6.7 Extra-oral damage

Some authors have expressed concern over detrimental effects to the facial profile as a result of orthodontics, particularly retraction of anterior teeth in conjunction with extractions. While a number of studies have shown little difference in profile between extraction and non-extraction treatment, it is important that when treatment planning to correct malocclusion, the impact on overall facial appearance is considered.

Contact dermatitis is reported in approximately 1% of the population and allergic reactions may be seen on facial skin in response to components of appliances, usually nickel. This may be managed by covering metal components with tape to prevent contact, or alternative treatment methods may be sought depending in the severity of the reaction.

Recoil injury from the elastic components of headgear poses a rare but potentially severe risk of damage to the eyes. This is discussed in more detail in Chapter 15 (see Section 15.5.3). Iatrogenic skin damage, such as burns from acid etch or hot instruments, are avoidable using the usual precautions employed in other fields of dentistry.

1.6.8 Relapse

Relapse is defined as the return of features of the original malocclusion following correction. Retention is a method to retain the teeth in their corrected position, and it is now accepted that without retention there is a significant risk the teeth will move. The extent of relapse is highly variable and difficult to predict but any undesirable tooth movement following orthodontic treatment will reduce the net benefit of orthodontic treatment. Relapse and retention are covered in detail in Chapter 16.

1.6.9 Failure to achieve treatment objectives

When deciding whether orthodontic treatment is likely to be beneficial it is important to consider the effectiveness of appliance therapy in correcting the malocclusion. There are a number of operator- and patient-related factors that may prevent treatment achieving a worthwhile improvement (Table 1.4).

Errors in diagnosis, treatment planning, and delivery can lead to poor selection of appliances and ineffective treatment. It is essential to determine whether planned tooth movements are attainable within the constraints of the skeletal and growth patterns of the individual patient, as excessive tooth movement or failure to anticipate adverse growth changes will reduce the chances of success (Chapter 7). There is evidence that orthodontic treatment is more likely to achieve a pleasing and successful result if the operator has had some postgraduate

Table 1.4 Failure to achieve treatment objectives

Operator factors	Patient factors
Errors of diagnosis	Poor oral hygiene/diet
Errors of treatment planning	Failure to wear appliances/elastics
Anchorage loss	Repeated appliance breakages
Technique errors	Failure to attend appointments
Poor communication	Unexpected unfavourable growth
Inadequate experience/training	

training in orthodontics, as this supports appropriate appliance selection and use.

Patient co-operation is essential to achieve a successful outcome. Patients must attend appointments, look after their teeth and appliances, and comply with wear and care instructions. Patients are more likely to co-operate if they, and their family, fully understand the process and their role from the outset. This should be explicitly stated during the consent process. It is important to establish that the patient and family feel willing and able to adhere to the agreed treatment plan before commencing treatment. Long-term effectiveness of treatment depends on patients' commitment to life-long retainer wear and this must be stressed at the beginning of discussions about orthodontic treatment (see Chapter 16).

1.7 Discussing orthodontic treatment need

It is important that patients and families are involved in the discussion about whether orthodontic treatment is needed and justified. Patients and their families have a key role in providing information about the impact of malocclusion, expectations from treatment, and their desired outcome. The clinician's role is to provide unbiased information about the potential risks and benefits of treatment based on best available evidence and their own clinical experience. General information should be tailored to the individual's clinical presentation and personal circumstance. Patients and families should be supported to participate in the decision about whether treatment is likely to provide sufficient benefit to outweigh any risks. Patients also have a vital role in determining whether they are likely to be able to comply with treatment adequately to achieve a satisfactory outcome. Treatment planning and consent are covered in more detail in Chapter 7.

Key points

- The decision whether to embark on orthodontic treatment is essentially a risk–benefit analysis.
- The perceived benefits of orthodontic intervention should outweigh any potential risks associated with treatment.
- Patients and families have an important role in determining whether treatment is likely to address issues caused by the malocclusion.

Relevant Cochrane reviews

Benson, P. E., Parkin, N., Dyer, F., Millett, D.T., Furness, S., and Germain, P. (2013). Fluorides for the prevention of early tooth decay (demineralised white lesions) during fixed brace treatment. *Cochrane Database of Systematic Reviews*, Issue 12. Art. No.: CD003809. DOI: 10.1002/14651858.CD003809.pub3. https://www.cochranelibrary.com/cdsr/doi/10.1002/14651858.CD003809.pub3/full

The authors report that (1) fluoride varnish applied every 6 weeks provided moderate-quality evidence of around 70% reduction in demineralized white lesions, and (2) no difference was found between different formulations of fluoride toothpaste and mouth rinse on white spot index, visible plaque index, and gingival bleeding index.

Principal sources and further reading

American Journal of Orthodontics and Dentofacial Orthopedics, 1992, **101**(1).
This is a special issue dedicated to the results of several studies set up by the American Association of Orthodontists to investigate the link between orthodontic treatment and the temporomandibular joint.

Davies, S. J., Gray, R. M. J., Sandler, P. J., and O'Brien, K. D. (2001). Orthodontics and occlusion. *British Dental Journal*, **191**, 539–49. [DOI: 10.1038/sj.bdj.4801229] [PubMed: 11767855]
This concise article is part of a series of articles on occlusion. It contains an example of an articulatory examination.

DiBiase, A. T. and Sandler, P. J. (2001). Malocclusion, orthodontics and bullying. *Dent Update*, **28**, 464–6. [DOI: 10.12968/denu.2001.28.9.464] [PubMed: 11806190]
An interesting discussion around bullying and the 'victim type'.

Egermark, I., Magnusson, T., and Carlsson, G. E. (2003). A 20-year follow-up of signs and symptoms of temporomandibular disorders in subjects with and without orthodontic treatment in childhood. *Angle Orthodontist*, **73**, 109–15. [DOI: 10.1043/0003-3219(**2003**)73<109:AYFOSA>2.0.CO] [PubMed: 12725365].
A long-term cohort study, which found no statistically significant difference in TMD signs and symptoms between subjects with or without previous experience of orthodontic treatment.

Guzman-Armstrong, S., Chalmers, J., Warren, J. J. (2011). Readers' forum: White spot lesions: prevention and treatment. *American Journal of Orthodontics and Dentofacial Orthopedics*, **138**, 690–6. [DOI: 10.1016/j.ajodo.2010.07.007] [PubMed: 21171493]
An interesting and informative read on decalcification during orthodontic treatment.

Helm, S. and Petersen, P. E. (1989). Causal relation between malocclusion and caries. *Acta Odontologica Scandinavica*, **47**, 217–21. [DOI: 10.3109/00016358909007704] [PubMed: 2782059]
A historic paper that demonstrates no link between malocclusion and caries.

Joss-Vassalli, I., Grebenstein, C., Topouzelis, N., Sculean, A., and Katsaros, C. (2010). Orthodontic therapy and gingival recession: a systematic review. *Orthodontics and Craniofacial Research*, **13**, 127–41. [DOI: 10.1111/j.1601-6343.2010.01491.x] [PubMed: 20618715]

Kenealy, P. M., Kingdon, A., Richmond, S., and Shaw, W. C. (2007). The Cardiff dental study: a 20-year critical evaluation of the psychological health gain from orthodontic treatment. *British Journal of Health Psychology*, **12**, 17–49. [DOI: 10.1348/135910706X96896] [PubMed: 17288664]
An interesting paper highlighting the complexities of self-esteem.

Luther, F. (2007). TMD and occlusion part I. Damned if we do? Occlusion the interface of dentistry and orthodontics. *British Dental Journal*, **202**, E2.

Luther, F. (2007). TMD and occlusion part II. Damned if we don't? Functional occlusal problems: TMD epidemiology in a wider context. *British Dental Journal*, **202**, E3.
These two articles are well worth reading.

Maaitah, E. F., Adeyami, A. A., Higham, S. M., Pender, N., and Harrison, J. E. (2011). Factors affecting demineralization during orthodontic treatment: a post-hoc analysis of RCT recruits. *American Journal of Orthodontics and Dentofacial Orthopedics*, **139**, 181–91. [DOI: 10.1016/j.ajodo.2009.08.028] [PubMed: 21300246]
A useful study that concludes that pre-treatment age, oral hygiene, and status of the first permanent molars can be used as a guide to the likelihood of decalcification occurring during treatment.

Mizrahi, E. (2010). Risk management in clinical practice. Part 7. Dento-legal aspects of orthodontic practice. *British Dental Journal*, **209**, 381–90. [DOI: 10.1038/sj.bdj.2010.926] [PubMed: 20966997].

Murray, A. M. (1989). Discontinuation of orthodontic treatment: a study of the contributing factors. *British Journal of Orthodontics*, **16**, 1–7. [DOI: 10.1179/bjo.16.1.1] [PubMed: 2647133].

Nguyen, Q. V., Bezemer, P. D., Habets, L., and Prahl-Andersen, B. (1999). A systematic review of the relationship between overjet size and traumatic dental injuries. *European Journal of Orthodontics*, **21**, 503–15. [DOI: 10.1093/ejo/21.5.503] [PubMed: 10565091].

Petti, S. (2015). Over two hundred million injuries to anterior teeth attributable to large overjet: a meta-analysis. *Dental Traumatology*, **31**, 1–8. [DOI: 10.1111/edt.12126] [PubMed: 25263806]
Two systematic reviews that demonstrate the relationship between increased overjet and dental trauma.

Roberts-Harry, D. and Sandy, J. (2003). Orthodontics. Part 1: who needs orthodontics? *British Dental Journal*, **195**, 433. [DOI: 10.1038/sj.bdj.4810592] [PubMed: 14576790]
A summary of the potential benefits of orthodontic treatment.

Seehra, J., Newton, J. T., and Dibiase A. T. (2011). Bullying in schoolchildren – its relationship to dental appearance and psychosocial implications: an update for GDPs. *British Dental Journal*, **210**, 411–15. [DOI: 10.1038/sj.bdj.2011.339] [PubMed: 21566605]
A useful summary of bullying and its relationship to malocclusion.

Steele, J., White, D., Rolland, S., and Fuller, E. (2015). *Children's Dental Health Survey 2013. Report 4: The burden of dental disease in children: England, Wales and Northern Ireland*. Leeds: Health and Social Care Information Centre.

Tsakos, G., Hill, K., Chadwick B., and Anderson, T. (2015). *Children's Dental Health Survey 2013. Report 1: Attitudes, behaviours and Children's Dental Health: England, Wales and Northern Ireland*. Leeds: Health and Social Care Information Centre.
The reports from the 2013 Child Dental Health Survey, highlighting orthodontic treatment need.

Travess, H., Roberts-Harry, D., and Sandy, J. (2004). Orthodontics. Part 6: Risks in orthodontic treatment. *British Dental Journal*, **196**, 71–7. [DOI: 10.1038/sj.bdj.4810891] [PubMed: 14739957]
A follow-up to the previous article by the same authors to outline the risks of orthodontic treatment, illustrated with cases.

Weltman, B., Vig, K. W., Fields, H. W., Shanker, S., and Kaizar, E. E. (2010). Root resorption associated with orthodontic tooth movement: a systematic review. *American Journal of Orthodontics and Dentofacial Orthopedics*, **137**, 462–76. [DOI: 10.1016/j.ajodo.2009.06.021] [PubMed: 20362905]

Wheeler, T. T., McGorray, S. P., Yurkiewicz, L., Keeling, S. D., and King, G. J. (1994). Orthodontic treatment demand and need in third and fourth grade schoolchildren. *American Journal of Orthodontics and Dentofacial Orthopedics*, **106**, 22–33. [DOI: 10.1016/S0889-5406(94)70017-6] [PubMed: 8017346]
Contains a good discussion on the need and demand for treatment.

Zhang, M., McGrath, C., and Hägg, U. (2006). The impact of malocclusion and its treatment on quality of life: a literature review. *International Journal of Paediatric Dentistry*, **16**, 381–7. [DOI: 10.1111/j.1365-263X.2006.00768.x] [PubMed: 17014535]

References for this chapter can also be found at: **www.oup.com/uk/orthodontics5e**. Where possible, these are presented as active links that direct you to the electronic version of the work to help facilitate onward study. If you are a subscriber to that work (either individually or through an institution), and depending on your level of access, you may be able to peruse an abstract or the full article if available.

2

The aetiology and classification of malocclusion

L. Mitchell

Chapter contents

2.1 The aetiology of malocclusion

An ideal occlusion is defined as an anatomically perfect arrangement of the teeth. While previously orthodontists may have concentrated on achieving a static, anatomically correct occlusion, it is now accepted that a functional occlusion is more important (see Box 2.1). It is important to realize that malocclusion is not in itself a disease; rather, it describes variation around the ideal.

The aetiology of malocclusion is a fascinating subject about which there is still much to elucidate and understand. Theoretically, malocclusion can occur as a result of genetically determined factors which are inherited, or environmental factors, or a combination of both inherited and environmental factors acting together. For example, failure of eruption of an upper central incisor may arise as a result of dilaceration following an episode of trauma during the deciduous dentition which led to intrusion of the primary predecessor—an example of environmental aetiology. Failure of eruption of an upper central incisor can also occur as a result of the presence of a supernumerary tooth—a scenario which questioning may reveal also affected the patient's parent, suggesting an inherited problem. However, if in the latter example, caries (an environmental factor) has led to early loss of many of the deciduous teeth then forward drift of the first permanent molar teeth may also lead to superimposition of the additional problem of crowding.

While it is relatively straightforward to trace the inheritance of syndromes such as cleft lip and palate (see Chapter 24), it is more difficult to determine the aetiology of features which are in essence part of normal variation, and the picture is further complicated by the compensatory mechanisms that exist. Evidence for the role of inherited factors in the aetiology of malocclusion has come from studies of families and twins. The facial similarity of members of a family, for example, the prognathic mandible of the Hapsburg royal family, is easily appreciated. However, more direct testimony is provided in studies of twins and triplets, which indicate that skeletal pattern and tooth size and number are largely genetically determined.

Examples of environmental influences include digit-sucking habits and premature loss of teeth as a result of either caries or trauma. Soft tissue pressures acting upon the teeth for more than 6 hours per day can also influence tooth position. However, because the soft tissues including the lips are by necessity attached to the underlying skeletal framework, their effect is also mediated by the skeletal pattern.

Crowding is extremely common in Caucasians, affecting approximately two-thirds of the population. As was mentioned above, the size of the jaws and teeth are mainly genetically determined; however, environmental factors, for example, premature deciduous tooth loss, can precipitate or exacerbate crowding. In evolutionary terms both jaw size and tooth size appear to be reducing. However, crowding is much more prevalent in modern populations than it was in prehistoric times. It has been postulated that this is due to the introduction of a less abrasive diet, so that less interproximal tooth wear occurs during the lifetime of an individual. However, this is not the whole story, as a change from a rural to an urban lifestyle can also apparently lead to an increase in crowding after about two generations.

Although this discussion may at first seem rather theoretical, the aetiology of malocclusion is a vigorously debated subject. This is because if one believes that the basis of malocclusion is genetically determined, then it follows that orthodontics is limited in what it can achieve. However, the opposite viewpoint is that every individual has the potential for ideal occlusion and that orthodontic intervention is required to eliminate those environmental factors that have led to a particular malocclusion. It is now acknowledged that the majority of malocclusions are caused by both inherited polygenic and environmental factors and the interplay between them. Malocclusion is not a single disease, but a collection of abnormal traits. These traits can be the result of complex interactions between different genes, interactions between genes and the environment (epigenetics), and distinct environmental factors.

When planning treatment for an individual patient, it is often helpful to consider the role of the following in the aetiology of their malocclusion. Further discussion of these factors will be considered in the forthcoming chapters covering the main types of malocclusion:

1. Skeletal pattern—in all three planes of space
2. Soft tissues
3. Dental factors.

Of necessity, the above is a brief summary, but it can be appreciated that the aetiology of malocclusion is a complex subject. The reader seeking more information is advised to consult the publications listed in the section on 'Principal sources and further reading' at the end of this chapter.

Box 2.1 Functional occlusion

- An occlusion which is free of interferences to smooth gliding movements of the mandible with no pathology.
- Orthodontic treatment should aim to achieve a functional occlusion.
- *But* there is a lack of evidence to indicate that if an ideal functional occlusion is not achieved that there are deleterious long-term effects on the temporomandibular joints.

2.2 Classifying malocclusion

The categorization of a malocclusion by its salient features is helpful for describing and documenting a patient's occlusion. In addition, classifications and indices allow the prevalence of a malocclusion within a population to be recorded, and also aid in the assessment of need, difficulty, and success of orthodontic treatment.

Malocclusion can be recorded qualitatively and quantitatively. However, the large number of classifications and indices which have been devised are testimony to the problems inherent in both these approaches. All have their limitations, and these should be borne in mind when they are applied (Box 2.2).

2.2.1 Qualitative assessment of malocclusion

Essentially, a qualitative assessment is descriptive and therefore this category includes the diagnostic classifications of malocclusion. The main drawback to a qualitative approach is that malocclusion is a continuous variable so that clear cut-off points between different categories do not always exist. This can lead to problems when classifying borderline malocclusions. In addition, although a qualitative classification is a helpful shorthand method of describing the salient features of a malocclusion, it does not provide any indication of the difficulty of treatment.

Qualitative evaluation of malocclusion was attempted historically before quantitative analysis. One of the better-known classifications was devised by Angle in 1899, but other classifications are now more widely used, for example, the British Standards Institute (1983) classification of incisor relationship.

> **Box 2.2 Important attributes of an index**
>
> - Validity—can the index measure what it was designed to measure?
> - Reproducibility—does the index give the same result when recorded on two different occasions and by different examiners?
> - Acceptability—is the index acceptable to both professionals and patients?
> - Ease of use—is the index straightforward to use?

2.2.2 Quantitative assessment of malocclusion

In quantitative indices, two differing approaches can be used:

- Each feature of a malocclusion is given a score and the summed total is then recorded (e.g. the Peer Assessment Rating (PAR) Index).
- The worst feature of a malocclusion is recorded (e.g. the Index of Orthodontic Treatment Need (IOTN)).

2.3 Commonly used classifications and indices

2.3.1 Angle's classification

Angle's classification was based upon the premise that the first permanent molars erupted into a constant position within the facial skeleton, which could be used to assess the anteroposterior relationship of the arches. In addition to the fact that Angle's classification was based upon an incorrect assumption, the problems experienced in categorizing cases with forward drift or loss of the first permanent molars have resulted in this particular approach being superseded by other classifications. However, Angle's classification is still used to describe molar relationship, and the terms used to describe incisor relationship have been adapted into incisor classification.

Angle described three groups (Fig. 2.1):

- *Class I or neutrocclusion*—the mesiobuccal cusp of the upper first molar occludes with the mesiobuccal groove of the lower first molar. In practice, discrepancies of up to half a cusp width either way were also included in this category.
- *Class II or distocclusion*—the mesiobuccal cusp of the lower first molar occludes distal to the Class I position. This is also known as a postnormal relationship.
- *Class III or mesiocclusion*—the mesiobuccal cusp of the lower first molar occludes mesial to the Class I position. This is also known as a prenormal relationship.

2.3.2 British Standards Institute classification

This is based upon incisor relationship and is the most widely used descriptive classification. The terms used are similar to those of Angle's classification, which can be a little confusing as no regard is taken of molar relationship. The categories defined by British Standard 4492 are shown in Box 2.3 (see also Figs 2.2, 2.3, 2.4, and 2.5).

As with any descriptive analysis, it is difficult to classify borderline cases. Some workers have suggested introducing a Class II intermediate category for those cases where the upper incisors are upright and the overjet increased to between 4 and 6 mm. However, this approach has not gained widespread acceptance.

2.3.3 Index of Orthodontic Treatment Need (IOTN)

The IOTN was developed as a result of a government initiative. The purpose of the index was to help determine the likely impact of a malocclusion on an individual's dental health and psychosocial well-being. It comprises two elements.

Dental health component

This was developed from an index used by the Dental Board in Sweden designed to reflect those occlusal traits which could affect the function

Box 2.3 British Standards incisor classification

- *Class I*—the lower incisor edges occlude with or lie immediately below the cingulum plateau of the upper central incisors.
- *Class II*—the lower incisor edges lie posterior to the cingulum plateau of the upper incisors. There are two subdivisions of this category:
  - *Division 1*—the upper central incisors are proclined or of average inclination and there is an increase in overjet.
  - *Division 2*—the upper central incisors are retroclined. The overjet is usually minimal or may be increased.
- *Class III*—the lower incisor edges lie anterior to the cingulum plateau of the upper incisors. The overjet is reduced or reversed.

Permission to reproduce extracts from British Standards is granted by BSI. British Standards can be obtained in PDF or hard copy formats from the BSI online shop: www.bsigroup.com/Shop or by contacting BSI Customer Services for hardcopies only: Tel: +44 (0)20 8996 9001, Email: cservices@bsigroup.com

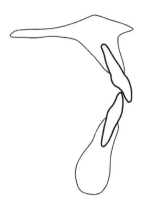

Fig. 2.2 Incisor classification—Class I.

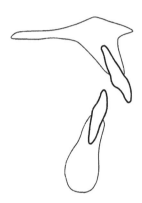

Fig. 2.3 Incisor classification—Class II division 1.

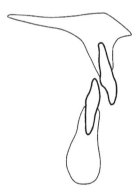

Fig. 2.4 Incisor classification—Class II division 2.

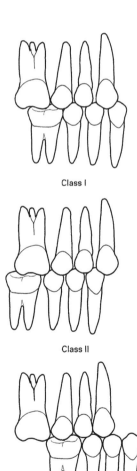

Class I

Class II

Class III

Fig. 2.1 Angle's classification.

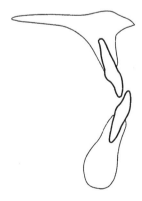

Fig. 2.5 Incisor classification—Class III.

and longevity of the dentition. The single worst feature of a malocclusion is noted (the index is not cumulative) and categorized into one of five grades reflecting need for treatment (Box 2.4):

- *Grade 1*—no need
- *Grade 2*—little need
- *Grade 3*—moderate need
- *Grade 4*—great need
- *Grade 5*—very great need.

A ruler has been developed to help with assessment of the dental health component (Fig. 2.6), and these are available commercially. As only the single worst feature is recorded, an alternative approach is to look consecutively for the following features (known as MOCDO):

- Missing teeth
- Overjet
- Crossbite
- Displacement (contact point)
- Overbite.

Aesthetic component

This aspect of the index was developed in an attempt to assess the aesthetic handicap posed by a malocclusion and thus the likely psychosocial impact upon the patient—a difficult task (see Chapter 1). The aesthetic component comprises a set of ten standard photographs (Fig. 2.7), which are also graded from score 1, the most aesthetically pleasing, to score 10, the least aesthetically pleasing. Colour photographs are available for assessing a patient in the clinical situation and black-and-white photographs for scoring from study models alone. The patient's teeth (or study models), in occlusion, are viewed from the anterior aspect and the appropriate score determined by choosing the photograph that is thought to pose an equivalent aesthetic handicap. The scores are categorized according to need for treatment as follows:

- Score 1 or 2—none
- Score 3 or 4—slight
- Score 5, 6, or 7—moderate/borderline
- Score 8, 9, or 10—definite.

An average score can be taken from the two components, but the dental health component alone is more widely used. The aesthetic component has been criticized for being subjective—particular difficulty is experienced in accurately assessing Class III malocclusions or anterior open bites, as the photographs are composed of Class I and Class II cases, but studies have indicated good reproducibility.

2.3.4 Peer Assessment Rating (PAR)

The PAR index was developed primarily to measure the success (or otherwise) of treatment. Scores are recorded for a number of parameters (listed below), before and at the end of treatment using study models. Unlike IOTN, the scores are cumulative; however, a weighting is accorded to each component to reflect current opinion in the UK as to their relative importance. The features recorded are listed as follows, with the current weightings in parentheses:

- Crowding—by contact point displacement (×1)
- Buccal segment relationship—in the anteroposterior, vertical, and transverse planes (×1)
- Overjet (×6)
- Overbite (×2)
- Centrelines (×4).

The difference between the PAR scores at the start and on completion of treatment can be calculated, and from this the percentage change in PAR score, which is a reflection of the success of treatment, is derived. A high standard of treatment is indicated by a mean percentage reduction of greater than 70%. A change of 30% or less indicates that no appreciable improvement has been achieved. The size of the PAR score at the beginning of treatment gives an indication of the severity of a malocclusion. Obviously it is difficult to achieve a significant reduction in PAR in cases with a low pre-treatment score.

2.3.5 Index of Complexity, Outcome and Need (ICON)

This index incorporates features of both the IOTN and the PAR. The following are scored and then each score is multiplied by its weighting:

- Aesthetic component of IOTN (×7)
- Upper arch crowding/spacing (×5)
- Crossbite (×5)
- Overbite/open bite (×4)
- Buccal segment relationship (×3).

The total sum gives a pre-treatment score, which is said to reflect the need for, and likely complexity of, the treatment required. A score of more than 43 is said to indicate a demonstrable need for treatment. Following treatment, the index is scored again to give an improvement grade and thus the outcome of treatment.

Improvement grade = pre-treatment score − (4 × post-treatment score)

This ambitious index has been criticized for the large weighting given to the aesthetic component and has not gained widespread acceptability.

2.3.6 Index of Orthognathic Functional Treatment Need (IOFTN)

Although the IOTN has proved a reliable method of assessing malocclusion, like any index, it does have its limitations. Many of these relate to

Box 2.4 The Index of Orthodontic Treatment Need

Grade 5 (Very Great)

5a	Increased overjet greater than 9 mm.
5h	Extensive hypodontia with restorative implications (more than one tooth missing in any quadrant) requiring pre-restorative orthodontics.
5i	Impeded eruption of teeth (with the exception of third molars) due to crowding, displacement, the presence of supernumerary teeth, retained deciduous teeth, and any pathological cause.
5m	Reverse overjet greater than 3.5 mm with reported masticatory and speech difficulties.
5p	Defects of cleft lip and palate.
5s	Submerged deciduous teeth.

Grade 4 (Great)

4a	Increased overjet 6.1–9 mm.
4b	Reversed overjet greater than 3.5 mm with no masticatory or speech difficulties.
4c	Anterior or posterior crossbites with greater than 2 mm discrepancy between retruded contact position and intercuspal position.
4d	Severe displacement of teeth, greater than 4 mm.
4e	Extreme lateral or anterior open bites, greater than 4 mm.
4f	Increased and complete overbite with gingival or palatal trauma.
4h	Less extensive hypodontia requiring pre-restorative orthodontic space closure to obviate the need for a prosthesis.
4l	Posterior lingual crossbite with no functional occlusal contact in one or both buccal segments.
4m	Reverse overjet 1.1–3.5 mm with recorded masticatory and speech difficulties.
4t	Partially erupted teeth, tipped and impacted against adjacent teeth.
4x	Supplemental teeth.

Grade 3 (Moderate)

3a	Increased overjet 3.6–6 mm with incompetent lips.
3b	Reverse overjet 1.1–3.5 mm.
3c	Anterior or posterior crossbites with 1.1–2 mm discrepancy.
3d	Displacement of teeth 2.1–4 mm.
3e	Lateral or anterior open bite 2.1–4 mm.
3f	Increased and complete overbite without gingival trauma.

Grade 2 (Little)

2a	Increased overjet 3.6–6 mm with competent lips.
2b	Reverse overjet 0.1–1 mm.
2c	Anterior or posterior crossbite with up to 1 mm discrepancy between retruded contact position and intercuspal position.
2d	Displacement of teeth 1.1–2 mm.
2e	Anterior or posterior open bite 1.1–2 mm.
2f	Increased overbite 3.5 mm or more, without gingival contact.
2g	Prenormal or postnormal occlusions with no other anomalies; includes up to half a unit discrepancy.

Grade 1 (None)

1	Extremely minor malocclusions including displacements less than 1 mm.

0	3 i 2 c	4	5			
2						
3		4				
4 - ms - 5						

5 Defect of CLP
5 Non-eruption of teeth
5 Extensive hypodontia
4 Less extensive hypodontia
4 Crossbite >2 mm discrepancy
4 Scissors bite
4 O.B. with G + P trauma

3 O.B. with NO G + P trauma
3 Crossbite 1.2 mm discrepancy
2 O.B. > ————
2 Dev. From full interdig
2 Crossbite < 1 mm discrepancy

IOTN Manchester (clinical)

Displacement
open bite

V

| | | |
| 4 | 3 | 2 | 1 |

Fig. 2.6 IOTN ruler. The Index of Orthodontic Treatment Need (IOTN) is the property of The University of Manchester. © The University of Manchester 2018. All rights reserved. Reproduced by kind permission of The University of Manchester. The SCAN scale was first published in 1987 by the European Orthodontic Society (Ruth Evans and William Shaw, Preliminary evaluation of an illustrated scale for rating dental attractiveness. *European Journal of Orthodontics* 9: 314–318).

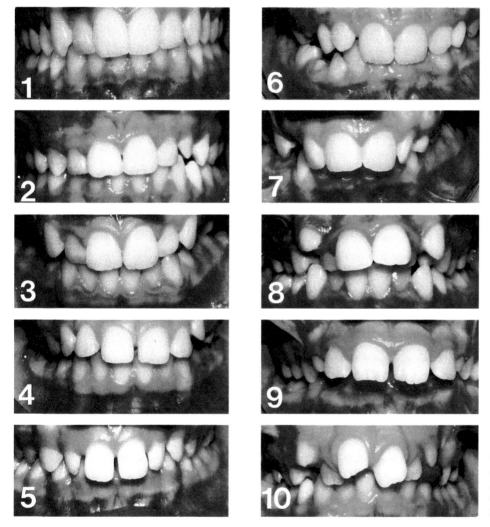

Fig. 2.7 Aesthetic component of IOTN. Reproduced from Evans, R. and Shaw, W. C., A preliminary evaluation of an illustrated scale for rating dental attractiveness. *European Journal of Orthodontics*, **9**: 314–318. Copyright (1987) with permission from Oxford University Press.

severe malocclusions which are not amenable to routine orthodontic appliances alone. For example, many severe Class III malocclusions have dento-alveolar compensation, that is, retroclination of the lower incisors and/or proclination of the upper incisors which masks the severity of the underlying skeletal discrepancy. As a result, when assessed with the IOTN these malocclusions may only score dental health component grade 3. Also, significant, unsightly excessive upper incisor show, which can lead to potential gingival and periodontal problems, is not reflected in the scoring parameters.

A new index was developed from the IOTN with the aim of trying to address these concerns and to reflect the functional issues that arise with these severe surgical cases. Like IOTN, it is based on a 5-point scale with Grade 5 reflecting a 'Very Great Need to Treatment' and Grade 1 'No Need for Treatment' (see Box 2.5).

Box 2.5 The Index of Orthognathic Functional Treatment Need

5. Very Great Need for Treatment

5.1	Defects of cleft lip and palate and other craniofacial anomalies.
5.2	Increased overjet greater than 9 mm.
5.3	Reverse overjet ≥ 3mm.
5.4	Open bite ≥ 4 mm.
5.5	Complete scissors bite affecting whole buccal segment(s) with signs of functional disturbance and/or occlusal trauma.
5.6	Sleep apnoea not amenable to other treatments such as MAD or CPAP (as determined by sleep studies).
5.7	Skeletal anomalies with occlusal disturbance as a result of trauma or pathology.

4. Great Need for Treatment

4.1	Increased overjet ≤ 6 mm and ≥ 9 mm.
4.2	Reversed overjet ≥ 0 mm and < 3 mm with functional difficulties.
4.3	Open bites < 4 mm with functional difficulties.
4.8	Increased overbite with evidence of dental or soft tissue trauma.
4.9	Upper labial segment gingival exposure ≥ 3 mm at rest.
4.10	Facial asymmetry associated with occlusal disturbance.

3. Moderate Need for Treatment

3.3	Reverse overjet ≥ 0 mm and < 3 mm with no functional difficulties.
3.4	Open bite < 4 mm with no functional difficulties.
3.9	Upper labial segment gingiva exposure < 3 mm at rest, but with evidence of gingival/periodontal effects.
3.10	Facial asymmetry with no occlusal disturbance.

2. Mild Need for Treatment

2.8	Increased overbite but no evidence of dental or soft tissue trauma.
2.9	Upper labial segment gingival exposure < 3 mm at rest with no evidence of gingival periodontal effects.
2.11	Marked occlusal cant with no effect on the occlusion.

1. No Need for Treatment

1.12	Speech difficulties.
1.13	Treatment purely for TMD.
1.14	Occlusal features not classified above.

2.4 Andrews' six keys

Andrews analysed 120 'normal' occlusions to evaluate those features which were key to a good occlusion (it has been pointed out that these occlusions can more correctly be described as 'ideal'). He found six features, which are described in Box 2.6. These six keys are not a method of classifying occlusion as such, but serve as a goal. Occasionally, at the end of treatment it is not possible to achieve a good Class I occlusion—in such cases it is helpful to look at each of these features in order to evaluate why.

Andrews used this analysis to develop the first pre-adjusted bracket system, which was designed to place the teeth (in three planes of space) to achieve his six keys (see Box 2.6). This prescription is called the Andrews' bracket prescription. For further details of pre-adjusted systems, see Chapter 18.

Box 2.6 Andrews' six keys

Correct molar relationship: the mesiobuccal cusp of the upper first molar occludes with the groove between the mesiobuccal and middle buccal cusp of the lower first molar. The distobuccal cusp of the upper first molar contacts the mesiobuccal cusp of the lower second molar.

Correct crown angulation: all tooth crowns are angulated mesially.

Correct crown inclination: incisors are inclined towards the buccal or labial surface. Buccal segment teeth are inclined lingually. In the lower buccal segments this is progressive.

No rotations.
No spaces.
Flat occlusal plane.

Reprinted from *American Journal of Orthodontics*, Volume 62, Issue 3, Lawrence F. Andrews, The six keys to normal occlusion, pp. 296–309, Copyright (1972), with permission from Elsevier.

Principal sources and further reading

Andrews, L. F. (1972). The six keys to normal occlusion. *American Journal of Orthodontics*, **62**, 296–309. [DOI: 10.1016/S0002-9416(72)90268-0] [PubMed: 4505873]

Angle, E. H. (1899). Classification of malocclusion. *Dental Cosmos*, **41**, 248–64.

British Standards Institute (1983). *Glossary of Dental Terms (BS 4492)*. London: BSI.

Daniels, C. and Richmond, S. (2000). The development of the Index of Complexity, Outcome and Need (ICON). *Journal of Orthodontics*, **27**, 149–62. [DOI: 10.1093/ortho/27.2.149] [PubMed: 10867071]

Flemming, P. S. (2008). The aetiology of malocclusion. *Orthodontic Update*, **1**, 16–21.
An easy-to-understand discussion of aetiology.

Harradine, N. W. T., Pearson, M. H., and Toth, B. (1998). The effect of extraction of third molars on late lower incisor crowding: a randomized controlled clinical trial. *British Journal of Orthodontics*, **25**, 117–22. [DOI: 10.1093/ortho/25.2.117] [PubMed: 9668994]

Ireland, A. J. (2014). An index of Orthognathic Functional Treatment Need (IOFTN). *Journal of Orthodontics*, **41**, 77–83. [DOI: 10.1179/1465313314Y.0000000100] [PubMed: 24951095]
Article describing the rationale for and development of the IOFTN.

Markovic, M. (1992). At the crossroads of oral facial genetics. *European Journal of Orthodontics*, **14**, 469–81. [DOI: 10.1093/ejo/14.6.469] [PubMed: 1486933]
A fascinating study of twins and triplets with Class II/2 malocclusions.

Proffit, W. R. (1978). Equilibrium theory revisited: factors influencing position of the teeth. *Angle Orthodontist*, **48**, 175–86. [DOI: 10.1043/0003-3219(1978)048<0175:ETRFIP>2.0.CO;2] [PubMed: 280125]
Further reading for those wishing to learn more.

Richmond, S., Shaw, W. C., O'Brien, K. D., Buchanan, I. B., Jones, R., Stephens, C. D., et al. (1992). The development of the PAR index (Peer Assessment Rating): reliability and validity. *European Journal of Orthodontics*, **14**, 125–39. [DOI: 10.1093/ejo/14.2.125] [PubMed: 1582457]
The PAR index, part 1.

Richmond, S., Shaw, W. C., Roberts, C. T., and Andrews, M. (1992). The PAR index (Peer Assessment Rating): methods to determine the outcome of orthodontic treatment in terms of improvements and standards. *European Journal of Orthodontics*, **14**, 180–7. [DOI: 10.1093/ejo/14.3.180] [PubMed: 1628684]
The PAR index, part 2.

Shaw, W. C., O'Brien, K. D., and Richmond, S. (1991). Quality control in orthodontics: indices of treatment need and treatment standards. *British Dental Journal*, **170**, 107–12. [DOI: 10.1038/sj.bdj.4807429] [PubMed: 2007067]
An interesting paper on the role of indices, with good explanations of the IOTN and the PAR index.

Tang, E. L. K. and Wei, S. H. Y. (1993). Recording and measuring malocclusion: a review of the literature. *American Journal of Orthodontics and Dentofacial Orthopedics*, **103**, 344–51. [DOI: 10.1016/0889-5406(93)70015-G] [PubMed: 8480700]
Useful for those researching the subject.

 References for this chapter can also be found at: **www.oup.com/uk/orthodontics5e**. Where possible, these are presented as active links which direct you to the electronic version of the work, to help facilitate onward study. If you are a subscriber to that work (either individually or through an institution), and depending on your level of access, you may be able to peruse an abstract or the full article if available.

3

Management of the developing dentition

L. Mitchell

Chapter contents

Learning objectives for this chapter

- Gain an appreciation of normal development.
- Be able to recognize deviations from normal development.
- Gain an understanding of the management of commonly occurring mixed dentition problems.

Many dental practitioners find it difficult to judge when to intervene in a developing malocclusion and when to let nature take its course. This is because experience is only gained over years of careful observation and decisions to intercede are often made in response to pressure exerted by the parents 'to do something'. It is hoped that this chapter will help impart some of the former, so that the reader is better able to resist the latter.

3.1 Normal dental development

It is important to realize that 'normal' in this context means average, rather than ideal. An appreciation of what constitutes the range of normal development is essential. One area in which this is particularly pertinent is eruption times (Table 3.1).

3.1.1 Calcification and eruption times

Knowledge of the calcification times of the permanent dentition is invaluable if one wishes to impress patients and colleagues. It is also helpful for assessing dental as opposed to chronological age; for determining whether a developing tooth not present on radiographic examination can be considered absent; and for estimating the timing of any possible causes of localized hypocalcification or hypoplasia (termed in this situation chronological hypoplasia).

3.1.2 The transition from primary to mixed dentition

The eruption of a baby's first tooth is heralded by the proud parents as a major landmark in their child's development. This milestone is described in many baby-care books as occurring at 6 months of age, which can lead to unnecessary concern as it is normal for the mandibular incisors to erupt at any time in the first year. Dental textbooks often dismiss 'teething', ascribing the symptoms that occur at this time to the diminution of maternal antibodies. Any parent will be able to correct this fallacy!

Eruption of the primary dentition (Fig. 3.1) is usually completed around 3 years of age. The deciduous incisors erupt upright and spaced—a lack of spacing strongly suggests that the permanent successors will be crowded. Overbite reduces throughout the primary dentition until the incisors are edge to edge, which can contribute to marked attrition.

The mixed dentition phase is usually heralded by the eruption of either the first permanent molars or the lower central incisors. The lower labial segment teeth erupt before their counterparts in the upper arch and develop lingual to their predecessors. It is usual for there to be some crowding of the permanent lower incisors as they emerge into the mouth, which reduces with intercanine growth. As a result, the lower incisors often erupt slightly lingually placed and/or rotated (Fig. 3.2), but will usually align spontaneously if space becomes available. If the arch is inherently crowded, this space shortage will not resolve with intercanine growth.

Table 3.1 Average calcification and eruption times

Primary dentition	Calcification commences (weeks *in utero*)	Eruption (months)
Central incisors	12–16	6–7
Lateral incisors	13–16	7–8
Canines	15–18	18–20
First molars	14–17	12–15
Second molars	16–23	24–36

Root development complete 1–1½ years after eruption

Permanent dentition	Calcification commences (months)	Eruption (years)
Mand. central incisors	3–4	6–7
Mand. lateral incisors	3–4	7–8
Mand. canines	4–5	9–10
Mand. first premolars	21–24	10–12
Mand. second premolars	27–30	11–12
Mand. first molars	Around birth	5–6
Mand. second molars	30–36	12–13
Mand. third molars	96–120	17–25
Max. central incisors	3–4	7–8
Max. lateral incisors	10–12	8–9
Max. canines	4–5	11–12
Max. first premolars	18–21	10–11
Max. second premolars	24–27	10–12
Max. first molars	Around birth	5–6
Max. second molars	30–36	12–13
Max. third molars	84–108	17–25

Root development complete 2–3 years after eruption.

The upper permanent incisors also develop lingual to their predecessors. Additional space is gained to accommodate their greater width because they erupt onto a wider arc and are more proclined than the primary incisors. If the arch is intrinsically crowded, the lateral incisors will not be able to move labially following eruption of the central incisors and therefore may erupt palatal to the arch. Pressure from the developing lateral incisor often gives rise to spacing between the central incisors which resolves as the laterals erupt. They in turn are tilted distally by the canines lying on the distal aspect of their root. This latter stage of development used to be described as the 'ugly duckling' stage of development (Fig. 3.3), although it is probably diplomatic to describe it as normal dental development to concerned parents. As the canines

erupt, the lateral incisors usually upright themselves and the spaces close. The upper canines develop palatally, but migrate labially to come to lie slightly labial and distal to the root apex of the lateral incisors. In normal development, they can be palpated buccally from as young as 8 years of age.

The combined width of the deciduous canine, first molar, and second molar is greater than that of their permanent successors, particularly in the lower arch. This difference in widths is called the leeway space (Fig. 3.4) and in general is of the order of 1–1.5 mm in the maxilla and 2–2.5 mm in the mandible (in Caucasians). This means that if the deciduous buccal segment teeth are retained until their normal exfoliation time, there will be sufficient space for the permanent canine and premolars.

The deciduous second molars usually erupt with their distal surfaces flush anteroposteriorly. The transition to the stepped Class I molar relationship occurs during the mixed dentition as a result of differential mandibular growth and/or the leeway space.

3.1.3 Development of the dental arches

Intercanine width is measured across the cusps of the deciduous/permanent canines, and during the primary dentition an increase of around 1–2 mm is seen. In the mixed dentition, an increase of about 3 mm occurs, but this growth is largely completed around a developmental stage of 9 years with some minimal increase up to age 13 years. After this time, a gradual decrease is the norm.

Arch width is measured across the arch between the lingual cusps of the second deciduous molars or second premolars. Between the ages of 3 and 18 years, an increase of 2–3 mm occurs; however, for clinical purposes arch width is largely established in the mixed dentition.

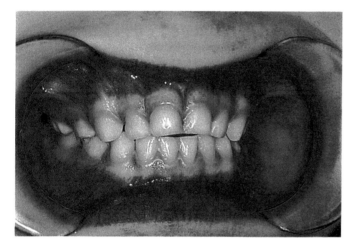

Fig. 3.1 Primary dentition.

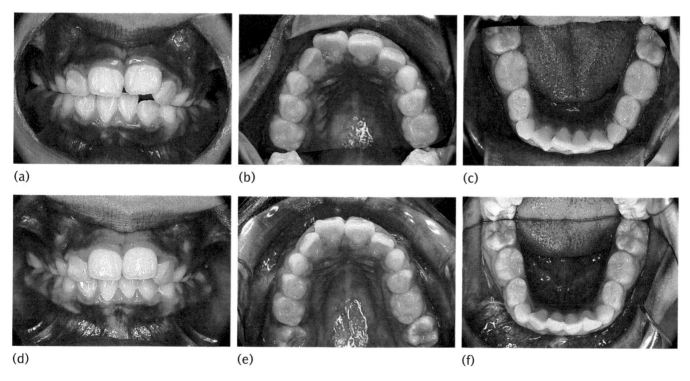

(a) (b) (c)

(d) (e) (f)

Fig. 3.2 Crowding of the labial segment reducing with growth in intercanine width: (a–c) age 8 years; (d–f) age 9 years.

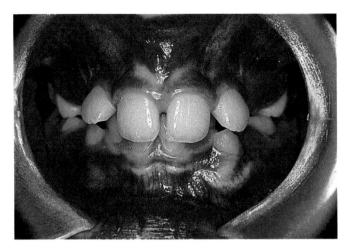

Fig. 3.3 'Ugly duckling' stage.

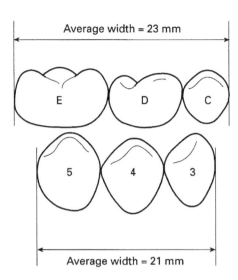

Fig. 3.4 Leeway space.

Arch circumference is determined by measuring around the buccal cusps and incisal edges of the teeth to the distal aspect of the second deciduous molars or second premolars. On average, there is little change with age in the maxilla; however, in the mandible, arch circumference decreases by about 4 mm because of the leeway space. In individuals with crowded mouths a greater reduction may be seen.

In summary, on the whole there is little change in the size of the arch anteriorly after the establishment of the primary dentition, except for an increase in intercanine width which results in a modification of arch shape. Growth posteriorly provides space for the permanent molars, and considerable appositional vertical growth occurs to maintain the relationship of the arches during vertical facial growth.

3.2 Abnormalities of eruption and exfoliation

3.2.1 Screening

Early detection of any abnormalities in tooth development and eruption is essential to give the opportunity for interceptive action to be taken. This requires careful observation of the developing dentition for evidence of any problems, for example, deviations from the normal sequence of eruption (see Fig. 3.5). If an abnormality is suspected, then further investigation including radiographs is indicated. Around 9–10 years of age it is important to palpate the buccal sulcus for the permanent maxillary canines in order to detect any abnormalities in the eruption path of this tooth. By the age of 10 the permanent maxillary canines will be palpable buccally in 70% of cases, by the age of 11, these teeth are palpable buccally in 95% of patients.

3.2.2 Natal teeth

A tooth, which is present at birth, or erupts soon after, is described as a natal tooth. Neonatal teeth are teeth that erupt within the first few weeks after birth. These most commonly arise anteriorly in the mandible and are typically a lower primary incisor which has erupted prematurely (Fig. 3.6). Because root formation is not complete at this stage, natal teeth can be quite mobile, but they usually become firmer relatively quickly. If the tooth (or teeth) interferes with breastfeeding or is so mobile that there is a danger of inhalation, removal is indicated and this

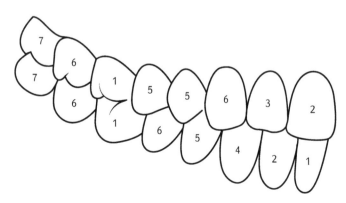

Fig. 3.5 Most common sequence of eruption.

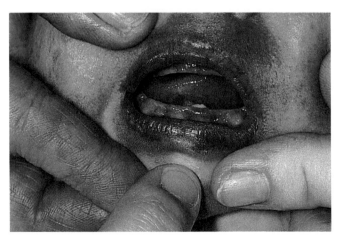

Fig. 3.6 Natal tooth present at birth.

can usually be accomplished with topical anaesthesia. If the tooth is symptomless, it can be left *in situ*.

3.2.3 Eruption cyst

An eruption cyst is caused by an accumulation of fluid or blood in the follicular space overlying the crown of an erupting tooth (Fig. 3.7). They usually rupture spontaneously, but very occasionally marsupialization may be necessary.

3.2.4 Failure of/delayed eruption

There is a wide individual variation in eruption times, which is illustrated by the patients in Fig. 3.8. Where there is a generalized tardiness in tooth eruption in an otherwise fit child, a period of observation is indicated. However, the following may be indicators of some abnormality and therefore warrant further investigation (Fig. 3.9). See also Box 3.1:

- A disruption in the normal sequence of eruption.
- An asymmetry in eruption pattern between contralateral teeth. If a tooth on one side of the arch has erupted and 6 months later there is still no sign of its equivalent on the other side, radiographic examination is indicated.

Localized failure of eruption is usually due to mechanical obstruction—this is advantageous as if the obstruction is removed then the affected tooth/teeth has/have the potential to erupt. More rarely, there is an abnormality of the eruption mechanism, which results in primary failure

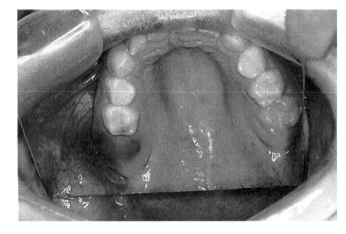

Fig. 3.7 Eruption cyst.

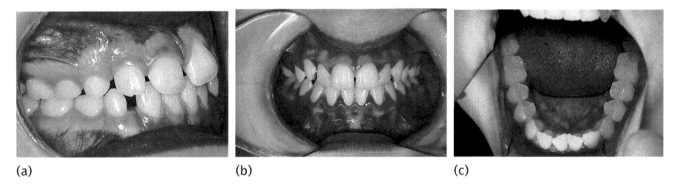

(a) (b) (c)

Fig. 3.8 Normal variation in eruption times: (a) patient aged 12.5 years with deciduous canines and molars still present; (b, c) patient aged 9 years with all permanent teeth to the second molars erupted.

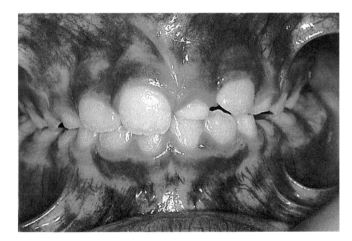

Fig. 3.9 Disruption of normal eruption sequence as 21/2 erupted, but /1 unerupted.

Box 3.1 **Causes of delayed eruption**

Generalized causes

- Hereditary gingival fibromatosis
- Down syndrome
- Cleidocranial dysostosis
- Cleft lip and palate
- Rickets.

Localized causes

- Congenital absence
- Crowding
- Delayed exfoliation of primary predecessor
- Supernumerary tooth
- Dilaceration
- Abnormal position of crypt
- Primary failure of eruption.

of eruption (the tooth does not erupt into the mouth) or arrest of eruption (the tooth erupts, but then fails to keep up with eruption/development). This problem usually affects molar teeth and unfortunately for the individuals concerned, all teeth distal to the affected tooth in that quadrant may also be involved. Extraction of the affected teeth is often necessary.

3.3 Mixed dentition problems

3.3.1 Premature loss of deciduous teeth

The major effect of early loss of a primary tooth, whether due to caries, premature exfoliation, or planned extraction, is localization of pre-existing crowding. In an uncrowded mouth this will not occur. However, where some crowding exists and a primary tooth is extracted, the adjacent teeth will drift or tilt around into the space provided. The extent to which this occurs depends upon the degree of crowding, the patient's age, and the site. Obviously, as the degree of crowding increases so does the pressure for the remaining teeth to move into the extraction space. The younger the child is when the primary tooth is extracted, the greater is the potential for drifting to ensue. The effect of the site of tooth loss is best considered by tooth type, but it is important to bear in mind the increased potential for mesial drift in the maxilla (see also Box 3.2).

- **Deciduous incisor:** premature loss of a deciduous incisor has little impact, mainly because they are shed relatively early in the mixed dentition.
- **Deciduous canine:** unilateral loss of a primary canine in a crowded mouth will lead to a centreline shift (Fig. 3.10). To avoid this when unilateral premature loss of a deciduous canine is necessary, consideration should be given to balancing with the extraction of the contralateral tooth.
- **Deciduous first molar:** unilateral loss of this tooth may result in a centreline shift, particularly in cases of crowding. In most cases, an automatic balancing extraction is not necessary, but the centreline should be kept under observation and, if indicated, a tooth on the opposite side of the arch removed.
- **Deciduous second molar:** if a second primary molar is extracted, the first permanent molar will drift forwards (Fig. 3.11). This is particularly marked if loss occurs before the eruption of the permanent tooth and for this reason it is better, if at all possible, to try to preserve the second deciduous molar at least until the first permanent molar has appeared. In most cases, balancing or compensating extractions of other sound second primary molars is not necessary unless they are also of poor long-term prognosis.

It should be emphasized that the above are suggestions, not rules, and at all times a degree of common sense and forward planning should be applied—in essence a risk–benefit analysis needs to be worked through for each child/tooth. For example, if extraction of a carious first primary molar is required and the contralateral tooth is also doubtful, then it might be preferable in the long term to extract both. Also, in children with an absent permanent tooth (or teeth), early extraction of the primary buccal segment teeth may be advantageous to encourage forward movement of the first permanent molars if space closure (rather than space opening) is planned.

The effect of early extraction of a primary tooth on the eruption of its successor is variable and will not necessarily result in a hastening of eruption.

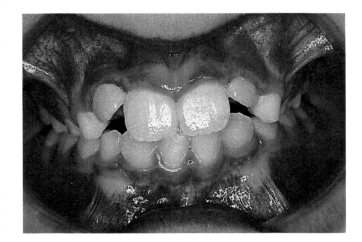

Fig. 3.10 Centreline shift to patient's left due to early unbalanced loss of lower left deciduous canine.

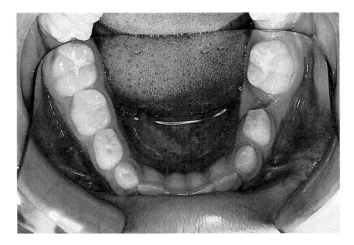

Fig. 3.11 Loss of a lower second deciduous molar leading to forward drift of first permanent molar.

Box 3.2 Balancing and compensating extractions

Balancing extraction is the removal of the contralateral tooth—*rationale is to avoid centreline shift problems.*

Compensating extraction is the removal of the equivalent opposing tooth—*rationale is to maintain occlusal relationships between the arches.*

Space maintenance

It goes without saying that the best space maintenance is a tooth—particularly as this will preserve alveolar bone. Much has been written in paedodontic texts about using space maintainers to replace extracted deciduous teeth, but in practice, most orthodontists avoid this approach in the mixed dentition because of the implications for dental health and to minimize straining patient cooperation (which may be needed for definitive orthodontic treatment later). The exception to this is where preservation of space for a permanent successor will avoid subsequent appliance treatment.

3.3.2 Retained deciduous teeth

A difference of more than 6 months between the shedding of contralateral teeth should be regarded with suspicion. Provided that the permanent successor is present, retained primary teeth should be extracted, particularly if they are causing deflection of the permanent tooth (Fig. 3.12).

3.3.3 Infra-occluded (submerged) primary molars

Infra-occlusion is now the preferred term for describing the process where a tooth fails to achieve or maintain its occlusal relationship with adjacent or opposing teeth. Most infra-occluded deciduous teeth erupt into occlusion but subsequently become 'submerged' because bony growth and development of the adjacent teeth continues (Fig. 3.13). Estimates vary, but this anomaly would appear to occur in around 1–9% of children.

Resorption of deciduous teeth is not a continuous process. In fact, resorption is interchanged with periods of repair, although in most cases the former prevails. If a temporary predominance of repair occurs, this can result in ankylosis and infra-occlusion of the affected primary molar.

The results of recent epidemiological studies have suggested a genetic tendency to this phenomenon and also an association with other dental anomalies including ectopic eruption of first permanent molars, palatal displacement of maxillary canines, and congenital absence of premolar teeth. Therefore, it is advisable to be vigilant in patients exhibiting any of these features.

Where a permanent successor exists, and in a good position, the phenomenon is usually temporary, and studies have shown no difference in the age at exfoliation of a submerged primary molar compared with an unaffected contralateral tooth. Therefore, provided the permanent successor is present and in a good position, extraction of a submerged primary tooth is only necessary under the following conditions:

- There is a danger of the tooth disappearing below gingival level (Fig. 3.14).
- Root formation of the permanent tooth is nearing completion (as eruptive force reduces markedly after this event).

In the buccal segments, if the permanent successor is missing, preservation of the primary molar will preserve bone, therefore consideration should be given to building up the occlusal surface to maintain occlusal relationships. If this is not practicable then extraction may be indicated.

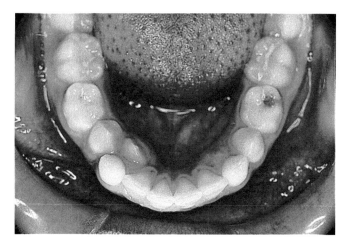

Fig. 3.12 Retained primary tooth contributing to deflection of the permanent successor.

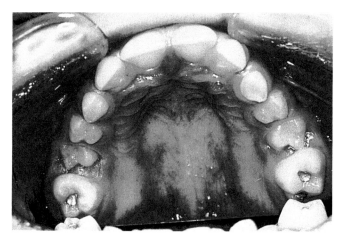

Fig. 3.13 Ankylosed primary molars.

3.3.4 Impacted first permanent molars

Impaction of a first permanent molar tooth against the second deciduous molar occurs in approximately 2–6% of children and is indicative of crowding. It most commonly occurs in the upper arch (Fig. 3.15). Spontaneous disimpaction may occur, but this is rare after 8 years of age. Mild cases can sometimes be managed by tightening a brass separating wire around the contact point between the two teeth over a period of about 2 months. This can have the effect of pushing the permanent molar distally, thus letting it jump free. In more severe cases of impaction, an appliance can be used to distalize the permanent molar and disimpact it. Alternatively, it can be kept under observation, although extraction of the deciduous tooth may be indicated if it becomes abscessed or the permanent tooth becomes carious and restoration is precluded by poor access. The resultant space loss can be dealt with in the permanent dentition.

3.3.5 Dilaceration

Dilaceration is a distortion or bend in the root of a tooth. It usually affects the upper central and/or lateral incisor.

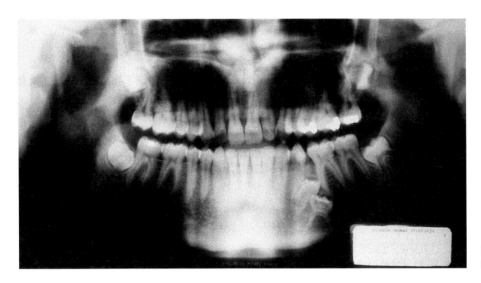

Fig. 3.14 Marked submergence of deciduous molar (with second premolar affected).

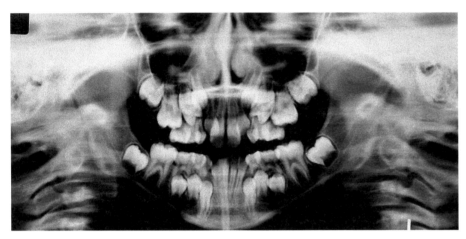

Fig. 3.15 Impacted bilateral upper first permanent molars.

Aetiology

There appear to be two distinct aetiologies:

- Developmental: this anomaly usually affects an isolated central incisor and occurs more often in females than males. The crown of the affected tooth is turned upward and labially and no disturbance of enamel and dentine is seen (Fig. 3.16).
- Trauma: intrusion of a deciduous incisor leads to displacement of the underlying developing permanent tooth germ. Characteristically, this causes the developing permanent tooth crown to be deflected palatally, and the enamel and dentine forming at the time of the injury are disturbed, giving rise to hypoplasia. The sexes are equally affected and more than one tooth may be involved depending upon the extent of the trauma.

Management

Dilaceration usually results in failure of eruption. Where the dilaceration is severe, there is often no alternative but to remove the affected tooth. In milder cases, it may be possible to expose the crown surgically and apply traction to align the tooth, provided that the root apex will be sited within cancellous bone at the completion of crown alignment.

3.3.6 Supernumerary teeth

A supernumerary tooth is one that is additional to the normal series. This anomaly occurs in the permanent dentition in approximately 2% of the population and in the primary dentition in less than 1%, though a supernumerary in the deciduous dentition is often followed by a supernumerary in the permanent dentition. The aetiology is not completely understood, but appears to have a genetic component. It occurs more commonly in males than females. Supernumerary teeth are also commonly found in the region of the cleft in individuals with a cleft of the alveolus.

Supernumerary teeth can be described according to their morphology or position in the arch.

Morphology

- Supplemental: this type resembles a tooth and occurs at the end of a tooth series, for example, an additional lateral incisor, second premolar, or fourth molar (Fig. 3.17).
- Conical: the conical or peg-shaped supernumerary most often occurs between the upper central incisors (Fig. 3.18). It is said to be more commonly associated with displacement of the adjacent teeth, but can also cause failure of eruption or not affect the other teeth.

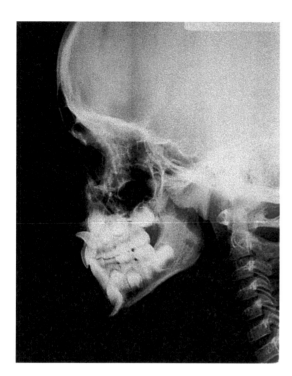

Fig. 3.16 A dilacerated central incisor.

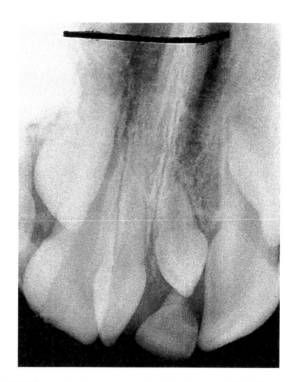

Fig. 3.18 Two conical supernumeraries lying between 1/1 with /A retained.

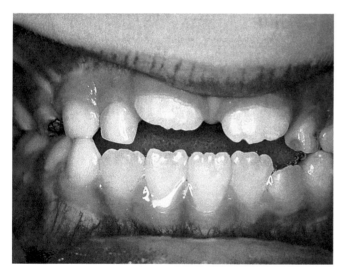

Fig. 3.17 A supplemental lower lateral incisor.

- Tuberculate: this type is described as being barrel shaped, but usually any supernumerary which does not fall into the conical or supplemental categories is included. Classically, this type is associated with failure of eruption (Fig. 3.19).

- Odontome: this variant is rare. Both compound (a conglomeration of small tooth-like structures) and complex (an amorphous mass of enamel and dentine) forms have been described.

Position

Supernumerary teeth can occur within the arch, but when they develop between the central incisors they are often described as a mesiodens.

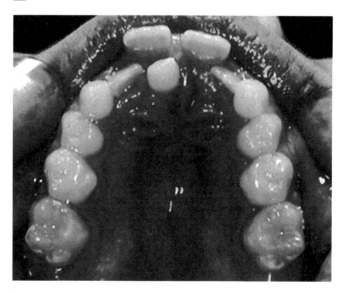

Fig. 3.19 A supernumerary which erupted palatal to upper incisors.

A supernumerary tooth distal to the arch is called a distomolar, and one adjacent to the molars is known as a paramolar. Eighty per cent of supernumeraries occur in the anterior maxilla.

Effects of supernumerary teeth and their management

Failure of eruption

The presence of a supernumerary tooth is the most common reason for the non-appearance of a maxillary central incisor. However, failure of eruption of any tooth in either arch can be caused by a supernumerary.

Management of this problem involves removing the impediment to eruption, the supernumerary, and ensuring that there is sufficient space to accommodate the unerupted tooth in the arch. If the tooth does not erupt spontaneously within 1 year, then a second operation to expose it and apply orthodontic traction may be required. Management of a patient with this problem is illustrated in Fig. 3.20.

Displacement

The presence of a supernumerary tooth can be associated with displacement or rotation of an erupted permanent tooth (Fig. 3.21). Management involves firstly removal of the supernumerary, usually followed by fixed appliances to align the affected tooth or teeth. It is said that this type of displacement has a high tendency to relapse following treatment, but this may be a reflection of the fact that the malposition

is usually in the form of a rotation or an apical displacement which, in themselves, are particularly liable to relapse.

Crowding

This is caused by the supplemental type and is treated by removing the most poorly formed or more displaced tooth (Fig. 3.22).

No effect

Occasionally, a supernumerary tooth (usually of the conical type) is detected as a chance finding on a radiograph of the upper incisor region (Fig. 3.23). Provided that the extra tooth will not interfere with any planned movement of the upper incisors, it can be left *in situ* under radiographic observation. In practice, these teeth usually remain symptomless and do not give rise to any problems. Some conical supernumeraries erupt palatally to the upper incisors, in which case their removal is straightforward.

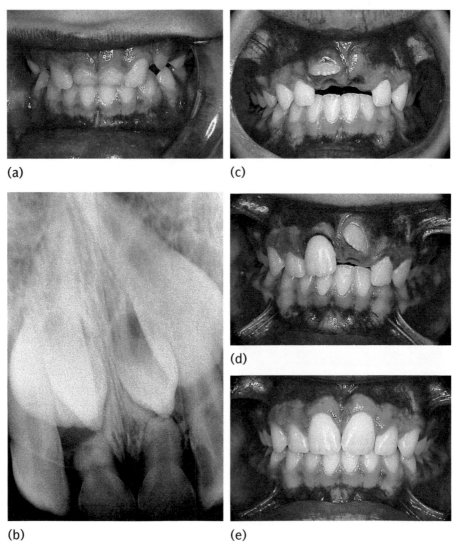

(a)

(c)

(b)

(d)

(e)

Fig. 3.20 Management of a patient with failure of eruption of the upper central incisors due to the presence of two supernumerary teeth: (a) patient on presentation aged 10 years; (b) radiograph showing unerupted central incisors and associated conical supernumerary teeth; (c) following removal of the supernumerary teeth an upper removable appliance was fitted to open space for the central incisors, until 1/ erupted 10 months later; (d) 7 months later /1 erupted and a simple appliance was used to align /1; (e) occlusion 3 years after initial presentation.

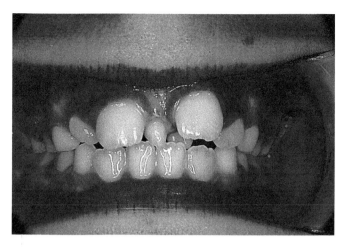

Fig. 3.21 Displacement of 1/1 caused by two erupted conical supernumerary teeth.

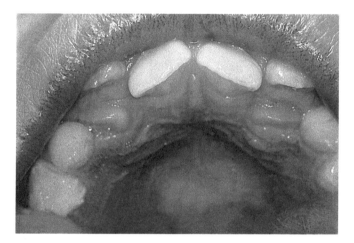

Fig. 3.22 Crowding due to the presence of two supplemental upper lateral incisors.

3.3.7 Habits

The effect of a habit will depend upon the frequency and intensity of indulgence. This problem is discussed in greater detail in Chapter 9, Section 9.1.4.

3.3.8 First permanent molars of poor long-term prognosis

The integrity of the first permanent molars is often compromised due to caries and/or hypoplasia secondary to a childhood illness. Treatment planning for a child with poor-quality first permanent molars is always difficult because several competing factors have to be considered before a decision can be reached for a particular individual. First permanent molars are rarely the first tooth of choice for extraction as their position within the arch means that little space is provided anteriorly for relief of crowding or correction of the incisor relationship unless appliances are used. Removal of maxillary first molars often compromises anchorage in the upper arch, and a good spontaneous result in the lower arch following extraction of the first molars is rare. However, patients for whom enforced extraction of the first molars is required are often the least able to support complicated treatment. Finally, it has to be remembered that, unless the caries rate is reduced, the premolars may be similarly affected a few years later. Nevertheless, if a two-surface restoration is present or required in the first permanent molar of a child, the prognosis for that tooth and the remaining first molars should be considered as the planned extraction of first permanent molars of poor quality may be preferable to their enforced extraction later on (Fig. 3.24).

Factors to consider when assessing first permanent molars of poor long-term prognosis

It is impossible to produce hard and fast rules regarding the extraction of first permanent molars, and therefore the following should only be considered a starting point:

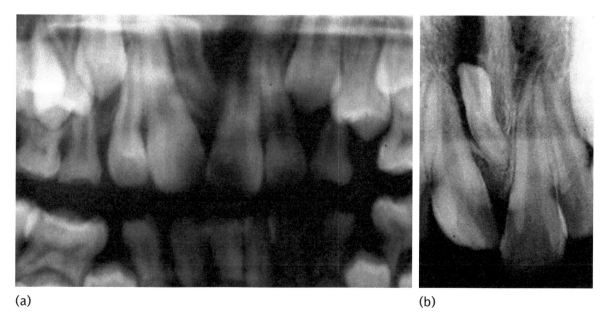

(a)   (b)

Fig. 3.23 Chance finding of a supernumerary on routine radiographic examination.

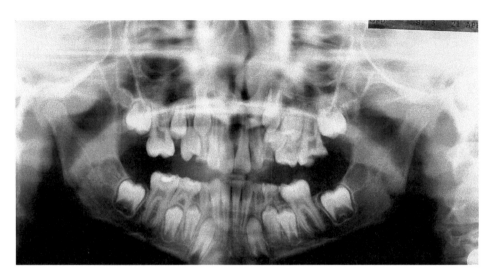

Fig. 3.24 All four first permanent molars were extracted in this patient because of the poor long-term prognosis for 6̄| and |6̲.

- Check for the presence of all permanent teeth. If any are absent, extraction of the first permanent molar in that quadrant should be avoided.

- If the dentition is uncrowded, extraction of first permanent molars should be avoided as space closure will be difficult.

- Remember that in the maxilla there is a greater tendency for mesial drift and so the timing of the extraction of upper first permanent molars is less critical if aiming for space closure.

- In the lower arch, a good spontaneous result is more likely if:
  (a) the lower second permanent molar has developed as far as its bifurcation
  (b) the angle between the long axis of the crypt of the lower second permanent molar and the first permanent molar is between 15° and 30°
  (c) the crypt of the second molar overlaps the root of the first molar (a space between the two reduces the likelihood of good space closure).

- Extraction of the first molars alone will relieve buccal segment crowding, but will have little effect on a crowded labial segment.

- If space is needed anteriorly for the relief of labial segment crowding or for retraction of incisors (i.e. the upper arch in Class II cases or the lower arch in Class III cases), then it may be prudent to delay extraction of the first molar, if possible, until the second permanent molar has erupted in that arch. The space can then be utilized, in conjunction with appliance therapy, for correction of the labial segment.

- Serious consideration should be given to extracting the opposing upper first permanent molar, should extraction of a lower molar be necessary. If the upper molar is not extracted, it will over-erupt and prevent forward drift of the lower second molar (Fig. 3.25).

- A compensating extraction in the lower arch (when extraction of an upper first permanent molar is necessary) should be avoided where possible as a good spontaneous result in the mandibular arch is less likely.

- Impaction of the third permanent molars is less likely, but not impossible, following extraction of the first molar.

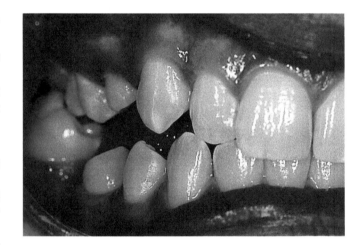

Fig. 3.25 Over-eruption of 6̲/ preventing forward movement of the lower right second permanent molar.

3.3.9 Median diastema

Prevalence

Median diastema occurs in around 98% of 6-year-olds, 49% of 11-year-olds, and 7% of 12–18-year-olds.

Aetiology

Factors which have been considered to lead to a median diastema include the following:

- Physiological (normal dental development)
- Familial or racial trait
- Small teeth in large jaws (a spaced dentition)
- Missing teeth
- Midline supernumerary tooth/teeth
- Proclination of the upper labial segment
- Prominent fraenum.

A median diastema is normally present between the maxillary permanent central incisors when they first erupt. As the lateral incisors and then the canines emerge, the diastema usually closes. Therefore, a midline diastema is a normal feature of the developing dentition; however, if it persists after eruption of the canines, it is unlikely that it will close spontaneously.

In the deciduous dentition, the upper midline fraenum runs between the central incisors and attaches into the incisive papilla area. However, as the central incisors move together with eruption of the lateral incisors, it tends to migrate round onto the labial aspect. In a spaced upper arch, or where the upper lateral incisors are missing (see Chapter 8, Fig. 8.5), this recession of the fraenal attachment is less likely to occur and in such cases it is obviously not appropriate to attribute the persistence of a diastema to the fraenum itself. However, in a small proportion of cases, the upper midline fraenum can contribute to the persistence of a diastema. Factors, which may indicate that this is the case, include the following.

- When the fraenum is placed under tension there is blanching of the incisive papilla.
- Radiographically, a notch can be seen at the crest of the interdental bone between the upper central incisors (Fig. 3.26).
- The anterior teeth may be crowded.

Management

It is advisable to take a periapical radiograph to exclude the presence of a midline supernumerary tooth prior to planning treatment for a midline diastema.

In the developing dentition, a diastema of less than 3 mm rarely warrants intervention; in particular, extraction of the deciduous canines should be avoided as this will tend to make the diastema worse. However, if the diastema is greater than 3 mm and the lateral incisors are present, it may be necessary to consider appliance treatment to approximate the

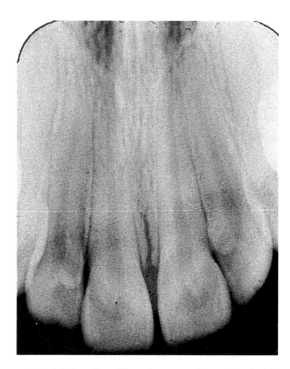

Fig. 3.26 Notch in interdental bone between 1/1 associated with a fraenal insertion running between 1/1 into the incisive papilla.

central incisors to provide space for the laterals and canines to erupt. However, care should be taken to ensure that the roots of the teeth being moved are not pressed against any unerupted crowns as this can lead to root resorption. If the crowns of the teeth are tilted distally, an upper removable appliance can be used to approximate the teeth, but usually fixed appliances are required. Closure of a diastema has a notable tendency to relapse, therefore long-term retention is required. This is most readily accomplished by placement of a bonded retainer.

3.4 Planned extraction of deciduous teeth

3.4.1 Serial extraction

Serial extraction is a historic approach involving a planned sequence of extractions (initially the deciduous canines, then the deciduous first molars) designed to allow crowded incisor segments to align spontaneously during the mixed dentition by shifting labial segment crowding to the buccal segments where it could be dealt with by first premolar extractions. The disadvantages to this approach are that it involves putting the child through several sequences of extractions and, as intercanine growth is occurring during this time, it is difficult to assess accurately how crowded the dentition will be, at the stage when serial extraction is usually embarked upon. In some Class I cases with moderate crowding and all permanent teeth present in a good position, extraction of only the first premolars upon eruption will produce an acceptable result.

3.4.2 Indications for the extraction of deciduous canines

There are a number of occasions where the timely extraction of the deciduous canines may avoid more complicated treatment later:

- In a crowded upper arch, the erupting lateral incisors may be forced palatally. In a Class I malocclusion, this will result in a crossbite and in addition the apex of the affected lateral incisor will be palatally positioned, making later correction more difficult. Extraction of the deciduous canines while the lateral incisors are erupting often results in them being able to escape spontaneously labially into a better position.
- In a crowded lower labial segment, one incisor may be pushed through the labial plate of bone, resulting in a compromised labial

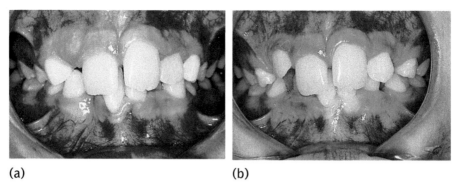

(a)   (b)

Fig. 3.27 (a) In this patient, all four deciduous canines were extracted to relieve the labial segment crowding; (b) note how the periodontal condition of the lower right central incisor has improved 6 months later.

periodontal attachment. Relief of crowding by extraction of the lower deciduous canines usually results in the lower incisor moving back into the arch and improving periodontal support (Fig. 3.27).

- Extraction of the lower deciduous canines in a Class III malocclusion can be advantageous.

3.5 What to refer and when

Most orthodontic problems are more appropriately referred and treated in the early permanent dentition. However, earlier referral is indicated in the following circumstances:

3.5.1 Deciduous dentition

- Cleft lip and/or palate (if patient not under the care of a cleft team).
- Other craniofacial anomalies (if patient not under the care of a multidisciplinary team).

3.5.2 Mixed dentition

- Severe Class III skeletal problems which would benefit from orthopaedic treatment.
- Delayed eruption of the permanent incisors.
- Presence of a supplemental incisor and the decision as to which to extract is not clear-cut.

- To provide space for appliance therapy in the upper arch, for example, correction of an instanding lateral incisor, or to facilitate eruption of an incisor prevented from erupting by a supernumerary tooth.
- To improve the position of a displaced permanent canine (see Chapter 14).

- Impaction or failure of eruption of the first permanent molars.
- First permanent molars of poor long-term prognosis where forced extraction is being considered.
- Ectopic maxillary canines.
- Hypodontia.
- Marked mandibular displacement on closure and/or anterior crossbites which compromise periodontal support.
- Patients with medical problems where monitoring of the occlusion would be beneficial.
- Pathology (e.g. cysts).

Growth modification in skeletal Class II malocclusions is more successful if carried out in early permanent dentition, therefore referral should be timed accordingly. The exceptions to this are patients with increased overjets who are being psychologically affected by severe teasing and those whose upper incisors are at risk of trauma (usually due to grossly incompetent lips).

Principal sources and further reading

Bishara, S. E. (1997). Arch width changes from 6 weeks to 45 years of age. *American Journal of Orthodontics and Dentofacial Orthopedics*, **111**, 401–9. [DOI: 10.1016/S0889-5406(97)80022-4] [PubMed: 9109585]
As it says on the tin.

Bjerklin, K., Kurol, J., and Valentin, J. (1992). Ectopic eruption of maxillary first permanent molars and association with other tooth and development disturbances. *European Journal of Orthodontics*, **14**, 369–75. [DOI: 10.1093/ejo/14.5.369] [PubMed: 1397075]
The results of this study suggest a link between ectopic eruption of first permanent molars, infra-occlusion of deciduous molars, ectopic maxillary canines, and absent premolars. Given this association, the wise practitioner will be alerted to other anomalies in patients presenting with any of these features.

British Orthodontic Society. Advice Sheet: Dummies and Digit Sucking (http://www.bos.org.uk/MembersAdviceSheets).
Unfortunately this advice sheet is only available to British Orthodontic Society members so you will need to approach a member to get a copy.

British Orthodontic Society. Managing the developing occlusion (http://www.bos.org.uk/Professionals-Members/Members-Area-Publications-General-Guidance/BOS-Publications).
This booklet contains much useful information but again is only available to British Orthodontic Society members so you will need to approach a member to get a copy.

British Orthodontic Society. Quick reference guide to orthodontic assessment and treatment need (http://bos.org.uk/Information-for-Dentists/Quick-Reference-Guide-to-Orthodontic-Assessment-and-Treatment).

A very useful two-page download that includes further information on what to refer and when.

Cobourne, M., Williams, A., and Harrison, M. (2017). *A Guideline for the Extraction of First Permanent Molars in Children*. London: Faculty of Dental Surgery of the Royal College of Surgeons of England (https://www.rcseng.ac.uk/dental-faculties/fds/publications-guidelines/clinical-guidelines/).
An excellent résumé of the available evidence on this important topic.

Gorlin, R. J., Cohen, M. M., and Levin, L. S. (1990). *Syndromes of the Head and Neck* (3rd edn). Oxford: Oxford University Press.
Source of calcification and eruption dates (and a vast amount of additional information not directly related to this chapter).

Kurol, J. and Bjerklin, K. (1986). Ectopic eruption of maxillary first permanent molars: a review. *Journal of Dentistry for Children*, **53**, 209–15. [PubMed: 3519711]
All you need to know about impacted first permanent molars.

Welbury, R. R., Duggal, M. S., and Hosey, M-T. (2012). *Paediatric Dentistry* (4th edn). Oxford: Oxford University Press.

Yacoob, O., O'Neill, J., Patel, S., Seehra, J., Bryant, C., Noar, J., and Gregg, T. (2016). Management of unerupted maxillary incisors. Faculty of Dental Surgery of the Royal College of Surgeons of England (https://www.rcseng.ac.uk/dental-faculties/fds/publications-guidelines/clinical-guidelines/).

 References for this chapter can also be found at: **www.oup.com/uk/orthodontics5e**. Where possible, these are presented as active links which direct you to the electronic version of the work, to help facilitate onward study. If you are a subscriber to that work (either individually or through an institution), and depending on your level of access, you may be able to peruse an abstract or the full article if available.

4

Craniofacial growth and the cellular basis of tooth movement

F. R. Jenkins

4.1 Introduction

Growth can be defined as an increase in size by natural development. Orthodontic treatment is often carried out on growing children, so knowledge of facial growth and development is essential for the dental professional to understand the optimum timing of treatment, predictors for success, potential pitfalls, and the stability of the finished result.

Craniofacial growth, including growth of the cranium and the facial bones is still not fully understood. The areas where growth occurs in the craniofacial bones and how this changes the shape of the bones and the face are, however, well described. Facial development will be described from the earliest development in the embryo to the reduction of growth to adult levels.

The ability to move teeth within the bones of the jaws is the basis of orthodontic treatment. This movement relies on the ability of the bone to remodel around the moving tooth and periodontal ligament (PDL). The cellular basis of tooth movement will be described.

4.2 Early craniofacial development

Craniofacial growth problems account for three-quarters of all birth defects. Knowledge of early formation of facial tissues can help us understand how problems in craniofacial growth can occur.

The fertilized egg divides rapidly into a ball of cells, or blastocyst. From day 4 after fertilization to around week 8 *in utero* (i.u.), the cells of the blastocyst differentiate and organize into different tissues and organ systems. This differentiation into various tissue types and patterning into the human shape is under tight genetic control and results from a myriad of complex interactions between the different tissues. During the fetal stage, from week 8 i.u. until birth, continued development is predominantly growth, without significant further differentiation.

4.2.1 Neural crest

Many of the tissues of the craniofacial region are derived from neural crest cells, including the cartilage and bone of the skull, cartilages of the pharyngeal arches, bones of the facial skeleton, and odontoblasts (tooth-forming cells). Neural crest cells are also responsible for other specialized tissues throughout the body. They migrate to the facial area from the tips of the neural crests, which join to form a tube around the primitive spinal cord in very early embryonic development, around week 3 i.u.

4.2.2 Pharyngeal arches

Pharyngeal arches form as part of the highly preserved genetic segmental patterning that occurs in many different species. There are six pairs of pharyngeal arches and they develop between the developing brain and heart. Each arch is separated by a groove, or cleft, on the outside and a pouch on the inside. Each arch contains cartilage, muscle, blood supply, and a nerve. The first pharyngeal arch goes on to form the maxilla, mandible, and the associated muscles and nerves. The cartilage of the first pharyngeal arch, known as 'Meckel's cartilage', does not directly form the bone of the mandible, but serves as a support and template for the developing mandible. First arch structures also include some of the bones of the middle ear and the external ear.

4.2.3 Facial development

See Fig. 4.1.

The development of the face begins around the end of the fourth week i.u. with the appearance of five swellings, or processes, around the stomodeum (primitive mouth). The maxillary and mandibular swellings, both derived from the first pharyngeal arch, appear laterally, on either side of the stomodeum. The mandibular swellings form the lower border and the fifth, frontonasal process, forms the upper border of the stomodeum. The maxillary swellings continue to grow forwards and move closer together toward the midline. Two thickenings develop on the frontonasal process, called nasal placodes. Nasal pits form at the centre of these and the raised rim around each nasal pit divides into lateral and medial nasal processes. At around the end of week 5 i.u., the mandibular swellings merge to form the primitive lower lip. The deepened nasal pits merge to form a single nasal sac, or primitive nasal cavity. The medial nasal processes merge with each other and from 6 to 7 weeks i.u. they develop into the intermaxillary process. The maxillary processes grow mesially toward the intermaxillary process. Between 7 and 10 weeks i.u. the maxillary processes merge in front of the intermaxillary process, forming the philtrum and completing the primitive upper lip. Failure of the maxillary swellings to fuse on either or both sides leads to unilateral or bilateral cleft lip respectively (see Chapter 24). The maxillary and mandibular swellings merge to create the cheeks, reducing the mouth to its final width.

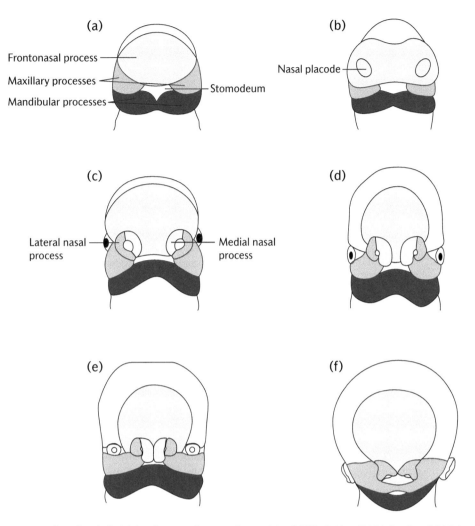

Fig. 4.1 Diagrammatic representation of early facial development from week 4 to 10 i.u. (a) Week 4 i.u.; (b) 28 days i.u.; (c) 32 days i.u.; (d) week 5 i.u.; (e) 48 days i.u.; (f) week 10 i.u. Further detail is given in the text: see Section 4.2.3. Redrawn from a previously available electronic source: http://www.biomed2.man.ac.uk/ugrad/biomedical/calpage/sproject/rob/glossary.html.

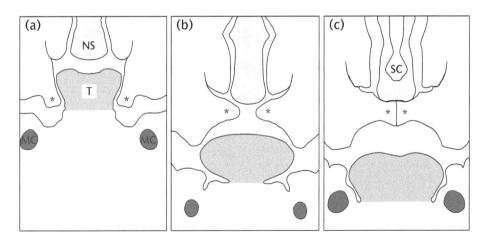

Fig. 4.2 Diagrammatic representation of palatal shelf elevation and fusion. (a) During week 7 i.u., the palatal shelves begin to develop and lie on either side of the tongue. (b) During week 8 i.u., the palatine shelves elevate rapidly due to the internal shelf-elevating force and developmental changes in the face. (c) During week 9 i.u., the shelves fuse with each other, the primary palate, and the nasal septum. MC = Meckel's cartilage; NS = nasal septum; SC = septal cartilage; T = tongue; * = palatal shelves.

4.2.4 Formation of the palate

See Fig. 4.2.

The intermaxillary process goes on to form the primary palate and then the pre-maxilla, a small part of the anterior palate, including the four upper incisor teeth. It also forms the nasal septum, which divides the nasal cavity vertically in two and the floor of the primitive nasal cavity.

At the beginning of week 7 i.u. the inner walls of the maxillary processes begin to develop thin extensions or 'palatine shelves', which form initially on either side of the developing tongue. As the tongue lowers, the palatine shelves rotate upwards toward the midline and grow toward each other. During week 8 and 9 i.u., the shelves fuse with each other, and also to the primary palate and the lower border of the nasal septum. Any disturbance in this process of elevation and fusion can cause a cleft of the palate (see Chapter 24).

4.3 Mechanisms of bone formation and growth

The process of new mineralized bone formation is known as ossification. This can occur in two ways:

- Intramembranous ossification—formation of bone in a membrane.
- Endochondral ossification—bony replacement of a cartilage model.

Once mature, the bone is the same for both types of ossification. A single bone may be formed by both intramembranous and endochondral ossification, merging almost indistinguishably.

Intramembranous ossification occurs during embryonic development in sheet-like osteogenic membranes. The bones of the calvarium, facial bones, most of the mandible, and the clavicle are formed by intramembranous ossification.

Endochondral ossification occurs in all other bones of the skeleton. It begins in ossification centres in cartilage models of the bones and spreads out from these primary ossification centres. Growth at primary ossification centres causes expansion. A synchondrosis is a cartilage-based growth centre with ossification and bony growth occurring in both directions. The bones on either side move apart as the bone grows, although growth is not necessarily even on both sides. At birth, there are three synchondroses in the cranial base. The most significant, in terms of influence on facial growth, is the synchondrosis between the sphenoid and occipital bones, the spheno-occipital synchondrosis. This will be discussed in Section 4.5.2.

Bone does not grow from the middle. It grows by depositing new bone around the outside edges and removing, or resorbing other bone to maintain shape. The periosteum covering the bone surface initiates the complex pattern of deposition and resorption, or remodelling. Resorption on one side of a bone and deposition on the other can give the appearance, over time, of a change in position or drift of the bone.

The bones of the face and skull touch together at sutures. Bony infill at the sutures occurs in response to forces separating the bones on either side. For example, an increase in the size of the growing brain leads to the bones of the calvarium being pushed apart and sutural bony growth to maintain the integrity of the bony casing. Growth which causes a mass of bone to be moved relative to its neighbours is known as displacement. Both remodelling and displacement can occur in the same bone at the same time, but the relative contribution of each is difficult to determine. The cartilage in the mandibular condyle is formed from a different type of cartilage to that found in most other joints in the body. The role of the condylar cartilage in facial growth is not yet fully understood, but it appears to grow in response to the growth of other facial structures.

4.4 Control of craniofacial growth

The mechanisms controlling facial growth are poorly understood, but involve a combination of genetic and environmental factors. Studies suggest that genetic control is greater in anteroposterior growth than vertical growth, for example, the heritability of Class III occlusion and prevalence in different racial groups.

There are two main theories:

- Some researchers believe that there is tight genetic control of facial growth at primary growth cartilages in the facial skeleton, the nasal septal cartilage for maxillary growth, and the condylar cartilage for mandibular growth. Although these cartilages are necessary for facial growth they do not appear to be primary growth centres.
- Other researchers believe that growth occurs due to growth of surrounding soft tissues, the 'functional matrix' theory.

It is likely that both theories play a part in the control of craniofacial growth. If we believe environmental factors play a role in facial growth, then it should be possible for clinicians to alter facial growth with orthodontic appliances.

4.5 Postnatal craniofacial growth

Growth studies clearly show that overall as the face enlarges, it grows forwards and downwards away from the cranial base (Fig. 4.3). The calvarium, the cranial base, the maxilla, and the mandible all grow at different rates and at different times and are under the influence of different genetic and environmental factors. A harmonious facial form relies on a harmonious pattern of facial development. Variations in facial development can lead to variations in facial form and jaw relationships.

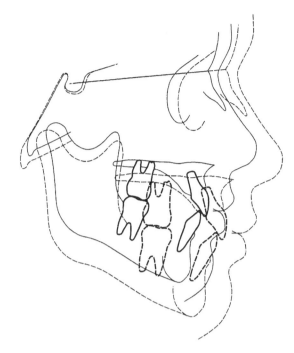

Fig. 4.3 Superimpositions on the cranial base showing overall downwards and forwards direction of facial growth. Solid line 8 years, broken line 18 years of age.

Facial growth in the first few years of life is determined principally by the growth of the brain (neural growth). There is rapid growth of the calvarium, eyes, and the bony orbits surrounding and protecting the eyes. This slows until the age of about 7 years, when growth of this area is almost complete. The face of a child represents a much smaller proportion of the skull than the face of an adolescent or adult (Fig. 4.4).

The rest of the face grows as the child increases in height, slowing down around puberty. Growth during puberty, the 'pubertal growth spurt', is rapid. Although there is significant variation in the timing of

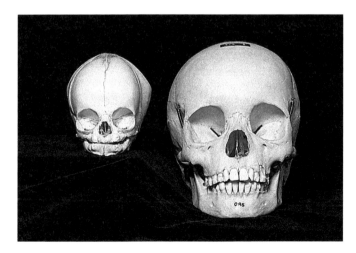

Fig. 4.4 The face in the newborn represents a much smaller proportion of the skull than the face of the adolescent

the pubertal growth spurt, this is reported to occur around the age of 10–12 years old in girls and 12–15 years old in boys. The maxilla follows a pattern of growth closer to neural growth and declines to adult levels around the age of 12. The mandible follows a pattern of growth more closely related to the rest of the body (somatic growth). Somatic growth increases significantly during puberty and continues until growth declines to adult levels around the age of 16 in girls and 18–20 in boys. Small growth spurts have been reported for males in their early twenties. Facial growth never completely stops, but reduces to adult levels, with subtle long-term changes throughout life.

4.5.1 Calvarium

The growth of the calvarium, the part of the skull that surrounds the brain, directly follows the growth of the brain. It is formed from several pairs of bones: frontal, parietal, occipital, and part of the temporal bones. The bones develop by intramembranous ossification. Ossification centres for each bone develop in the outer membrane of the brain during week 8 i.u. Bone formation spreads until the bone-forming fronts reach adjacent bones and sutures are formed. Where more than two bones meet, the intersecting areas are known as fontanelles. Six fontanelles are present at birth and close by 18 months. Continuing sutural growth allows expansion of the calvarium with resorption on the inside of the cranial bones and deposition on the outside. Growth of the skull is almost complete by 7 years of age. Eventually all the sutures undergo varying degrees of fusion.

4.5.2 Cranial base

The cranial base develops by endochondral ossification. Condensations of cartilage develop in three regions of the cranial base from around week 6 i.u. Several separate ossification centres appear between 3 and 5 months i.u. Most of the growth of the cranial base is influenced by the growth of the brain, with half of the postnatal growth complete by 3 years of age. Remodelling and sutural infilling occur as the brain enlarges. There are also primary cartilaginous growth sites in the cranial base, the synchondroses. Of these, the spheno-occipital synchondrosis makes an important contribution to the growth of the cranial base in childhood. It continues to grow until the age of 13–15 in females and 15–17 in males, fusing at about 20 years. The other two synchondroses in the anterior cranial base fuse around the age of 7 years. There is no further growth in this area after the age of 7. This means that the anterior cranial base can be used as a relatively stable structure to superimpose lateral cephalogram radiographs and to analyse changes in facial form due to growth and orthodontic treatment (see Chapter 6, Section 6.10).

Growth at the spheno-occipital synchondrosis, which lies between the anterior cranial base and the temporomandibular joint (TMJ), influences the overall skeletal pattern (Fig. 4.5). Growth at this site increases the length of the cranial base, effectively moving the TMJs and the lower jaw further back, away from the maxilla. A Class II skeletal pattern is often associated with a long cranial base. The shape, or angle, of the cranial base also affects the jaw relationship. A small, or acute, angle is more likely to produce a Class III skeletal pattern; a larger or more obtuse angle, a Class II skeletal pattern (Fig. 4.6).

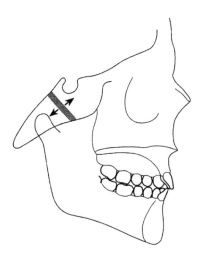

Fig. 4.5 Anteroposterior growth at the spheno-occipital synchondrosis affects the anteroposterior relationship of the jaws.

4.5.3 Maxillary complex

The maxillary complex or middle third of the facial skeleton is a complex structure including the maxilla, palatal, zygomatic, ethmoid, vomer, and nasal bones. These separate bones join with each other and the anterior cranial base at sutures. Clinical orthodontic practice is concerned primarily with the teeth and the associated supporting alveolar bone. Growth of the maxillary complex is clearly an important factor in the position of the upper teeth relative to the lower teeth and the final maxillary position and facial appearance. Until the age of 7 years, growth of the maxillary complex occurs by downward and forward displacement and by drift and remodelling (Fig. 4.7). As growth of the brain and calvarium slows so does maxillary growth. Forward displacement of the maxillary complex allows space for the maxilla to grow backwards, lengthening the dental arch posteriorly in the area of the tuberosities and allowing room for the permanent molars to erupt. Downward growth also occurs by drift of the hard palate and vertical development of the alveolar processes as the teeth erupt and complete

root formation. Lateral growth occurs by displacement of the two halves of the maxilla and infill at the mid-palatal suture. Complex patterns of surface remodelling maintain and develop the shape of the bones of the midfacial skeleton.

After the age of 7 years, growth of the maxillary complex slows. Orthodontic interventions to advance the maxilla, for example, with protraction headgear in Class III cases, are reported to be more successful before the age of 10 when the sutures around the maxilla are more amenable to displacement (see Chapter 11, Section 11.4.2). Interventions to expand the maxilla by rapid maxillary expansion are reported to be more successful before the age of 16 and progressive bony fusion of the mid-palatal suture (see Chapter 13, Section 13.4.6). Growth of the maxillary complex slows to adult levels at around 12 years.

4.5.4 Mandible

Most mandibular growth occurs by periosteal activity. The shape of the angle of the mandible and the coronoid process develop in reaction to forces from the attached muscles. The alveolar processes add to vertical growth with the eruption and development of the teeth. The mandible is displaced forward, by growth of the tongue. Growth at the condylar cartilage fills in posteriorly and periosteal remodelling maintains the shape of the mandible (Fig. 4.8). The role of the condylar cartilage in mandibular growth remains unclear, but it is not a primary growth centre. It appears to grow in response to other influences. Backward drift of the ramus as it remodels allows lengthening of the dental arch posteriorly and creates room for the permanent molars to erupt. Remodelling increases the width of the mandible posteriorly and lengthening of the mandible and remodelling causes the chin to appear more prominent. As with the maxilla, complex patterns of surface remodelling maintain and develop the shape of the mandible. Growth occurs at a steady rate of 2–3 mm per year in length of the body of the mandible until puberty when growth rates double. Mandibular growth slows to adult levels at around 17 years in girls and around 19 years in boys.

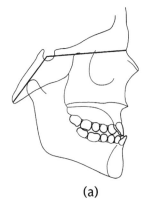

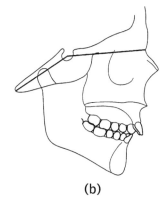

(a)

(b)

Fig. 4.6 (a) Low cranial base angle associated with Class III skeletal pattern. (b) High cranial base angle associated with a Class II skeletal pattern. Reprinted from Enlow, D. H. *Facial Growth*, Copyright (1990) with permission from Elsevier.

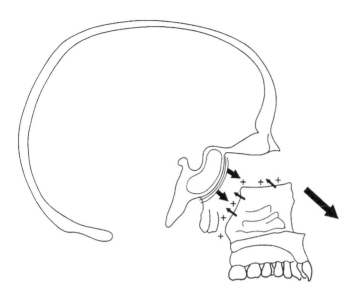

Fig. 4.7 Forward and downward displacement of the maxillary complex associated with deposition of bone at sutures. Reprinted from Enlow, D. H. and Hans M. G. *Essentials of facial growth*, 2nd edition. Copyright (2008) with permission from Elsevier. After Enlow, D. H. *Facial Growth*, Copyright (1990) with permission from Elsevier.

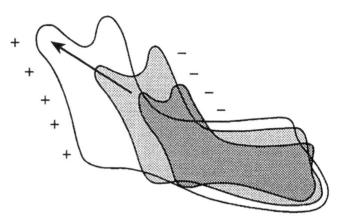

Fig. 4.8 Growth at the condylar cartilage 'fills in' for the mandible following anterior displacement, while its shape is maintained by remodelling, including posterior drift of the ramus. After Enlow, D. H. *Facial Growth*, Copyright (1990) with permission from Elsevier.

4.6 Growth rotations

Growth studies clearly show that overall as the face enlarges, it grows forwards and downwards. Research by Björk shows that the direction of facial growth is curved, giving a rotational effect. Growth rotations are most obvious in the mandible. They are dependent on differential growth of different structures contributing to posterior and anterior face height. Posterior face height is determined by several factors, including the direction of growth at the condyles (Fig. 4.9), vertical growth at the spheno-occipital synchondrosis, and the influence of the attached muscles on the ramus of the mandible. Anterior face height is determined by the eruption of the teeth, and vertical growth of the soft tissues of the anterior neck.

Forward growth rotations are more common than backward rotations, with the average being a mild forward rotation which produces a harmonious facial appearance. A marked forward growth rotation tends to result in reduced anterior facial proportions and an increased overbite (Fig. 4.10). A marked backward rotation tends to result in an increased anterior vertical facial proportion and a reduced overbite or anterior open bite (Fig. 4.11). Growth rotations play an important part in the aetiology of some malocclusions, as well as the stability

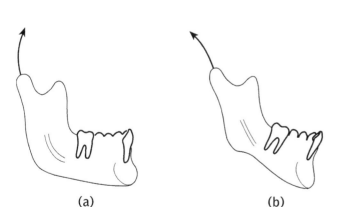

Fig. 4.9 Direction of condylar growth and mandibular growth rotations: (a) forward rotation; (b) backward rotation.

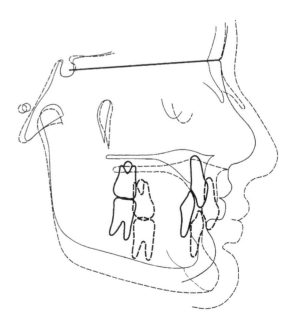

Fig. 4.10 Forward growth rotation. Solid line 11 years, broken line 18 years of age.

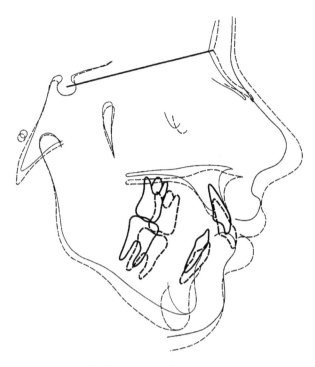

Fig. 4.11 Backward growth rotation. Solid line 12 years, broken line 19 years of age.

of the result. Correction of a Class II malocclusion will be helped by a forward growth rotation but made more difficult by a backward rotation. Forward growth rotations will tend to increase an overbite; backward growth rotations reduce an overbite or result in an open bite.

It is possible to assess the general direction of mandibular growth clinically with an examination of the anterior facial proportion and the mandibular plane angle. It is not possible to predict the extent and direction of growth rotations with any degree of accuracy.

4.7 Growth of the soft tissues

Facial form can be masked or accentuated by the facial soft tissues. The teeth are positioned in an area of relative stability between the tongue on one side, and the lips and cheeks on the other. Soft tissues are important in both the aetiology of malocclusion and stability of the orthodontic result after treatment.

Facial muscles are well developed at birth to allow the newborn child to suckle and maintain their airway. Facial expression, swallowing patterns, chewing, and speech develop later. The lips, tongue, and cheeks guide the erupting teeth toward each other to achieve an occlusion. The pressure of the soft tissues may compensate for a skeletal discrepancy, bringing the teeth as close together as possible within the confines of the dental bases; for example, proclination of the upper incisors and retroclination of the lower incisors in a Class III skeletal pattern.

During growth the brows become more prominent, the eye sockets become deeper, and flattening of the cheeks occurs in both males and females. The lips increase in length and thickness in both males and females, although the growth in both dimensions is greater for males and continues for longer. Increase in lip length during orthodontic treatment may aid stability in the treatment of patients with increased overjet. The nose grows most in adolescence. Nasal growth peaks in females at 12 years and continues until 16 years. In males, nasal growth peaks between 13 and 14 years and continues for longer, with significant ongoing growth as an adult. The soft tissues covering the chin follow the development of the underlying bones, becoming more prominent in males. Greater differential nasal growth leads to a relative flattening or retrusion of the lips, accentuated again by the increased prominence of the chin in males. This should be considered during orthodontic treatment planning, notably for individuals with a Class II malocclusion, where moving the upper incisors back to meet the lower incisors may accentuate the flattening of the profile.

4.8 Growth prediction

It would be useful to predict how the facial growth of any individual child will progress, to help plan future orthodontic treatment. Attempts to predict future facial growth from measurements on cephalometric radiographs have so far had limited success. Assessment of height and secondary sex characteristics help indicate whether the patient has entered and completed the pubertal growth spurt, which may be important if functional appliances are being considered. The stage of maturation of the bones on hand–wrist radiographs have been used as an indication of the onset of puberty, but the correlation with jaw growth has been found to be poor. More success has been achieved by assessing the stage of maturation of cervical vertebrae seen on lateral cephalograms.

At the present time, it is difficult to consistently predict the amount, direction, and timing of growth of the facial skeleton with any degree of precision.

4.9 The cellular basis of tooth movement

The ability of the PDL to respond to mechanical load by remodelling of the alveolar bone and allowing movement of the tooth through bone is the basis of orthodontic treatment. The cells of the PDL are responsible for sensing the load, then initiating and orchestrating the remodelling. When optimum force is applied, bone is laid down where the PDL is under tension. Bone is resorbed from areas where the PDL is compressed. Some of the complex molecular and cellular interactions that allow this apparently simple movement will be described.

4.9.1 The periodontal ligament

The PDL consists of several different cell types surrounded by type 1 collagen and oxytalan fibres and a ground substance consisting of proteoglycans and glycoproteins. There are four main cell types:

- Fibroblasts: responsible for producing and degrading the PDL fibres.
- Cementoblasts: responsible for producing cementum.
- Osteoblasts: responsible for bone production and coordination of bone deposition and resorption.
- Osteoclasts: responsible for bone resorption.

There are also some small islands of cells, known as the cell rests of Malassez, which are left following original root formation and macrophages, responsible for dealing with dead cells and debris.

The PDL has a high turnover rate and requires a good blood supply. This is derived from the superior and inferior alveolar arteries and forms a dense network of capillaries, or plexus, within the PDL around the tooth, occupying up to half of the periodontal space.

4.9.2 Cells involved in bone homeostasis

There are three main cell types involved in bone homeostasis:

- Osteoblasts: orchestrate the production of the inorganic matrix of bone and its mineralization. They recruit and activate osteoclasts and are the main regulators of bone homeostasis. It has been established that during normal function there is balance between bone resorption and deposition, controlled by the osteoblast. They can become surrounded by mineralized bone and become osteocytes.

- Osteocytes: continue to communicate with each other via cytoplasmic extensions in canaliculi in the bone. They are thought to be responsible for detecting mechanical load on the bone.

- Osteoclasts: large multinucleate cells responsible for resorption of bone. They are found on bone surfaces undergoing active resorption in pits called Howship's lacunae.

The organic matrix of bone consists of type 1 collagen fibres, proteoglycans, and many growth factors. Bone contains more growth factors than any other tissue, which may in part explain its capability for regeneration, repair, and remodelling. Many of the growth factors and signalling molecules shown to be associated with bone homeostasis play an active role in the bone remodelling associated with orthodontic tooth movement. See Table 4.1.

4.9.3 Cellular events in response to mechanical loading

Application of mechanical load, for example, a force on a tooth from an orthodontic appliance, affects the PDL by causing fluid movement in the PDL space and by stretching and compressing of the collagen fibres and extracellular matrix (ECM). This leads to deformation of the alveolar bone. The distortions in the PDL and alveolar bone are detected by the cells (fibroblasts, osteoblasts, and osteocytes), which are connected to the ECM by proteins known as integrins in their cell walls. There is also evidence that cell shape influences activity, with rounded cells exhibiting catabolic (destructive or resorptive) behaviour and flat cells exhibiting anabolic (building or depositing) behaviour. It is possible that changes in cell shape in the PDL is at least partly responsible for the chain of events seen when the PDL is under compression (Box 4.1) or tension (Box 4.2)

Four basic stages of tooth movement have been described:

1. Matrix strain and fluid flow in the PDL and alveolar bone.
2. Cell strain, secondary to matrix strain and fluid flow.
3. Cell activation and differentiation.
4. Remodelling of the PDL and alveolar bone.

See Fig. 4.12.

Table 4.1 Factors, terms, and cell types used in the explanation of bone remodelling during orthodontic tooth movement

Bone morphogenetic proteins (BMPs)	A group of growth factors known to induce the formation of bone and cartilage
Cathepsin K (CTSK)	An enzyme involved in bone remodelling and resorption, expressed predominantly in osteoclasts
Colony stimulating factor (macrophage colony stimulating factor) (CSF-1 (M-CSF))	Polypeptide growth factor found in bone matrix and produced by osteoblasts. Acts directly on osteoclast precursor cells to control proliferation and differentiation into osteoclasts
Extracellular signal-related kinase (ERK)	Intracellular messenger that provides a key link between external signals received by the cell and changes in patterns of gene expression within the cell, changing cell activity
Hydrogen ions	The presence of hydrogen ions (H^+) creates an acidic environment, actively demineralizing the inorganic bone
Integrins	Proteins that straddle the cell membrane, linking the internal cytoskeleton of the cell to external stimuli
Interleukin-1(IL-1)	Potent stimulator of bone resorption and inhibitor of bone deposition
Leukotrienes	Found in sites of inflammation. Produced by cells in response to mechanical loading. Active in both bone destruction and bone formation
Macrophages	Large cells usually responsible for removing debris. Stimulated to produce IL-1 partly responsible for signalling to and recruitment of osteoclasts
Matrix metalloproteinases (MMPs)	Range of enzymes produced to break down unmineralized ECM, e.g. collagenase and gelatinase
Monocyte	A type of white blood cell, which coalesce to form osteoclasts
Osteoid	Narrow layer of unmineralized bone matrix covering the surface of bone
Osteopontin	Helps osteoclasts to adhere to the bone surface
Osteoprotogerin (OPG)	Produced by osteoblasts in response to RANKL, to decrease the activity of osteoclasts to regulate bone resorption
Prostaglandin E-2 (PGE-2)	Mediator of bone resorption. Produced in sites of inflammation. Produced by cells in response to mechanical loading. Increases production of intracellular messengers
Receptor activator of nuclear factor (RANKL)	Produced by osteoblasts. Essential stimulatory factor for the differentiation, fusion, activation and survival of osteoclasts.
RUNX-2	Important gene, vital for cellular differentiation into osteoblasts
Tissue inhibitors of metalloproteinases (TIMPs)	Produced by various cell types to bind to MMPs to inhibit or reduce their activity

---

Box 4.1 Possible chain of cellular events when the periodontal ligament is subjected to a compressive load

- The mechanical load causes strain in the ECM of the PDL and in alveolar bone, causing fluid flow in both tissues.

- The strain in ECM is sensed by PDL cells due to their connection to the ECM via integrins. Osteocytes in the bone also sense the mechanical force by fluid flow through the canaliculi (microscopic canals connecting the osteocytes).

- Osteocytes respond to mechanical deformation by producing bone morphogenetic proteins (BMPs) and other cytokines which activate osteoblasts. Fibroblasts respond by producing matrix metalloproteinases (MMPs). Osteoblasts respond by producing prostaglandins (e.g. PGE-2) and leukotrienes.

- Osteoblast production of PGE-2 and leukotrienes leads to an elevation of intracellular messengers. These cause the osteoblast to produce interleukin-1 (IL-1) and colony stimulating factor (CSF-1) and an increase in receptor activator of nuclear factor (RANKL).

- Macrophages respond to mechanical deformation by increasing production of IL-1.

- IL-1 production by osteoblasts and macrophages also increases the production of RANKL by the osteoblast.

- RANKL and CSF-1 cause increased attraction and proliferation of blood monocytes which fuse to form osteoclasts. RANKL also stimulates the osteoclasts to become active.

- The osteoblasts bunch up to expose the underlying osteoid and produce MMPs to degrade the osteoid and to give the osteoclasts access to the underlying mineralized bone. The osteoblasts also produce osteopontin (OPN) which causes the osteoclasts to attach to the exposed bone surface.

- The osteoclasts resorb the bone by excreting hydrogen ions into the matrix, softening the hydroxyapatite crystals, and then use proteases such as cathepsin K to break down the ECM.

- The osteoblasts also produce inhibitors of some enzymes and cytokines (e.g. TIMPs and OPG to ensure that bone resorption is carefully controlled).

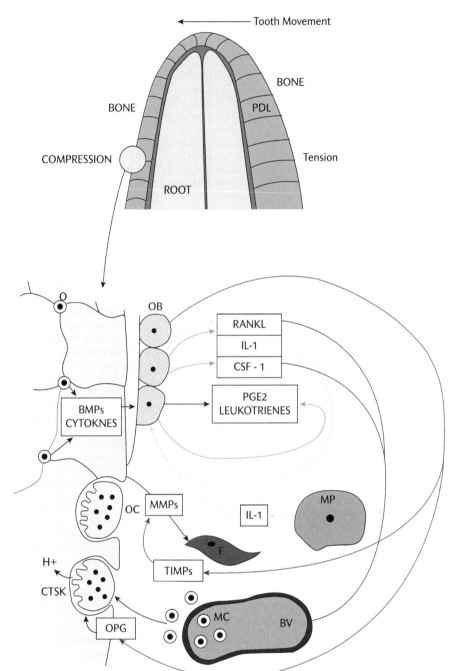

Fig. 4.12 Schematic diagram of cellular signalling involved in bone remodelling response to compressive load. All black arrows indicate up-regulation of factors. Red arrows indicate inhibition. Note the osteoblasts lining the bone surface (osteoid), the osteocytes within the bone detecting the mechanical load, and the monocytes exiting the blood vessel in response to RANKL and CSF-1. BV = blood vessel; F = fibroblast; MC = monocyte; MP = macrophage; O = osteocyte; OB = osteoblast; OC = osteoclast.

Box 4.2 Possible chain of cellular events when the periodontal ligament is subject to tension

- In areas of tension, the osteoblasts are flattened and the osteoid remains unexposed.
- Cells in the PDL increase the amount of a specific secondary messenger (extracellular signal-related kinase (ERK)) in response to tension.
- ERK signalling induces the expression of RUNX-2 which in turn causes an increase in osteoblast number, possibly by inducing differentiation of fibroblasts into osteoblasts.
- Osteoblasts clump into groups, secreting collagen and other proteins composing the organic matrix, then produce hydroxyapatite, which mineralizes the matrix resulting in new bone.

4.10 Cellular events associated with excess force

If the force applied to a tooth exceeds the pressure in the capillaries (30 mmHg, or around 50 g) the blood vessels will be occluded and the nutrient supply to the PDL will reduce. This causes cell death in the compressed PDL, and the PDL is described as 'hyalinized', as it takes on a glass-like appearance due to sterile necrosis. There are no osteoblasts to recruit osteoclasts to resorb the bone in the expected way. It takes several days for cells to migrate from undamaged areas. Eventually osteoclasts appear in the adjacent marrow spaces and resorb the bone from underneath the necrotic area. This is known as undermining resorption. Where hyalinization and undermining resorption occur, there is a delay in tooth movement of 10–14 days. The clinical implications of excessive force are more discomfort for the patient, an increased risk of root resorption, and the risk of loss of anchorage. Anchorage is defined as the resistance to unwanted tooth movement and is discussed in Chapter 15. Loss of anchorage may occur due to inadequate treatment planning, but may also occur due to excessive force levels being applied to the teeth. When an excessive force is applied to a tooth, it won't move initially; however, there is still force being applied to the teeth providing anchorage. This force on the anchorage teeth may be enough to produce unwanted movement, leading to loss of anchorage.

Table 4.2 Optimal force levels for different tooth movements

Type of tooth movement	Approximate force (grams)
Tipping	50–75
Bodily movement	100–150
Root uprighting	75–125
Extrusion	50–100
Intrusion	15–25

The optimum force for tooth movement will vary between different teeth and types of movement. It depends on the area of the PDL that the applied force is spread across. For example, a low force should be used to intrude a tooth, where the force is concentrated in a small area at the apex. A higher force can be used to bodily move teeth, where the force is spread across the whole side of a tooth root (Table 4.2).

4.11 Cellular events during root resorption

External apical root resorption is a complex inflammatory process that occurs in virtually all patients undergoing treatment with orthodontic appliances. The cells responsible for the resorption of mineralized dental tissue, odontoclasts, are similar, but not identical to, osteoclasts. In mild cases of orthodontically induced root resorption (OIRR), only small areas of cementum are resorbed and these areas are repaired with cellular cementum once the orthodontic force has stopped. In more severe cases, the apical portion of the root is removed by odontoclast activity and the root length is decreased. The remaining dentine will be recovered by cementum, but the root will remain shortened. There is increasing evidence to suggest that OIRR is more likely where force levels are excessive, especially in areas of compression.

4.12 Summary

4.12.1 Facial growth

- Facial development begins at the end of week 4 i.u. with the development of five swellings (frontonasal, two maxillary, and two mandibular) around the stomodeum (primitive mouth).
- The maxilla and the mandible derive from the first pharyngeal arch into which cranial neural crest cells have migrated.
- Bone formation occurs by either intramembranous or endochondral ossification.
- Bone growth occurs by remodelling and displacement.
- The calvarium ossifies intramembranously, closely following the growth of the brain. Growth is complete at 7 years.
- The cranial base ossifies endochondrally. Growth at the spheno-occipital synchondrosis occurs in two directions until the mid teens.
- The maxilla and the mandible ossify intramembraneously and undergo complex patterns of remodelling. They are displaced forwards and downwards in relation to cranial base. Growth occurs posteriorly at the tuberosities (maxilla) and the ramus (mandible) to accommodate the permanent dentition.
- The mandible experiences rotational growth with most individuals having an upward and forward direction of rotation.
- Facial growth continues at low levels in the adult. The decline to adult levels is seen first in the transverse dimension, followed by the anteroposterior dimension, and finally the vertical dimension. Growth continues for longer in boys in the anteroposterior and vertical dimensions.
- During puberty, there is a large increase in nasal dimensions and the lips lengthen and thicken, especially in boys. Soft tissue growth continues throughout adulthood.
- The control of facial growth is a combination of genetics and environmental factors. The latter offers the possibility of modification of growth with orthodontic appliances.
- Currently, it is not possible to accurately predict the timing, rate, or amount of facial growth.

4.12.2 Cellular basis of tooth movement

- Orthodontic treatment would not be possible without the ability of the alveolar bone to remodel.
- The cells of the PDL are responsible for the bone remodelling and, hence, tooth movement.
- The osteoblast is the bone-forming cell and is responsible also for the recruitment and activation of osteoclasts (bone-resorbing cells).
- Many different growth factors and signalling molecules are now known to be involved in bone turnover during orthodontic tooth movement with the RANK/RANKL/OPG osteoclast programme being the most important.

- Excessive force can cause cell death and hyalinization of the PDL. This leads to a time delay (10–14 days) before the bone is removed by undermining resorption and then tooth movement can continue. Clinically this can lead to pain, root resorption, inefficient tooth movement, and anchorage loss.

4.12.3 Root resorption

- Root resorption occurs in most patients undergoing orthodontic treatment.
- The cell responsible for the removal of cementum and dentine is the odontoclast.

Principal sources and further reading

Björk, A. and Skieller, V. (1983). Normal and abnormal growth of the mandible. A synthesis of longitudinal cephalometric implant studies over a period of 25 years. *European Journal of Orthodontics*, **5**, 1–46. [DOI: 10.1093/ejo/5.1.1] [PubMed: 6572593]
A summary of the implant work on mandibular growth rotations.

Enlow, D. H. and Hans M. G. (2008). *Essentials of Facial Growth* (2nd edn). Philadelphia, PA: Saunders.
The Bible of facial growth.

Henneman, S., Von den Hoff, J. W., and Maltha, J. C. (2008). Mechanobiology of tooth movement. *European Journal of Orthodontics*, **30**, 299–306. [DOI: 10.1093/ejo/cjn020] [PubMed: 18540017]
An up-to-date and easy-to-understand review of the biology of orthodontic tooth movement.

Houston, W. J. B. (1979). The current status of facial growth prediction: a review. *British Journal of Orthodontics*, **6**, 11–17. [PubMed: 396940].
An authoritative assessment of the value of growth prediction.

Houston, W. J. B. (1988). Mandibular growth rotations – their mechanism and importance. *European Journal of Orthodontics*, **10**, 369–73. [DOI: 10.1093/ejo/10.4.369] [PubMed: 3061834]
A concise review of the aetiology and clinical importance of growth rotations.

Sandy, J. R., Farndale, R. W., and Meikle, M. C. (1993). Recent advances in understanding mechanically induced bone remodelling and their relevance to orthodontic theory and practice. *American Journal of Orthodontics and Dentofacial Orthopedics*, **103**, 212–22. [DOI: 10.1016/0889-5406(93)70002-6] [PubMed: 8456777]
Still a key paper in understanding the cellular events behind orthodontic tooth movement.

References for this chapter can also be found at: **www.oup.com/uk/orthodontics5e**. Where possible, these are presented as active links which direct you to the electronic version of the work, to help facilitate onward study. If you are a subscriber to that work (either individually or through an institution), and depending on your level of access, you may be able to peruse an abstract or the full article if available.

5

Orthodontic assessment

S. J. Littlewood

Chapter contents

5.1 Introduction to orthodontic assessment

The purpose of an orthodontic assessment is to gather information about the patient to produce an accurate orthodontic diagnosis. This information is collected by:

- taking a full history
- undertaking a clinical examination
- collecting appropriate records.

The assessment will produce data identifying a list of the patient's orthodontic problems, and it is this problem list that will form the basis of the orthodontic diagnosis (Fig. 5.1). Problems can be divided into pathological problems and developmental problems. Pathological problems are problems related to diseases, such as caries and periodontal disease, and need to be addressed before any orthodontic treatment is undertaken. Developmental problems are those factors related to the malocclusion and will be the focus of this chapter.

Orthodontic treatment is nearly always elective, and so it is important that the orthodontic assessment identifies sufficient information not only to identify features that would benefit from treatment and those that don't need to be changed, but also to identify any potential risks of proposed treatment (see Chapter 1, Section 1.6). By understanding both the risks and benefits of treatment the patient can make an informed

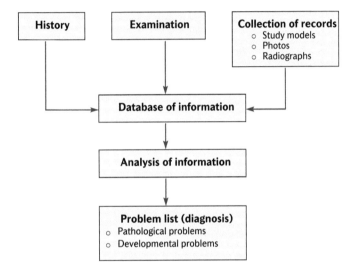

Fig. 5.1 The process of creating a problem list in orthodontics.

decision as to whether they would like to proceed with treatment or not. (Consent is discussed in more detail in Chapter 7, Section 7.8.)

5.2 Taking an orthodontic history

The patient should be given the chance to describe their problem in their own words and the clinician can then guide them through a series of questions to address the areas, as summarized in Box 5.1.

When the patient is a child, the parent or guardian may lead this discussion, but it is important to get the child's input, as the child is the one who may undergo treatment and would therefore need to be willing and able to comply with the treatment plan.

Box 5.1 Information to be gathered during the history-taking process

- Patient's complaint and expectations of treatment.
- Medical history—identifying any aspects that may affect orthodontic treatment.
- Dental history—any trauma, any previous or ongoing dental treatment, TMJ problems, any known inherited dental problems (e.g. hypodontia), and any previous orthodontic treatment.

- Habits—details of any digit-sucking habits or other habits involving the dentition.
- Physical growth status (identifying whether growth is complete or still ongoing may affect the timing and nature of future treatment).
- Patient (or parent's) motivation.
- Socio-behavioural factors—these may affect the patient's ability to complete the treatment.

Table 5.1 Orthodontic relevance of some medical conditions

Medical condition	Relevance to orthodontics
Epilepsy	• Epilepsy needs to be under control before starting treatment
	• Extra-oral headgear may present an unacceptably high risk
	• Stress may induce a seizure
	• The antiepileptic phenytoin may cause gingival hyperplasia
Latex allergy	• Confirm allergy with the patient's doctor
	• Use latex-free gloves and orthodontic products
Nickel allergy	• Intra-oral reactions are very rare
	• Use plastic-coated headgear to avoid contact with skin
	• If intra-oral allergy is confirmed, then use nickel-free orthodontic products
Diabetes	• Patient may be more prone to intra-oral infections and periodontal problems
	• Be aware of risk of hypoglycaemia if snacks or meals are missed, so schedule appointments appropriately
	• Treatment should be avoided in poorly controlled diabetics
Heart defects with a risk of infective endocarditis	• Antibiotic cover used to be prescribed routinely for patients with structural heart defects who were undergoing any form of dentogingival manipulation that could produce a bacteraemia
	• The guidelines have now changed as in many cases the risk of anaphylaxis caused by the antibiotic is greater than the risk of infective endocarditis
	• The clinician should refer to contemporary guidelines and contact the patient's doctor or cardiologist if in doubt
Bleeding disorders	• Generally orthodontic treatment is not contraindicated
	• Precautions and medical advice are required for dental extractions
	• Avoiding trauma to soft tissues from wires or sharp edges is even more important for these patients
Asthma	• The regular use of steroid-based inhalers may predispose to intra-oral candidal infections, so excellent oral hygiene, particularly when using appliances that cover the palate, is important
Bisphosphonates	• These may predispose to osteonecrosis and affect bone turnover
	• The patient's physician should be contacted for advice about any proposed treatment plan, particularly if extractions may be required
Learning difficulties or behavioural disorders	• These may affect the patient's ability to cope with treatment, and may affect the choice, process, and aims of treatment

It is also important to make a note of any medications that the patient is taking that may have an impact on tooth movement or general oral health
The reader is referred to the section on 'Principal sources and further reading' for more comprehensive information on this topic

5.2.1 Patient's perception of the problem

The patient should be given the opportunity to express, in their own words, what their problem is and what they would like corrected. They may perceive their problem as:

• aesthetics

• functional (speech or mastication difficulties)

• related to dental health (like a traumatic overbite).

It is important to recognize that the patient's perception of their problem may not always seem appropriate to the trained clinician. However, the patient is unlikely to be satisfied unless their problem is addressed as part of the treatment plan. Allowing the patient to describe their concerns will help to determine whether the patient's expectations are realistic and achievable (see Section 5.2.6).

5.2.2 Medical history

As with all aspects of dentistry, oral problems cannot be treated in isolation of the rest of the body. A clear understanding of a patient's medical problems and how this can affect potential orthodontic treatment is vital. Table 5.1 summarizes the key areas of the medical history of importance for orthodontic patients, and the section on 'Principal sources and further reading' provides more details.

5.2.3 Dental history

The patient should be asked about their previous dental experience. This will provide an idea of their attitude towards dental health, what treatment they have had experienced previously, and how this may affect their compliance with orthodontic treatment. In particular, it is important to determine any ongoing dental problems, history of jaw joint problems, and any history of trauma to the teeth. There may also be a history of relevant inherited disorders affecting the dentition (e.g. hypodontia or enamel defects) and previous orthodontic treatment.

5.2.4 Habits

The patient should be asked about any previous or ongoing habits that involve the dentition. The most important are digit-sucking habits and the clinician needs to know the duration and nature of the habit. Other habits such as nail biting may predispose to an increased risk of root resorption.

5.2.5 Physical growth status

For some orthodontic treatment, the patient's growth status is important. In some cases, orthodontic treatment is more successful if they are still growing—for example, when a patient has an underlying skeletal problem that could be improved using a process known as growth modification (see Chapters 7 and 19). In others, treatment planning is best undertaken when growth is complete (e.g. an adolescent with a severe Class III malocclusion). The patient, or their parents, can be asked questions to determine if they are still growing.

5.2.6 Motivation and expectations

Undergoing orthodontic treatment requires a great deal of active participation and cooperation from the patient. No matter how skilful the orthodontist, treatment will not be successful unless the patient is sufficiently motivated to comply with all aspects of their care. If a patient is not sufficiently motivated, then treatment should not be undertaken.

We have already explained the importance of finding out which features of their malocclusion a patient is unhappy with, and importantly, the result they are hoping for, or expect, at the end of treatment. Where possible, the clinician should formulate a plan that addresses the patient's area of concern. However, occasionally the patient's perception of their problem or their expectations may be unrealistic. The role of the orthodontist is then to counsel the patient carefully to explain what can or cannot be achieved. If a patient's expectations are unrealistic, then treatment should not be undertaken.

5.2.7 Socio-behavioural factors

Compliance for treatment is also affected by the patient's ability to attend regularly for appointments and any potential practical or social reasons that may make this impossible should be identified. Orthodontic treatment often requires long-term treatment with multiple appointments, and it is important to determine if the patient, and in the case of a child, their family or carer, are able to commit to the whole treatment and the retention that follows. In addition, the patient's ability to comply with treatment may be affected by some behavioural problems.

5.3 Clinical examination in three dimensions

The purpose of the clinical examination is to identify pathological and developmental problems and determine which (if any) diagnostic records are required. It is important to remember that the face and dentition should be examined in all three planes (anteroposteriorly, vertically, and transversely). Box 5.2 summarizes how the different aspects of orthodontic assessment relate to the three planes.

Box 5.2 The three dimensions of clinical examination

Anteroposterior

Extra-oral

Maxilla to mandible relationship (Class I, II, or III).

Intra-oral

Incisor classification.
Overjet.
Canine relationship.
Molar relationship.
Anterior crossbite.

Vertical

Extra-oral

Facial thirds.
Angle of lower border of mandible to the maxilla.

Intra-oral

Overbite, anterior open bite, or lateral open bite.

Transverse

Extra-oral

Facial asymmetry.

Intra-oral

Centrelines.
Posterior crossbites.

5.4 Extra-oral examination

An appreciation of a patient's underlying skeletal pattern and overlying soft tissues will help to identify the aetiology of a malocclusion. This will help the clinician appreciate the anatomical limitations of any proposed treatment. In addition, a key aim of all orthodontic treatment should be to produce an aesthetic smile. Simply aligning teeth and producing a good occlusion does not necessarily guarantee a great smile. An understanding of the relationship between the teeth and the lips is vital and an assessment of the smile aesthetics should form part of any orthodontic assessment.

The patient needs to be examined in a frontal view and in profile. To ensure an accurate assessment representing the true skeletal relationships, it is important to ensure that the patient is in the 'natural head position', which is the position the patient carries their head naturally. The patient should sit upright in the chair and be asked to focus on something in the distance. This same natural head position should also be used for any cephalometric radiographs to ensure consistency between all patient records (see Chapter 6, Section 6.1).

The key to the extra-oral assessment is an understanding of the normal proportions of the face and recognizing when patients deviate from these normal relationships. The patient is assessed extra-orally in the:

- frontal view (assessing in the vertical and transverse planes)
- profile view (assessing in the anteroposterior and vertical planes).

An assessment of the smile aesthetics, soft tissues (lips and tongue), and an examination of the temporomandibular joint (TMJ) should also be undertaken.

5.4.1 Anteroposterior assessment

This aims to assess the relationship between the tooth-bearing portions of the maxilla and mandible to each other, and also their relationships to the cranial base. The anteroposterior relationship can be assessed in the following three ways:

- Assessing the relationship of the lips to a vertical line, known as the zero meridian, dropped from soft tissue nasion (Fig. 5.2).
- Palpating intra-orally the anterior portion of the maxilla at A point and the mandible at B point (Fig. 5.3).
- Assessing the convexity of the face by determining the angle between the middle and lower thirds of the face in profile (Fig. 5.4).

5.4.2 Vertical assessment

The face can be assessed vertically in two ways:

- Using the rule of thirds.
- Measuring the angle of the lower border of the mandible to the maxilla.

The face can be split into thirds (Fig. 5.5). In a face with normal proportions, each third is approximately equal in size. Any discrepancy in these thirds may suggest a facial disharmony in the vertical plane. In particular, orthodontists are interested in any increase or decrease in the proportion of the lower third of the face. The lower third of the face

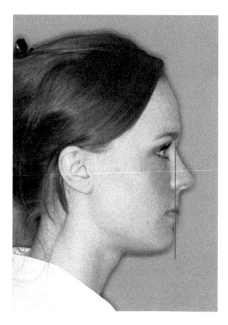

Fig. 5.2 Using zero meridian to estimate anteroposterior relationship. Zero meridian is the true vertical line dropped from the soft tissue nasion. In a Class I relationship (as shown here), the upper lip lies on or slightly anterior to this line and the chin point lies slightly behind it.

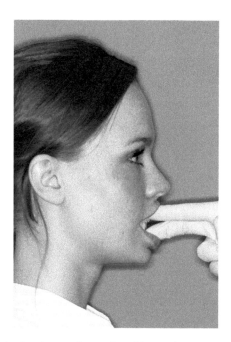

Fig. 5.3 Palpating the anterior portion of the maxilla at A point and the mandible at B point to determine the underlying skeletal anteroposterior relationship. In a normal (Class I) skeletal relationship, as shown here, the upper jaw lies 2–4 mm in front of the lower. In a Class II, the lower jaw would be greater than 4 mm behind the upper jaw. In a Class III, the lower jaw is less than 2 mm behind the upper (in more severe Class III cases, the lower jaw may be in front of the upper).

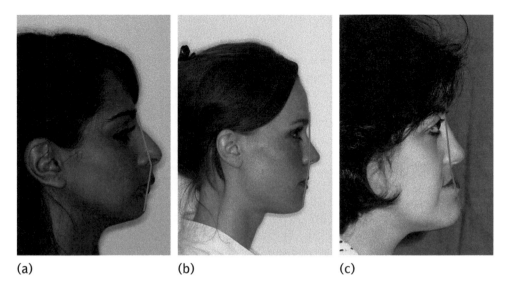

(a)   (b)   (c)

Fig. 5.4 The anteroposterior relationship of the jaws can also be assessed using the convexity of the face. This is assessed by the angle between the upper face (glabella to subnasale) and the lower face (subnasale to pogonion). The mean value is 12° ± 4°. (a) A patient with a convex profile with an increased angle of facial convexity indicating a Class II skeletal pattern. (b) A patient with a straighter profile with a normal angle of facial convexity indicating a Class I skeletal pattern. (c) A patient with a concave profile indicating a Class III skeletal pattern.

can also be split into thirds, with the upper lip lying in the upper third, and the lower lip lying in the lower two-thirds (Fig. 5.5).

Another clinical assessment that can be used to determine the vertical relationships is to assess the angle between the lower border of the mandible and the maxilla (Fig. 5.6). Placing a finger, or the handle of a dental instrument, along the lower border of the mandible gives an indication of the clinical mandibular plane angle.

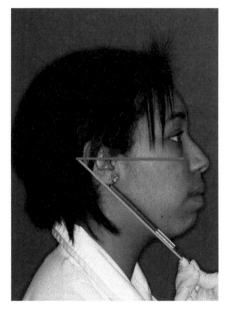

Fig. 5.6 The mandibular plane angle can be estimated clinically by looking at the point of contact of intersecting lines made up by the lower border of the mandible (in blue) and the Frankfort horizontal plane (in red). The Frankfort plane is actually measured on a lateral cephalogram (between porion and orbital), but can be estimated clinically by palpation of the lower border of the orbit. The angle is considered normal if the two lines intersect at the occiput. In this case, the lines intersect anterior to the occiput, which is consistent with an increased angle, suggesting increased vertical proportions. If the lines intersect posterior to the occiput, then the angle would be decreased, indicating reduced vertical proportions.

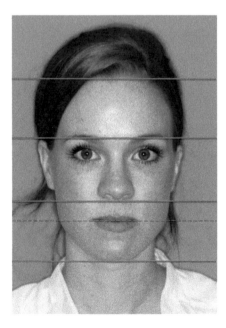

Fig. 5.5 The face can be divided into equal thirds: hairline to glabella between the eyebrows (forehead), glabella to subnasale (middle third), and subnasale to lowest part of the chin (lower third). The lower third can be further divided into the thirds, with the upper lip lying in the upper third and the lower lip lying at the top of the lower two-thirds.

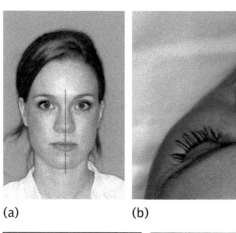
(a)

(b)

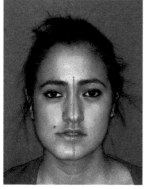
(c)

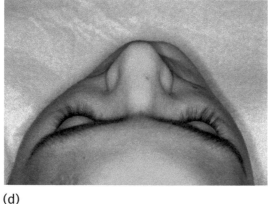
(d)

Fig. 5.7 The transverse examination of the face should be done from the front, and from above the patient (by standing behind and above the patient while they are seated in the dental chair). (a) The patient has a symmetrical face, with the facial midline showing alignment of the soft tissue nasion, middle part of the upper lip at the vermillion border, and the chin point. (b) The same patient viewed from behind, confirming the symmetry. (c, d) A patient with marked mandibular asymmetry to the right.

5.4.3 Transverse assessment

The transverse proportions of the face can be examined from the frontal view, but also by looking down on the face, by standing behind and above the patient (Fig. 5.7). No face is truly symmetrical, but any significant asymmetry should be noted. The soft tissue nasion, middle part of the upper lip at the vermillion border, and the chin point should all be aligned. The face can also be divided into fifths, with each section being approximately equal to the width of an eye (Fig. 5.8).

5.4.4 Smile aesthetics

Most patients seek orthodontic treatment to improve their smile, so it is important to recognize the various components of a smile that will improve the aesthetics (see section on 'Principal sources and further reading').

A normal smile should show the following (Fig. 5.9):

- The whole height of the upper incisors should be visible on full smiling, with only the interproximal gingivae visible. This smile line is usually 1–2 mm higher in females.

- The upper incisor edges should run parallel to the lower lip (smile arc).

- The upper incisors should be close to, but not touching, the lower lip.

- The gingival margins of the anterior teeth are important if they are visible in the smile. The margins of the central incisors and canines should be approximately level, with the lateral incisors lying 1 mm more incisally than the canines and central incisors.

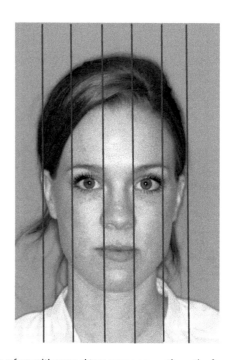

Fig. 5.8 In a face with normal transverse proportions, the face can divided into approximately five equal sections—each the width of an eye.

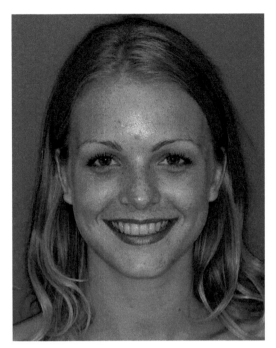

Fig. 5.9 The patient demonstrates many of the features of the normal smile: (1) the whole of the upper incisors is visible with only the interproximal gingivae visible; (2) the upper incisor edges are parallel to the lower lip—indicating a 'consonant' smile arc; (3) the upper incisors do not touch the lower lip; (4) the gingival margins of the central incisors and canines should be approximately level, with the lateral incisors lying 1 mm incisally; (5) the buccal corridors are visible, but minimal; and (6) symmetrical dental arrangement. In this case, the only aspect where the smile aesthetics deviate slightly from the normal is that the upper dental centreline is slightly to the right of the facial midline.

- The width of the smile should be such that buccal corridors should be visible, but minimal. The buccal corridor is the space between the angle of the mouth and the buccal surfaces of the most distal visible tooth.
- There should be a symmetrical dental arrangement.
- The upper dental midline should be coincident to the middle of the face.

Many aspects of facial or smile aesthetics cannot be influenced by orthodontics alone, or indeed cannot be influenced at all. This needs to be discussed with the patient, and if appropriate, surgical and restorative options may need to be considered.

5.4.5 Soft tissue examination

In addition to assessing the smile aesthetics, a soft tissue examination will also assess:

- lips (see Box 5.3)
- tongue.

Lips can be competent (i.e. meet together at rest), potentially competent (position of incisors prevents comfortable lip seal to be obtained at rest, but the patient can hold the lips together if required),

Box 5.3 Features of the lips to assess

- Lip competence
- Lip fullness
- Nasolabial angle
- Method of achieving an anterior seal.

or incompetent (require considerable muscular activity to obtain a lip seal). Lip incompetence is common in preadolescent children, but increases with age due to vertical growth of the soft tissues. The ability to achieve lip competence is particularly important when reducing an overjet in a Class II division 1 malocclusion, as the stability of the case is improved if the upper incisor position is under the control of competent lips at the end of treatment.

Lips should be everted at their base, with some vermillion border seen at rest. Protrusion of the lips does differ between different ethnic groups with patients of Afro-Caribbean origin being more protrusive than those of Caucasian origin (see Fig. 5.6). The use of Ricketts' esthetic line (E-line) provides a guide to the appropriate prominence of the lips within the face (see Chapter 6, Fig. 6.14).

The nasolabial angle is formed between the base of the nose and the upper lip and should be 90–110° (Fig. 5.10). It can be affected by the shape of the nose, but also the drape of the upper lip. The drape of the upper lip can be affected by the support of the upper incisor. If the shape of the nose is normal, a high nasolabial angle could therefore indicate a retrusive lip, whereas a low nasolabial angle could indicate lip protrusion.

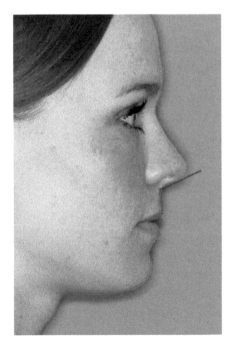

Fig. 5.10 The normal nasolabial angle is 90–110°. This is important to note as the angle can be affected by orthodontic movement of the upper incisors.

The reason why an assessment of the tongue is performed during the extra-oral examination is to determine the method by which patients achieve an anterior seal during swallowing, and the position of the tongue at rest. In some patients with incompetent lips, the tongue thrusts forward to contact with the lips to form an anterior seal. This is usually adaptive to the underlying malocclusion, so when the treatment is complete and normal lip competence can be achieved, the tongue thrust ceases. In some patients, there is a so-called endogenous tongue thrust, which will re-establish itself after treatment, leading to relapse. Being able to identify cases that may have this strong relapse potential would be helpful. It is, however, very difficult to confidently distinguish between an adaptive tongue thrust and an endogenous tongue thrust. Patients with an endogenous tongue thrust tend to show proclination of both the upper and lower incisors, an anterior open bite, an associated

lisp, and the tongue tends to sit between the incisors at rest. It is probably the resting position of the tongue, rather than the action of the tongue in function that is more important.

5.4.6 Temporomandibular joint examination

It is important to note the presence of any signs of pathology in the TMJ and muscles of mastication during the orthodontic assessment. Any tenderness, clicks, crepitus, and locking should be noted, as well as recording the range of movement and maximum opening. As mentioned in Chapter 1 (see Section 1.4.6), there is no strong evidence to suggest that TMJ disorders are either associated with malocclusions or cured by orthodontic treatment. However, if signs or symptoms are detected then they must be recorded and it may be worth referring the patient to a specialist before commencing orthodontic treatment.

5.5 Intra-oral examination

The intra-oral examination allows the clinician to assess the:

- stage of dental development (by charting the teeth present)
- soft tissues and periodontium for pathology
- oral hygiene
- overall dental health, including identifying any caries and restorations
- tooth position within each arch and between arches.

5.5.1 Assessment of oral health

It is key that any pathology is identified in the mucosal surfaces, periodontally or in the teeth themselves. Generally, any pathology needs to be treated and stabilized before any orthodontic treatment can be undertaken.

Periodontal disease is fortunately unusual in child patients, but is relatively common in adults. Any mucogingival or periodontal problems need to be carefully noted. Section 20.4 in Chapter 20 discusses the importance of identifying and stabilizing periodontal disease, allowing us to modify treatment planning and mechanics for these patients.

Excellent oral hygiene is essential for orthodontic treatment otherwise there is a high risk of decalcification and increased attachment loss. Treatment should not begin until a patient can demonstrate they can consistently maintain high levels of oral hygiene.

Dental pathology can have a significant influence on the treatment plan, and additional radiographs and special tests (such as vitality tests) may be required. We are particularly interested in detecting:

- caries
- areas of hypomineralization
- effects of previous trauma
- non-vital teeth
- tooth wear
- teeth of abnormal size or shape
- existing restorations which may change the way we bond to the tooth, as well determine the choice of extractions if space is required.

5.5.2 Assessment of each dental arch

Each arch is assessed individually for:

- crowding (see Box 5.4) or spacing
- alignment of teeth, including displacements or rotations of teeth
- inclination of the labial segments (proclined, upright, or retroclined)
- angulation of the canines (mesial, upright, or distal) as this affects anchorage assessment later
- arch shape and symmetry
- depth of curve of Spee (see Chapter 7, Section 7.7.1).

5.5.3 Assessment of arches in occlusion

The arches are now assessed in occlusion. The incisor relationships are assessed first: incisor classification, overjet or anterior crossbites (anteroposterior), overbite or open bite (vertical), and centrelines (transverse). Then the buccal relationships are assessed: canine and molar relationships (anteroposterior), any lateral open bites (vertical), and buccal crossbites (transverse).

Incisor classification

This is discussed in Chapter 2, Section 2.3.

Overjet

This is measured from the labial surface of the most prominent incisor to the labial surface of the mandibular incisor (Fig. 5.11). This would normally be 2–4 mm. If the lower incisor lies anterior to the upper incisors, then overjet is given a negative value.

> **Box 5.4 Describing the amount of crowding present**
>
> 0–4 mm = mild crowding.
> 4–8 mm = moderate crowding.
> > 8 mm = severe crowding.

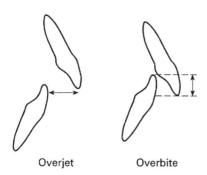

Fig. 5.11 Measurement of overjet and overbite.

Overbite

This measures how much the maxillary incisors overlap the mandibular incisors vertically (Fig. 5.11). There are three features to note when assessing the overbite:

- Amount of overlap.
- Whether the lower teeth are in contact with the opposing teeth or soft tissues (complete overbite) or if they are not touching anything (incomplete overbite).
- Whether any soft tissue damage is being caused (when it is described as traumatic).

A normal value would be one-third coverage of the crown of the lower incisor. If the overlap is greater than this, the overbite is described as increased, and if it is less than this, it is decreased. If there is no overlap at all, it is an anterior open bite.

Occasionally an overbite can be traumatic. This usually happens when the teeth occlude with the junction between the tooth and cervical gingivae. This could be labial to the lower incisors, or palatal to the upper incisors (Fig. 5.12).

Centrelines

The centrelines should ideally be coincident with each other and to the facial midline.

Canine relationship

This is discussed in Chapter 2, Section 2.3.

Molar relationship

This is discussed in Chapter 2, Section 2.3.

Crossbites

A crossbite is a discrepancy in the buccolingual relationship of the upper and lower teeth. These relationships are described in more detail in Chapter 13. They can be described by:

- location (anterior or posterior)
- nature of the crossbite (see Box 5.5).

It is very important to note whether there is a displacement of the mandible on closure when any crossbite is present. A displacement of the mandible is caused as a result of a premature contact on a particular tooth or teeth when the patient closes together. This premature contact may lead to the mandible being positioned further anteriorly, or

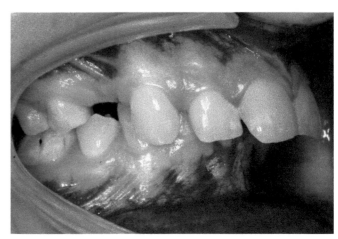

(a)

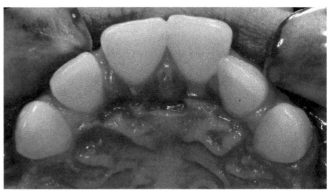

(b)

Fig. 5.12 Traumatic overbite. (a) A case with a very deep overbite; (b) demonstrates that the overbite is complete and traumatic (note damage associated with gingival stripping palatally of the upper central incisors).

to the left or right, to allow the patient to close into full intercuspation and obtain a more comfortable bite. As a result, there will be a discrepancy between the retruded contact position and intercuspal position (Fig. 5.13). It is vital that this displacement of the mandible is identified, because the crossbite is artificially holding the jaw in a different position, and as a result all the other measures of occlusion will be inaccurate. The orthodontic treatment plan should be based on the retruded contact position, as this is the position the jaw will return to when the displacement is removed when the crossbite is corrected.

Box 5.5 Description of crossbites

Buccal crossbite

The buccal cusps of the lower teeth occlude buccal to the buccal cusps of the upper teeth.

Lingual crossbite (or scissor bite)

The buccal cusps of the lower teeth occlude lingual to the lingual cusps of the upper teeth

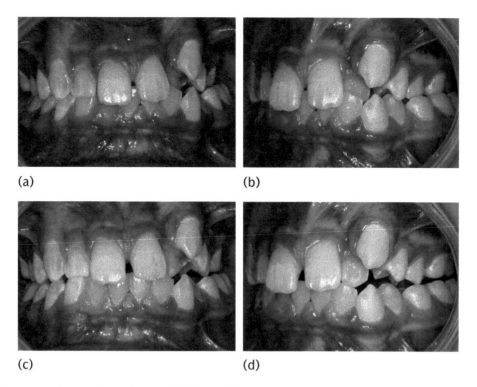

(a) (b)

(c) (d)

Fig. 5.13 This patient has an anterior crossbite on the upper left lateral incisor, and posterior crossbite affecting the upper left second premolar and upper left first molar. When examined carefully it is clear that the patient has a mandibular displacement forwards and to the left on closure, and this is caused by a premature contact on the upper left lateral incisor. (a, b) The patient with the teeth in maximum intercuspation (intercuspal position); (c, d) the patient before displacement off the lateral incisor. Note the difference in the occlusal relationships, particularly the centrelines, as a result of the displacement of the mandible.

5.6 Diagnostic records

Orthodontic records may be required for a number of possible purposes:

- Diagnosis and treatment planning
- Monitoring growth
- Monitoring treatment
- Medico-legal record
- Patient communication and education
- Audit and research.

5.6.1 Study models

Study models should show all the erupted teeth and be extended into the buccal sulcus. Traditionally, they are poured in dental stone and are typically produced from alginate impressions. They should be mounted in occlusion, using a wax or polysiloxane bite. They are produced using a technique known as Angle trimming, which allows models to be placed on a flat surface and viewed in the correct occlusion from varying angles (Fig. 5.14).

Digital versions of study models, which should not deteriorate with time, are easier to transfer, and do not take up physical space, are gradually replacing stone models. Virtual study models are discussed in the section on technology advances in orthodontic records in Section 5.6.5.

5.6.2 Photographs

These provide a key colour record. The usual views taken are as follows:
Four extra-oral (in natural head position):

- Full facial frontal at rest
- Full facial frontal smiling
- Facial three-quarters view
- Facial profile.

Five intra-oral:

- Frontal occlusion
- Buccal occlusion (left and right)
- Occlusal views of upper and lower arch.

Some operators take short video clips of the patient talking and smiling, as this may provide additional useful information about the dentition and smile in function.

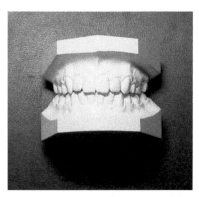

(a)

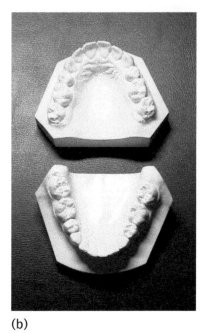

(b)

Fig. 5.14 Study models should be produced using a technique known as Angle's trimming. This means the models can be placed on a flat surface on different edges, so the correct occlusion can be viewed from different angles. (a) The teeth are shown in occlusion, on this occasion stood on their posterior trimmed base; (b) the two arches viewed independently.

5.6.3 Radiographs

Any radiograph carries a low but identifiable risk, so each radiograph must be clinically justified. A radiograph is only prescribed after a full clinical examination to ensure that information cannot be gained by a less invasive method (see Box 5.6). When considering interceptive or active orthodontic treatment, a radiograph may provide additional information on:

- presence or absence of teeth
- stage of development of permanent dentition
- root morphology of teeth, including root length and any existing root resorption

---

> **Box 5.6 Radiographs commonly used in orthodontic assessment**
>
> - Dental panoramic tomograph (DPT)
> - Cephalometric lateral skull radiograph
> - Upper standard occlusal radiograph
> - Periapical radiographs
> - Bitewing radiographs.

- presence of ectopic or supernumerary teeth
- presence of dental disease
- relationship of the teeth to the skeletal dental bases, and their relationship to the cranial base.

Dental panoramic tomograph (DPT)

This is useful for confirming the presence, position, and morphology of unerupted teeth, and a general overview of the teeth and their supporting structures. The focal trough is narrow in the incisor region, so additional views may be required for some patients in this region (Fig. 5.15).

A DPT should only be taken in the presence of specific signs and symptoms, so they should not be used as a method of screening clinically asymptomatic patients.

Cephalometric lateral skull radiograph

Sometimes referred to as a 'lateral ceph', this is discussed in more detail in Chapter 6.

Upper occlusal radiograph

This gives a view of the maxillary incisor region and is used to assess the root form of incisors, detect the presence of supernumerary teeth, and to locate ectopic canine teeth (Fig. 5.16). The location of teeth on radiographs often requires views to be taken at different angles using a technique known as parallax (see Chapter 14, Section 14.5).

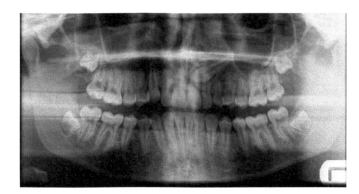

Fig. 5.15 A DPT showing an unerupted upper left canine and unerupted third permanent molars.

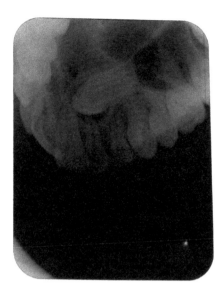

Fig. 5.16 Upper occlusal radiograph taken to investigate the impacted canine shown in Fig. 5.15. There is a suggestion of possible resorption of the root of the upper lateral incisor, associated with the crown of the palatally impacted upper left canine.

Periapical radiographs

These can be used in any part of the mouth and are useful for assessing root form and local pathology, and locating unerupted teeth (like the upper occlusal, they can be used with other radiographic views to identify the position of these teeth using parallax).

Bitewing radiographs

They may be useful in assessing caries and the condition of existing restorations.

5.6.4 Cone beam computed tomography (CBCT)

Conventional computed tomography (CT) imaging involves the use of rotating X-ray equipment, combined with a digital computer, to obtain images of the body. Using CT imaging, cross-sectional images of body organs and tissues can be produced. CBCT is a faster, more compact version of traditional CT with a lower dose of radiation. Through the use of a cone-shaped X-ray beam, the size of the scanner, radiation dosage, and time needed for scanning are all dramatically reduced. The three-dimensional (3D) views produced may be useful in certain orthodontic cases:

- Accurate location of impacted teeth and a more accurate assessment of any associated pathology, particularly resorption of adjacent teeth (Fig. 5.17).
- Assessment of alveolar bone coverage.
- Cleft palate.
- Assessment of alveolar bone height and volume (which may be relevant in potential implant cases).
- TMJ or airway analysis.
- Planning of some complex combined orthodontics and orthognathic surgery cases.

Although the radiation dose is considerably smaller than conventional CT scanning, the dose is still higher than for the conventional radiographs discussed in Section 5.6.3. At the present time, CBCT should therefore only be used when conventional radiography has failed to give, or is very unlikely to give, the necessary diagnostic information, for example, in cases of impacted teeth.

Other 3D imaging techniques are also being developed for use in orthodontics, such as optical laser scanning and stereo photogrammetry.

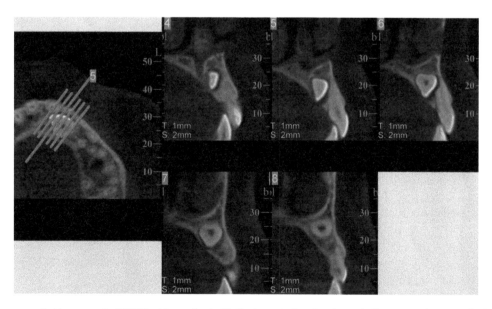

Fig. 5.17 Cone-beam computed tomography (CBCT) of the patient with the impacted canine shown in Figs 5.15 and 5.16, confirming that there is a small amount of root resorption occurring on the palatal aspect of the upper left lateral incisor, close to the apex of the tooth.

The use of 3D imaging in combined orthodontic and orthognathic surgery is covered in Chapter 22, Section 22.10.1.

The use of 3D imaging is one of the most rapidly developing fields in orthodontics and the reader is directed to the section on 'Principal sources and further reading' for more details.

5.6.5 Technological advances in orthodontic records and treatment

Digital photography and radiography have of course been available for many years. Computer software can be used to combine the two-dimensional hard and soft tissues information obtained from the photographs and radiographs to morph images to simulate the outcomes of orthodontic and/or surgical treatment. This aids treatment planning and can also help communication and providing informed consent for patients. This is discussed in more detail in Chapter 22. In more recent years, there has been a move towards 3D digital records for orthodontic patients.

Intra-oral scanning can now be used, instead of traditional impressions, to produce virtual study models. Software can be used to efficiently measure arch lengths, tooth size discrepancies, as well as provide 'virtual treatment set-ups' offering predictions of the likely occlusion at the end of treatment. When combined with the information gained from CBCT, this may allow a better 3D understanding of the relationships of the crowns to the roots and surrounding alveolar bone, helping

to define the biological bony limits of any orthodontic treatment. As technology improves, it will also help in predicting the effect of orthodontic treatment on the relationships of the teeth to the surrounding soft tissues (smile aesthetics), and the likely effect on facial appearance.

3D imaging in orthodontics has allowed the production of stereolithographic models, which can then be used to fabricate appliances. This has been particularly successful in the development of clear aligner therapy (see Chapter 21). It has also been used in the production of guides for fixation plates in orthognathic surgery (see Chapter 22).

Digital technology has also lead to the rise of CAD/CAM (computer-assisted design and manufacture) fixed appliances, producing customized appliances, personalized to the patient's individual dentition. This has been done in two ways:

- Using intra-oral scans of the patient's teeth with traditional brackets in place, to produce customized archwires bent by a robot (see 'Principal sources and further reading' section).
- Using intra-oral scans of the teeth to produce customized brackets with individualized bases and personalized prescriptions with the aim of producing more efficient and predictable results.

It is also possible to combine both customization of the wires and the brackets to produce fully customized CAD/CAM fixed appliances. This technology is more frequently used in lingual orthodontics and is discussed in more detail in Chapter 20, Section 20.6.3.

5.7 Forming a problem list

The information collected from the history, examination, and records produces a database identifying a list of problems. It is this list of problems that allows the clinician to form a diagnosis (Fig. 5.1). An example of an orthodontic patient assessment is given in Fig. 5.18.

Chapter 7 will discuss the process by which the problem list produces a list of aims of treatment. Once the aims of treatment are clear, various options for treatment can be discussed with the patient, considering the risks and benefits of each of the options. When the patient understands all the options, a definitive treatment plan can be agreed.

5.8 Case study: example case to demonstrate orthodontic assessment

(Case (LM) treated by Dr Taiyab Raja under the supervision of Simon Littlewood.)

Problem list for LM

Pathological problems

Oral hygiene is poor. The first permanent molars have large restorations and may therefore have a limited long-term prognosis.

Developmental (orthodontic) problems

Patient's concerns: LM is concerned about her prominent and crooked upper teeth. She has good motivation for treatment and realistic expectations.

Facial and smile aesthetics: the missing upper right lateral incisor is compromising her smile. This has caused an unusual gingival margin relationship and an asymmetric dental arrangement. Her mandible is slightly retrognathic, but acceptable. Her lips are incompetent at rest—competence can only be achieved by straining the lips.

Alignment and symmetry in each arch: the lower arch is symmetrical and U-shaped, with 7 mm of crowding. The upper arch is symmetrical and V-shaped with 1 mm of crowding. The upper right lateral incisor is developmentally absent and the upper left lateral incisor is peg shaped. The upper incisors are proclined at 120° and the upper left canine is severely rotated.

Skeletal and dental problems in the transverse plane: there is no skeletal asymmetry. The upper centreline is 2 mm to the right of the facial midline, and the lower centreline is correct. There is a crossbite tendency on the upper left second premolar.

Skeletal and dental problems in anteroposterior plane: the mandible is slightly retrognathic, but clinically acceptable. There is an increased overjet of 8 mm. The molars and canines are ¾ unit Class II bilaterally.

Skeletal and dental problems in the vertical plane: the patient presents with normal vertical skeletal proportions. There is an average overbite, with an increased curve of Spee in the lower arch of 3 mm.

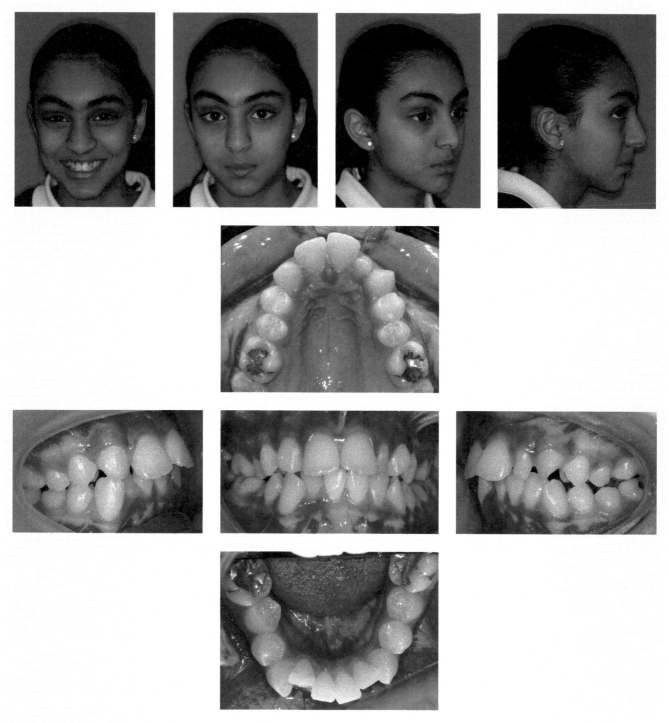

Fig. 5.18 (a) Initial photos for case LM.

Aims of treatment for LM

The **aims** of treatment are directly related to the problem list.

Patient's concerns: address the patient's concerns by reducing slightly the prominent upper incisors and aligning the teeth.

Facial and smile aesthetics: improve her smile by creating more normal gingival margin relationships, with the central incisors being higher than the adjacent tooth. Improve the symmetry of the smile by balancing the tooth proportions on the right and left in the upper labial segment. Allow her to obtain lip competence at rest by minimal retraction of the upper dentition.

Alignment and symmetry in each arch: relieve the crowding in both arches. Maintain the lower archform and make the upper

Orthodontic Assessment Form

Patient Details

Name ████████ █████████	Referrer:
Address ████████████████████ ████████	██████████████████
	Reason for referral
	Missing lateral incisor
Tel Contact: ████████████	
Date of birth: ████████ *Age 12 years 11 months*	

History

Patient's complaint	Habits
Upper teeth stick out & are crooked	*None noted*
	Growth status
	Still growing
Medical history	Motivation
Medically fit & well	*Very keen for treatment with realistic expectations for treatment*
Dental History (including trauma & previous treatments)	
No trauma history. Regular dental attender, with experience of restorations in adult teeth	Socio-behaviour factors *Supportive family able to attend appointments. No apparent behavioral problems*

Extra-oral examination

Anteroposterior	Smile Aesthetics
Mild Class II	*Smile aesthetic compromised by missing upper right lateral incisor – creating unusual gingival margin relationships and asymmetrical dental arrangement*
Vertical	
Average vertical proportions	
	Soft tissues
	Lips incompetent at rest with lower lip behind upper incisors at rest. Normal swallowing pattern
Transverse	
Symmetrical	TMJ
	No signs or symptoms reported

Intra-oral examination

Teeth present:	Lower arch
7 6 5 4 3 1 1 2 3 4 5 6 7 7 6 5 4 3 2 1 1 2 3 4 5 6 7	*Moderate crowding (approximately 7mm) Slightly mesially inclined lower canines*
Oral hygiene	
Unsatisfactory – needs to improve	
Periondontal health	Upper arch
Bleeding on probing in labial segments	*Absent upper right lateral and peg-shaped upper left lateral incisor. Very mild crowding with upper right canine rotated mesio-palatally by 90°*
Tooth quality	
Heavily restored first permanent molars	

Teeth in occlusion

Incisor relationship	Molars
Class II division 1	Right *¼ unit Class II* Left *¼ unit Class II*
Overjet = 8 mm	Canines Right *¼ unit Class II* Left *¼ unit Class II*
Overbite	
Increased & incomplete	Crossbites
Centre-lines	*Crossbite tendency upper left second premolar*
Upper centre-line 2mm to right of facial midline	Displacements
Lower centre-line correct to facial midline	*None detected*

Fig. 5.18 (b) Completed orthodontic assessment sheet for case LM. A blank version of this form is available at the end of this book (see 'Orthodontic Assessment Form').

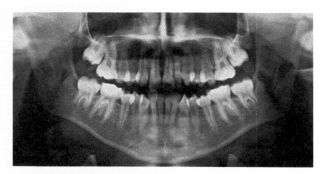

Fig. 5.18 (c) DPT for case LM. The DPT demonstrates the absence of the upper right lateral incisor and all third permanent molars. There are also large restorations in all first permanent molars, particularly the upper left and the lower right first permanent molars.

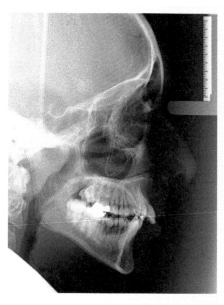

arch compatible with this. Improve the symmetry in the upper arch, reduce the prominence and proclination of the upper incisors, and align the teeth, including the rotated upper left canine.

Skeletal and dental problems in the transverse plane: correct the upper centreline to the facial midline, and expand the upper arch to remove the crossbite tendency on the upper left second premolar.

Skeletal and dental problems in the anteroposterior plane: reduce the overjet principally by retraction of the upper incisors. Some minimal proclination of the lower labial segment could be

Fig. 5.18 (d) Lateral ceph radiograph of LM. Analysis of this radiograph shows the following values: sella–nasion–A point angle (SNA) = 75°, (sella–nasion–B point angle) SNB = 73°, A point–nasion–B point angle (ANB) = 2°, upper incisor to maxilla = 120°, lower incisor to mandible = 90° and maxillary–mandibular planes angle = 28°. An Eastman correction on the ANB produces an ANB = 5°. Lateral ceph analysis will be explained further in Chapter 6. This radiograph confirms the clinical findings of a mild Class II skeletal pattern, with normal vertical proportions and proclined upper incisors.

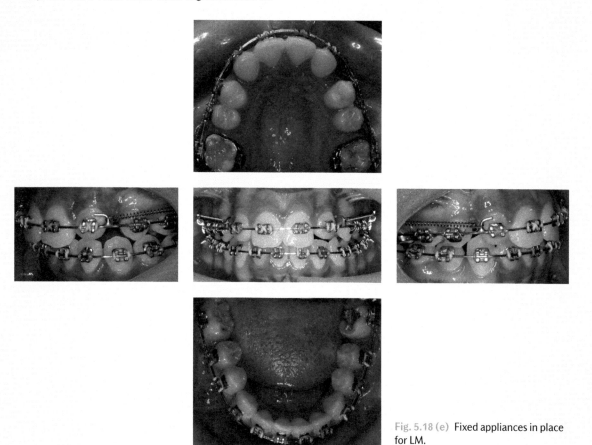

Fig. 5.18 (e) Fixed appliances in place for LM.

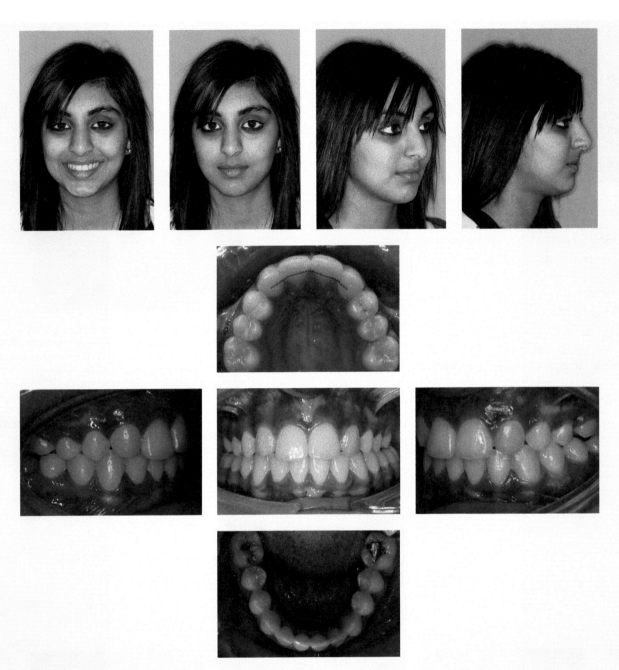

Fig. 5.18 (f) End of treatment records for LM.

accepted. The canines should be treated to a Class I relationship. The mandible is slightly retrognathic so the case can be treated by orthodontic camouflage.

Skeletal and dental problems in the vertical plane: flatten the curve of Spee in the lower arch.

Treatment plan for LM

(The treatment planning process is discussed in Chapter 7.)

- Improve oral hygiene to level suitable for orthodontic treatment.
- Extract peg-shaped upper left lateral incisor and all first permanent molars.

- Transpalatal arch connecting upper second permanent molars (see Chapter 15).
- Upper and lower fixed appliances—aiming to close spaces anteriorly and camouflaging upper canines as upper lateral incisors, and camouflaging upper first premolars as upper canines. This should give a more symmetrical and aesthetic smile.
- Pericision to upper left canine to reduce relapse (see Chapter 16, Section 16.7.1).
- Upper bonded retainer and upper and lower vacuum-formed retainers (see Chapter 16).

Key points about orthodontic assessment

- Orthodontic assessment involves taking a history, undertaking a clinical examination, and collecting appropriate diagnostic records.

- The history should include the patient's presenting complaint, medical history, dental history (including any history of trauma and previous treatment), habits, physical growth status, motivation, and any relevant socio-behavioural factors.

- The clinical examination should be a systematic assessment of the face and dentition in three dimensions.

- As well as assessing the patient extra-orally in three dimensions it is important to assess the smile aesthetics and soft tissues.

- The intra-oral examination should assess the overall dental health, each arch individually, and the arches in occlusion.

- The history and examination should determine which diagnostic records are required. This may include study models, photographs, and appropriate radiographs and possibly 3D imaging.

- Technological advances in digital orthodontics are changing the records collected in orthodontic assessment as well as influencing the approach to treatment.

Principal sources and further reading

Drage, N. (2018). Cone beam computed tomography in orthodontics. *Ortho Update*, **11**, 27–30. [DOI: 10.12968/ortu.2018.11.1.27]
This provides a contemporary overview of CBCT in orthodontics, focusing on selection criteria, dose reduction, and current guidance regarding reporting.

Isaacson, K. G., Thom, A. R., Atack, N. E., Horner, K., and Waites, E. (2015). *Guidelines for the Use of Orthodontic Radiographs in Clinical Orthodontics* (4th edn). London: British Orthodontic Society.
These radiographic guidelines have been specifically written for orthodontics and provide an excellent overview of appropriate use of radiographic records in orthodontics.

Larson, B. E., Vaubel, C. J., and Grunheid, T. (2013). Effectiveness of computer-assisted orthodontic treatment technology to achieve predicted outcomes. *Angle Orthodontist*, **83**, 557–62. [DOI: 10.2319/080612-635.1] [PubMed: 23181776]

Grauer, D. and Proffit, W. R. (2011). Accuracy in tooth positioning with a fully customized lingual orthodontic appliance. *American Journal of Orthodontics and Dentofacial Orthopedics*, **140**, 433–43. [DOI: 10.1016/j.ajodo.2011.01.020] [PubMed: 21889089]
These two papers provide the reader with an insight into the development and applications of technology advances in orthodontics.

Patel, A., Burden, D. J., and Sandler, J. (2009). Medical disorders and orthodontics. *Journal of Orthodontics*, **36**, 1–21. [DOI: 10.1179/14653120722851] [PubMed: 19934236].
This comprehensive article provides an excellent in-depth review of medical disorders that could affect orthodontic treatment.

Sarver, D. M. (2001). The importance of incisor positioning in the esthetic smile: the smile arc. *American Journal of Orthodontics and Dentofacial Orthopedics*, **120**, 98–111. [DOI: 10.1067/mod.2001.114301] [PubMed: 11500650].
This paper provides an overview of the important topic of smile aesthetics.

Sarver, D. M. (2016). Special considerations in diagnosis and treatment planning. In: Graber, L., Vanarsdall, R., Vig, K., and Huang, G. (eds) *Orthodontics: Current Principles and Techniques* (6th edn), pp. 245–88. St. Louis, MO: Elsevier.
This chapter provides a detailed overview of diagnosis and treatment planning in orthodontics, with an emphasis on aesthetics.

6
Cephalometrics
S. K. Barber

Chapter contents

Cephalometry is the analysis and interpretation of standardized radiographs of the facial bones. In practice, cephalometrics has come to be associated with a true lateral view (Fig. 6.1). An anteroposterior radiograph can also be taken in the cephalostat, but this view is more difficult to interpret and is usually only employed in cases with a skeletal asymmetry.

6.1 The cephalostat

Standardization is required to enable comparison of cephalometric radiographs from one patient at different time points or from different individuals. To achieve this, the cephalostat was developed by B. Holly Broadbent in the period after the First World War. The cephalostat consists of an X-ray machine set at a fixed distance from ear posts, which fit into the patient's external auditory meatus. The central beam of the machine is directed towards the ear posts, which also serve to stabilize the patient's head (Fig. 6.2). The position of the head in the vertical axis is standardized by ensuring that the Frankfort plane (for definition see Section 6.5.2) is horizontal. This can be done by manually positioning the patient or, alternatively, by placing a mirror some distance away level with the patient's head and asking him or her to look into their own eyes. This is called the natural head position. It is normal practice to cone down the area exposed so that the skull vault is not routinely included in the X-ray beam.

Difficulties in standardizing the distances from the tube to the patient (usually between 1.5 to 1.8 m) and from the patient to the film (usually around 30 cm) mean some magnification, usually around 7–8%, is inevitable with a lateral cephalometric film. To allow estimation of the magnification and thus the comparability of different films, it is helpful if a scale is included in the view. It is essential that the magnification for a particular cephalostat is standardized if comparison between radiographs is required. To give a better definition of the soft tissue outline of the face an aluminium wedge is positioned to attenuate the beam in that area, although this is required less frequently with newer digital systems.

6.1.1 Digital radiographs

Conventionally, following the exposure of the X-ray beam onto the radiographic film, the film is processed to give an individual radiograph. With digital radiographs, the image is stored electronically and viewed directly on a computer screen. This approach has the advantage that processing faults are eliminated and the storage and transfer of images is facilitated.

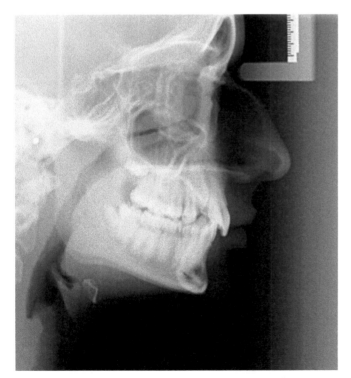

Fig. 6.1 A lateral cephalometric radiograph. An aluminium wedge has been positioned to attenuate the beam thereby enhancing the view of the soft tissues. The scale allows estimation of the magnification.

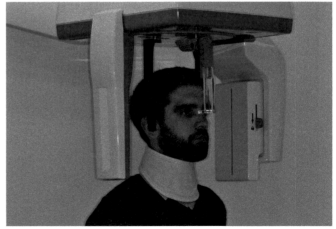

Fig. 6.2 A cephalostat machine with the patient in natural head position and ear posts stabilizing the head. A thyroid collar is used to reduce the risk of damage from the ionizing radiation.

Box 6.1 **Types of digital radiographs**

Direct digital radiography using solid-state sensors

- A sensor is used, which consists of either a charged couple device (CCD) or a complementary metal oxide semiconductor (CMOS) overlaid with a scintillation layer.
- X-ray energy strikes the scintillation layer and is converted into visible light, which interacts with the CCD/CMOS to create an electrical charge.
- For intra-oral X-rays, the sensor is placed in the mouth and for extra-oral X-rays, the sensor replaces the film.
- The sensor is connected by a cable to the computer, which converts the electrical charge into a digital image.
- Information is displayed in 'real time' on a computer screen.

Computed radiography using photostimulable phosphor (PSP) plates

- PSP is placed in cassette.
- Activation of phosphors by X-ray photons excites electrons to a higher energy level, which are stored until the plate is read.
- A laser beam scans the plate, releasing the stored energy as fluorescent light, which is then converted to a digital signal.
- This results in a delay in the image appearing on screen.

There are currently two main approaches used to produce digital radiographs (Box 6.1). The digital lateral cephalometric image can be digitized directly and the values noted or alternatively, a proprietary software package can be used for digitization and analysis of the computer image.

6.2 Indications for cephalometric evaluation

An increasing awareness of the risk of damage to human tissue associated with ionising radiation has led clinicians to reduce the use of lateral cephalometry. The following reasons are considered valid indications for taking a lateral cephalometric radiograph.

6.2.1 Aid to diagnosis and treatment planning

It is possible to carry out successful orthodontic treatment without taking a cephalometric radiograph, particularly in Class I malocclusions. However, cephalometric analysis may provide useful information for assessing the aetiology of malocclusion and for planning treatment. The benefit to the patient in terms of the additional information gained must be weighed against the radiation dose (Table 6.1). Pre-treatment lateral cephalometric radiographs may be best limited to patients with a skeletal discrepancy and/or where anteroposterior movement of the incisors is planned. In a small proportion of patients it may be helpful to monitor growth with serial cephalometric radiographs to optimize the planning and timing of treatment. Again, the additional radiation dosage to the patient must be justifiable and, where possible, other methods of growth monitoring that do not require ionising radiation should be used.

A further use for lateral views during diagnosis is to aid localization of unerupted displaced teeth and other pathologies (see Chapter 14, Fig. 14.2).

6.2.2 Pre-treatment record

A lateral cephalometric radiograph is useful in providing a baseline record prior to the placement of appliances, particularly where growth modification or movement of the upper and lower incisors is planned.

6.2.3 Monitoring treatment progress

In the management of severe malocclusions, where tooth movement is occurring in all three planes of space (e.g. treatments involving functional appliances or upper and lower fixed appliances), it may be helpful to take a lateral cephalometric radiograph during treatment to monitor incisor inclinations and anchorage requirements. A lateral cephalometric radiograph taken during treatment to assess treatment progress may also provide information about the movement of unerupted teeth and upper incisor root resorption. However, intra-oral images are preferred as greater detail is gained with lower radiation dose.

6.2.4 End of orthodontic treatment

For patients with severe malocclusions, a lateral cephalometric radiograph may be taken near the end of active treatment to check all

Table 6.1 Approximate effective dosages of different types of radiographs

Radiograph	Approximate effective dose (µSv)
Upper anterior occlusal	8
OPT	3–38
Lateral cephalogram	<6
CBCT: small volume (dento-alveolar) Large volume (craniofacial)	10–670 30–1100

treatment objectives have been met and to aid planning of retention. Post-treatment lateral cephalometric radiographs are usually restricted to patients where there is uncertainty around the stability of the outcome as a result of the treatment methods used, or a concern around future unfavourable growth.

6.2.5 Research purposes

A great deal of information has been obtained about growth and development by longitudinal studies, which involved taking serial cephalometric radiographs from birth to the late teens or beyond. While the data provided by previous investigations are still used for reference purposes, it is no longer ethically possible to repeat this type of study due to the risks associated with ionising radiation. However, views taken routinely during the course of orthodontic diagnosis and treatment for clinical care may be used to study the effects of growth and treatment if the necessary consent and ethical approval are obtained.

6.3 Evaluating a cephalometric radiograph

Before starting a tracing, it is important to examine the radiograph for any abnormalities or pathology. For example, a pituitary tumour could result in an increase in the size of the sella turcica.

6.3.1 Hand tracing

In order to be able to derive meaningful information, an accurate and systematic approach is required which also involves selecting the right conditions and equipment for the task.

- The tracing should be carried out in a darkened room on a light viewing box. All but the area being traced should be shielded to block out any extraneous light.
- Proprietary acetate sheets are the best medium as their transparency facilitates landmark identification.
- A sharp pencil should be used. A 0.3 mm leaded propelling pencil is recommended to remove the need for a pencil sharpener.
- The acetate sheet should be secured onto the film with masking tape, which does not leave a sticky residue when removed. The tracing should be oriented in the same position as the patient was when the radiograph was taken, that is, with the Frankfort plane horizontal.
- Stencils can be used to obtain a neat outline of the incisor and molar teeth. However, too much artistic licence can lead to inaccuracies, particularly if the crown root angle of a tooth is not 'average'.
- For landmarks which are bilateral, an average of the two should be taken unless they are directly superimposed.
- With a careful technique, tracing errors should be of the order of ± 0.5 mm for linear measurements and ± 0.5° for angular measurements.
- It is a valuable 'learning experience' to trace the same radiograph on two separate occasions and compare the tracings. This helps to reduce the temptation to place undue emphasis upon small variations from normal cephalometric values.

Definitions of the various points and reference planes are given in Section 6.5.

6.3.2 Digitization

Information from a conventional hard copy lateral cephalometric film can be entered into a computer by means of a digitizer, comprising an illuminated radiographic viewing screen connected to the computer and a cursor to record the horizontal and vertical (x, y) coordinates of cephalometric points and bony and soft tissue outlines. For digital radiographs the points can be entered directly by a mouse click. Specialized software can then be employed to produce a tracing and/or the analysis of choice. An example of a digitized tracing is shown in Fig. 6.3 and Table 6.2.

Studies have shown digitizing to be as accurate as tracing a radiograph by hand and with the increasing use of digital radiographs this has now become the norm. Digitizing is particularly useful for research, as any number of radiographs can be entered, superimposed, and/or compared statistically.

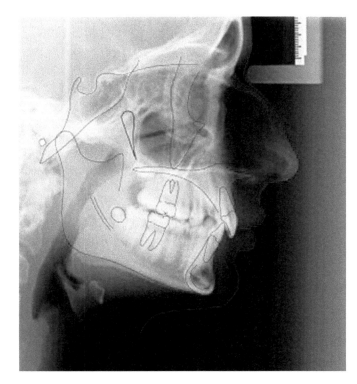

Fig. 6.3 A lateral cephalogram patient MH (female, aged 13 years) with digital tracing and values.

Table 6.2 Cephalometric values for patient MH (see Fig. 6.3)

	MH	Mean
SNA	83°	81° ± 3°
SNB	77°	78° ± 3°
ANB	6°	3° ± 2°
UInc to MxPl	103°	109° ± 6°
LInc to MnPl	96°	93° ± 6°
MMPA	20°	27° ± 4°
LInc to APog	−0.7 mm	1 mm ± 2 mm
LAFP	53.3%	55% ± 2%

6.4 Cephalometric analysis: general points

The extensive array of cephalometric analyses available in the orthodontic literature highlights that no single method is sufficient for all purposes and all methods have their drawbacks. In a book of this size, it is more appropriate to consider one analysis in depth. Therefore, one of the approaches used commonly in the UK will be considered, the Eastman cephalometric standard (Table 6.3). For details of other analyses, the reader is referred to the publications cited in the section 'Principal sources and further reading'.

Cephalometric analyses are based on comparison of the values obtained for a particular individual (or group of individuals) with the average values for their population (e.g. Caucasians). The range given by one standard deviation around the mean will include 66% of the population and two standard deviations will include 95%.

Cephalometric analysis is of value in identifying the component parts of a malocclusion and probable aetiological factors—it is useful when a tracing is finished to reflect why that individual has that particular malocclusion. However, it is important not to give more credence to cephalometric analysis than it actually merits; it should always be remembered that it is an adjunctive tool to clinical diagnosis and differences of cephalometric values from the average are not in themselves an indication for treatment, particularly as variations from normal in a specific value may be compensated for elsewhere in the facial skeleton or cranial base. In addition, cephalometric errors can occur due to incorrect positioning of the patient and incorrect identification of landmarks (see Section 6.11).

6.5 Commonly used cephalometric points and reference lines

The points and reference lines are shown in Fig. 6.4.

6.5.1 Points

A point (A): the point of deepest concavity on the anterior profile of the maxilla. It is also called the subspinale and is taken to represent the anterior limit of the maxilla. 'A' point can be tricky to locate accurately, however, tracing the outline of the root of the upper central incisor first and shielding all extraneous light can aid identification. 'A' point is located on alveolar bone and is liable to changes in position with tooth movement and growth.

Table 6.3 Cephalometric norms for Caucasians (Eastman Standard)

Measurement	Mean value	Standard deviation	Measurement	Mean value	Standard deviation
SNA	81°	3°	Inter-incisal angle	135°	10°
SNB	78°	3°	MMPA	27°	4°
ANB	3°	2°	Facial proportion	55%	2%
UInc to MxPl	109°	6°	LInc to APog line	+1 mm	2 mm
LInc to MnPl	93°	6°	SN to MxPl	8°	3°

For definitions see Section 6.5

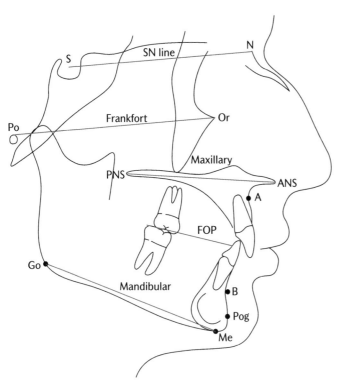

Fig. 6.4 Commonly used points and reference lines.

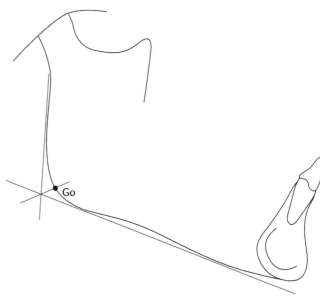

Fig. 6.5 Construction of gonion (Go): tangents are drawn to the posterior and inferior borders of the mandible. A line is then drawn from the angle formed by the tangents to bisect the angle of the mandible. Note—if two mandibular outlines are visible, the procedure is completed for both outlines and gonion is estimated to be midway between the two constructed gonion points

Anterior nasal spine (ANS): the tip of the anterior process of the maxilla, situated at the lower margin of the nasal aperture.

B point (B): the point of deepest concavity on the anterior surface of the mandibular symphysis. B point is also sited on alveolar bone and can alter with tooth movement and growth.

Gonion (Go): the most posterior inferior point on the angle of the mandible. This point can be 'guesstimated', or determined more accurately by bisecting the angle formed by the tangents from the posterior border of the ramus and the inferior border of the mandible (Fig. 6.5).

Menton (Me): the most inferior point on the mandibular symphysis.

Nasion (N): the most anterior point on the frontonasal suture. If it is difficult to locate the nasion, the point of deepest concavity at the intersection of the frontal and nasal bones can be used instead.

Orbitale (Or): the most inferior anterior point on the margin of the orbit. By definition, the left orbital margin should be used to locate this point. However, this can be a little tricky to determine radiographically, and so an average of the two images of left and right is usually taken.

Pogonion (Pog): the most anterior point on the mandibular symphysis.

Porion (Po): the uppermost outermost point on the bony external auditory meatus. This landmark can be obscured by the ear posts of the cephalostat, and some advocate tracing these instead. This is not recommended, however, as they do not approximate to the position of the external auditory meatus.

Posterior nasal spine (PNS): the tip of the posterior nasal spine of the maxilla. This point is often obscured by the developing third molars, but lies directly below the pterygomaxillary fissure.

Sella (S): the midpoint of the sella turcica.

6.5.2 Reference lines

SN line: the line connecting the midpoint of the sella turcica with the nasion, taken to represent the cranial base.

Frankfort plane: the line joining the porion and the orbitale. This plane is difficult to record accurately because of the problems inherent in determining the orbitale and porion.

Maxillary plane: the line joining the ANS with the PNS. Where it is difficult to determine the ANS and PNS accurately, a line parallel to the nasal floor can be used instead.

Mandibular plane: the line joining gonion and menton. This is only one of several definitions of the mandibular plane, but is probably the most widely used. Other definitions can be found in the publications listed in the section on 'Principal sources and further reading'.

Functional occlusal plane (FOP): a line drawn between the cusp tips of the permanent molars and premolars (or deciduous molars in mixed dentition). It can be difficult to decide where to draw this line, particularly if there is an increased curve of Spee or only the first permanent molars are in occlusion during the transition from mixed to permanent dentition. The functional plane can change orientation with growth and/or treatment and it is therefore not particularly reliable for longitudinal comparisons.

6.6 Anteroposterior skeletal pattern

6.6.1 Angle ANB

To enable comparison of the position of the maxilla and mandible, it is necessary to have a fixed point or plane. The skeletal pattern is often determined cephalometrically by comparing the relationship of the maxilla and mandible with the cranial base by means of angles SNA and SNB. The difference between these two measurements, angle ANB, is classified broadly as shown in Table 6.4.

Table 6.4 Classifications of ANB angle

ANB < 2°	Class III
2° ≤ ANB ≥ 4°	Class I
ANB > 4°	Class II

Table 6.5 Change in value of SNA, SNB, and ANB angle as nasion position changes (see Fig. 6.4)

Nasion in original position (black)	Nasion moved anteriorly (red)
SNA = 83°	SN*A = 80°
SNB = 77°	SN*B = 76°
ANB = 6°	AN*B = 4°

However, this approach has two assumptions: (1) the cranial base, as indicated by the line SN, is a reliable basis for comparison; and (2) points A and B are indicative of maxillary and mandibular basal bone. As previously indicated, A and B points can be affected by changes in incisor root position and this should be remembered when using SNA, SNB, and ANB to assess treatment changes. Variations in the position of nasion, particularly anteroposterior changes, affect angles SNA and SNB and thus their relationship in ANB (Fig. 6.6 and Table 6.5). Hence, an increase or reduction in SNA from the average value could be due to either a discrepancy in the position of the maxilla (point A) or nasion.

To compensate for the effect of an aberrant nasion position on ANB, a modification called the 'Eastman correction' is suggested (Fig. 6.7). This is only applied to cases with a change in the position of the nasion, indicated by a normal angle between the maxillary plane and sella–nasion line (8° ± 3°). An angle value outside this range indicates the position of the sella is at fault and because this affects the SNA and SNB values to the same extent, the ANB value does not require correction.

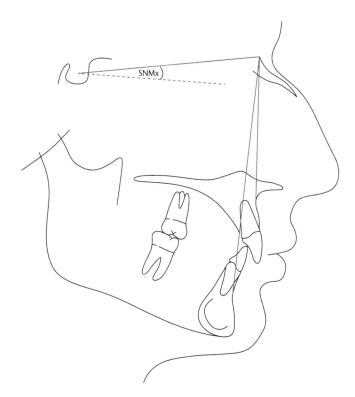

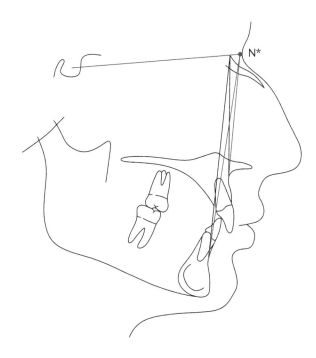

Fig. 6.6 Effect of variations in the position of nasion on angles SNA, SNB, and ANB. Nasion has been moved anteriorly (N*).

Fig. 6.7 Assessment of skeletal pattern using ANB derived from angles SNA and SNB, with application of the Eastman correction. SNA is increased and the angle between the SN line and maxillary plane is within normal range. Therefore the correction can be applied:

$$ANB + \frac{(81° - 83°)}{2} = 6° - 1° = 5°$$

The ANB difference of 6° suggests a mild Class II skeletal pattern. However, if the ANB difference is corrected, the new value of 5° suggests a Class I skeletal pattern based on the Eastman Standard values.

Table 6.6 Anteroposterior assessment of patient MH

	MH	Mean
SNA	83°	81° ± 3°
SNB	77°	78° ± 3°
SNMx	9°	8° ± 3°
ANB	6°	3° ± 2°

To perform the correction:

- If SNA is increased: for every degree that SNA is greater than 81°, subtract 0.5° from ANB.
- If SNA is reduced: for every degree that SNA is less than 81°, add 0.5° to ANB.

6.6.2 Nasion perpendicular

Another popular cephalometric method for assessing anteroposterior jaw relations arises from the McNamara analysis. A line is drawn inferiorly from the nasion perpendicular to the Frankfort plane (nasion–perpendicular) and this can be used to estimate maxillary and mandibular positions using point A and pogonion respectively. The method is as follows:

1. The nasion perpendicular is constructed by drawing a line perpendicular to the Frankfort plane, extending inferiorly from the nasion.
2. The distance from the point A perpendicular to this line is measured to assess the maxillary position (a).
3. The distance from the pogonion perpendicular to this line is measured to assess the mandibular position (b).

See Fig. 6.8 and Table 6.7. This method has similarities to the clinical assessment using the zero meridian (see Chapter 5, Section 5.4.1). The main limitations in using the nasion perpendicular arise from location of the Frankfort plane and the potential variation in the position of the nasion.

Alternatively, an approach that avoids the cranial base and nasion, for example, the Ballard conversion (see Section 6.6.3) or the Wits analysis (see Section 6.6.4) can be used to supplement the above analyses, particularly where the cephalometric findings are at variance with the clinical assessment.

6.6.3 Ballard conversion

Ballard's method uses the incisors as indicators of the relative position of the maxilla and mandible. The aim is to tilt the teeth to their normal angles (thus eliminating any dento-alveolar compensation) with the result that the residual overjet will indicate the relationship of the maxilla to the mandible. The method is as follows (Fig. 6.9):

1. Trace the outline of the maxilla, the mandibular symphysis, the incisors, and the maxillary and mandibular planes (shown in black).

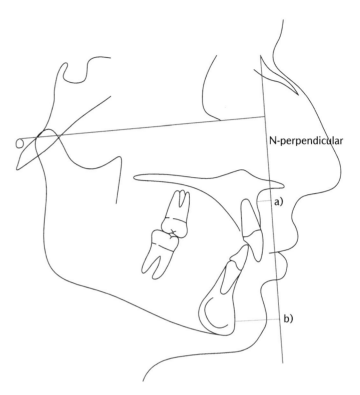

Fig. 6.8 Anteroposterior skeletal relationships assessed using nasion perpendicular.

Table 6.7 Average values for anteroposterior assessment using nasion perpendicular

	Composite norm
Nasion perpendicular to point A	0 mm to +1 mm
Pogonion to nasion perpendicular	–2 mm to +4 mm

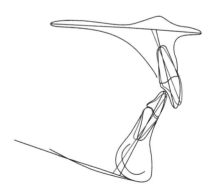

Fig. 6.9 Ballard conversion MH (female, aged 13 years): average upper incisor angle to maxillary plane, 109°; lower incisor angle to mandibular plane, 120° – 20° = 100°.

2. Mark the 'rotation points' of the incisors one-third of the root length away from the root apex.

3. Rotating around the point marked, reposition the upper incisor at an angle of 109° to the maxillary plane (shown in red).

4. Repeat for the lower incisor—in this case, reposition lower incisor to 100° to allow for the maxillary mandibular planes angle of 20° (shown in red). The residual overjet reflects the underlying skeletal pattern.

In the case shown in Fig. 6.9, the lower incisor edge lies distal to the cingulum plateau of the uppers with an increased overjet, indicating a mild Class II skeletal pattern.

The Ballard conversion should not be confused with a prognosis tracing (see Section 6.8.1, Fig. 6.13), which aims to assess the scope for orthodontic camouflage in patients with an underlying skeletal discrepancy.

6.6.4 Wits analysis

This analysis compares the relationship of the maxilla and mandible with the occlusal plane. There are several definitions of the occlusal plane, but for the purposes of the Wits analysis it is taken to be a line drawn between the cusp tips of the molars and premolars (or deciduous molars), known as the FOP. Perpendicular lines from both point A and point B are drawn to the FOP to give points AO and BO. The distance between AO and BO is then measured.

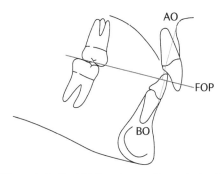

Fig. 6.10 Wits analysis. For MH (female, age 13 years), the distance from AO to BO for MH is 0.3 mm, suggesting a Class I skeletal pattern.

The method is as follows (Fig. 6.10):

1. The FOP is constructed.

2. A perpendicular line is drawn from point A and point B to the FOP to give points AO and BO.

3. The distance between AO and BO is measured. The average values are −1 mm (± 1.9 mm) for males and 0 mm (± 1.77 mm) for females.

The main drawback to the Wits analysis is that the FOP is not easy to locate, which affects the accuracy and reproducibility of the Wits analysis. A slight difference in the angulation of the FOP can have a marked effect on the relative positions of AO and BO.

6.7 Vertical skeletal pattern

There are many different ways of assessing vertical skeletal proportions. The more commonly used include the following.

- The maxillary–mandibular planes angle (MMPA) (Fig. 6.11 and Table 6.8). The average MMPA is 27 ± 4°.

- Frankfort mandibular planes angle (FMPA) (Fig. 6.11 and Table 6.8). The average angle is 28 ± 4°. However, the maxillary plane is easier to locate accurately and is therefore more widely used.

- The anterior facial proportion (Fig. 6.12). This is the ratio of the lower anterior facial height (maxillary plane to menton) to the total anterior facial height (nasion to menton) measured perpendicularly from the maxillary plane, calculated as a percentage:

$$\text{Anterior facial proportion} = \frac{\text{Lower anterior face height}}{\text{Total anterior face height}} \times 100$$

A discrepancy between the results for the MMPA and the facial proportion can arise from an altered posterior face height, as MMPA reflects both posterior lower facial height and anterior lower facial height (Fig. 6.12). For example, in the case of patient MH in Fig. 6.12

who has a decreased MMPA but an average facial proportion it would appear that the posterior lower facial height is increased (as opposed to a decreased anterior lower facial height).

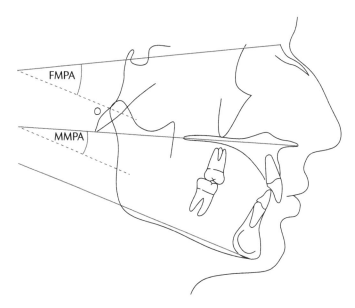

Fig. 6.11 Assessment of vertical skeletal pattern using the MMPA and FMPA for patient MH (female, aged 13 years). The MMPA is decreased. This may be due to either a decreased lower anterior face height or an increased lower posterior face height.

Table 6.8 Vertical assessment of patient MH

	MH	Mean
MMPA	20°	27° ± 4°
FMPA	25°	28° ± 4°

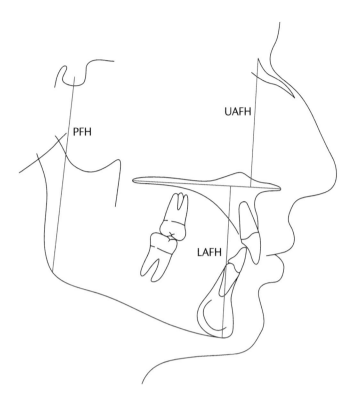

Fig. 6.12 The facial proportion can also be used to assess vertical components. For MH (female, aged 13 years) the lower anterior face height is in the normal range (53.3%).

$$\text{Upper Anterior Face Height}(N-M\times Pl)=44\,\text{mm}$$

$$\text{Lower Anterior Face Height}(M\times Pl-Me)=51.5\,\text{mm}$$

$$\text{Total Anterior Face Height}(LAFH+UAFH)=95.5\,\text{mm}$$

$$\text{Lower Anterior Facial Proportion}=\left(\frac{LAFH}{TAFH}\right)\times100=\left(\frac{51.5}{95.5}\right)\times100=53.3\%$$

This does not agree with the reduced vertical component indicated by the MMPA value 20°. A discrepancy may be noted between the anterior face height and the MMPA or FMPA if the posterior face height (S–Go) is outside the normal range.

For MH, the posterior face height is increased, suggesting a horizontal (forward) growth rotation.

$$\text{Posterior Face Height}(S-Go)=66.2\,\text{mm}$$

$$\text{Posterior: Anterior ratio}(\text{Jarabak's ratio})=\frac{PFH}{AFH}=\frac{66.2\,\text{mm}}{95.5\,\text{mm}}=69.3\%$$

> 65% indicates a forward growth rotation
< 62% indicates a backwards growth rotation

6.8 Incisor position

The average value for the angle formed between the upper incisor and the maxillary plane is 109 ± 6°, and for the lower incisor and the mandibular plane is 93 ± 6° in Caucasians. It should be remembered that there is ethnic variation in these norms and more proclination is expected for other racial groups. The inter-incisal angle, formed by intersecting the lines through the upper and lower incisors, is important for overbite correction (see Chapter 10).

The 'normal' value for the lower incisor angle is for an individual with an average MMPA of 27°. It has been suggested that there is a relationship between the MMPA and the lower incisor angle: as the MMPA increases, the lower incisors become more retroclined. As the sum of the average MMPA (27°) and the average lower incisor angle (93°) equals 120°, an alternative way of deriving the 'average' lower incisor angulation for an individual is to subtract the MMPA from 120°: Lower incisor angle = 120° – MMPA.

6.8.1 Prognosis tracing

Sometimes it is helpful to be able to determine the type and amount of incisor movement required to correct an increased or reverse overjet. Although the skeletal pattern will give an indication, on occasion, compensatory proclination or retroclination (known as dento-alveolar compensation) of the incisors, can create challenges when determining the scope for tooth movement. In such cases it may be helpful to carry out a prognosis tracing. This involves 'moving' the incisor(s) to mimic the movements achievable with different treatment approaches to help determine the best course of action for that patient. An example is shown in Fig. 6.13, where it can be seen that bodily retraction of the upper incisors would result in their being retracted out of the palatal bone. This is obviously not a practical treatment proposition and indicates alternative treatment methods are needed, in this case a surgical approach.

Another useful rough guide to assessing tooth movement is to assume that for 2.5° of angular movement (about a point of rotation one-third of the way down the root from the apex) the upper incisor edge will translate approximately 1 mm.

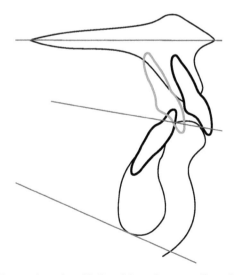

Fig. 6.13 Prognosis tracing: CP (female) aged 18 years. From this diagram it can be seen that bodily movement of the upper incisors to reduce this patient's overjet would not be feasible. Therefore, a surgical approach was recommended.

6.8.2 A–pogonion line

Raleigh Williams noted when he analysed the lateral cephalometric radiographs of individuals with pleasing facial appearances that one feature which they all had in common was that the tip of their lower incisor lay on or just in front of the line connecting point A with the pogonion. He advocated using this position of the lower incisor as a treatment goal to help ensure a good facial profile. While this line may be useful when planning orthodontic treatment, it must be remembered that it is only a guideline to good facial aesthetics and not an indicator of stability. If the lower incisors are moved from their pre-treatment position of labio-lingual balance there is a likelihood of appreciable relapse following removal of appliances.

6.9 Soft tissue analysis

Careful analysis of the soft tissues is important, particularly if changes to incisor position are planned and in diagnosis and planning prior to orthognathic surgery (see Chapter 22). As with other elements of cephalometric analysis, there are a large number of different analyses of varying complexity. Some of the more commonly used analyses include:

- the Holdaway line: a line from the soft tissue chin to the upper lip

- Rickett's E-plane: a line joining the soft tissue chin and the tip of the nose
- the facial plane: a line between soft tissue nasion and soft tissue chin.

These analyses are demonstrated in Fig. 6.14.

As with other aspects of cephalometrics, but perhaps more pertinently, these analyses should be supplementary to a clinical examination and it should also be remembered that beauty is in the eye of the beholder.

6.10 Assessing growth and treatment changes

The advantage of standardizing lateral cephalometric radiographs is the scope it gives for comparison of radiographs between (1) groups of patients for research purposes or (2) the same patient over time to evaluate growth and treatment changes. In some cases, it may be helpful to monitor growth of a patient over time before deciding upon a treatment plan, particularly if unfavourable growth would result in a malocclusion that could not be treated by orthodontics alone. During treatment, it can be helpful to determine the contributions that tooth movements and/or growth have made to orthodontic correction and to help ensure that, where possible, a stable result is achieved.

Hard and soft tissue changes can be assessed by simply comparing the values of sequential cephalograms, however, superimposition of the

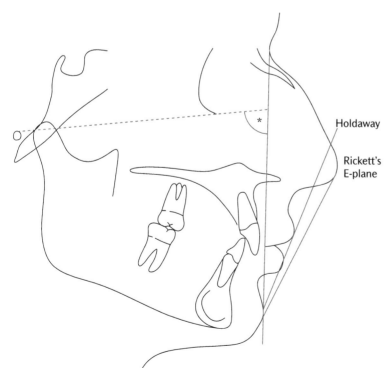

Holdaway

Rickett's E-plane

Fig. 6.14 Commonly used soft tissue analyses. The Holdaway line: a line from the soft tissue chin to the upper lip. In a well-proportioned face, this line, if extended, should bisect the nose. Rickett's E-plane: a line joining soft tissue chin and tip of the nose. In a balanced face, the lower lip should lie 2 mm (± 2 mm) anterior to this line with the upper lip positioned a little further posteriorly to the line. The facial plane: a line between soft tissue nasion and soft tissue chin. In a well-balanced face, the Frankfort plane should bisect the facial plane at an angle of about 86° (indicated by *) and point A should lie on it.

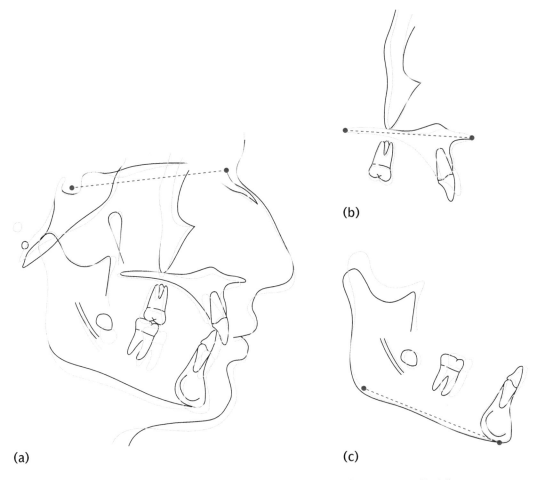

(b)

(a)

(c)

Fig. 6.15 Cephalometric superimposition provides a detailed picture of changes due to growth or treatment. Black lines = pre-treatment; blue lines = post treatment. The structures used for the superimposition will determine the changes that can be assessed. (a) Superimposition on the cranial base using the SN line. This allows evaluation of overall facial change relative to the cranial base. (b) Maxillary superimposition using the maxillary plane. This enables evaluation of dental and skeletal changes in the maxilla. (c) Mandibular superimposition using the mandibular plane. This enables assessment of dental and skeletal changes in the mandible.

cephalometric tracings provides a more detailed picture of the changes (Fig. 6.15). To enable accurate comparison of radiographs it is necessary to have a fixed point or reference line, which does not change with time or growth. This poses a dilemma, as there are no natural fixed points or planes within the face and skull. This should be borne in mind when interpreting the differences seen on superimposed cephalometric radiographs.

The lack of natural stable reference points within the face and skull was overcome in the historical studies by Björk, where metal markers were inserted in the facial skeleton to provide a fixed reference point. Whilst this approach is obviously not applicable in the management of patients, it did provide considerable information on patterns of facial growth. Björk's 'Structural Method' for undertaking cephalometric superimposition is based on the anatomical structures known to be most stable and this is generally accepted to be the

most accurate approach. A reference for a comprehensive guide to superimpositions is provided in the section on 'Principal sources and further reading'.

6.10.1 Cranial base

The SN line is taken in cephalometrics to be an approximation of the cranial base. However, growth does occur at the nasion, and therefore superimpositions on this line for the purpose of evaluating changes over time should be based at the sella. Unfortunately, growth at the nasion does not always conveniently occur along the SN line and if the nasion moves upwards or downwards with growth, this will introduce a rotational error in comparisons of tracings superimposed on the SN. It is more accurate to use the outline of the cranial base (called de Coster's line) as little change occurs in the anterior cranial base after 7 years of age (see Chapter 4). This method is more difficult and a clear radiograph and good knowledge of anatomy are required to do this reliably.

6.10.2 The maxilla

Growth of the maxilla occurs on all surfaces by periosteal remodelling. For the purpose of interpretation of growth and/or treatment changes, the least affected surface is the anterior contour of the zygomatic process. This is the preferred structure for superimposition, however, the maxillary plane registered at the PNS is commonly used as it is easier to identify.

6.10.3 The mandible

The mandibular plane is sometimes used for superimposition of the mandible; however, this can be highly erroneous due to significant remodelling in the lower border and angle of mandible. The landmarks that change least with growth and are therefore preferred for superimposition are as follows (in order of usefulness):

- The innermost surface of the cortical bone of inferior border of the symphysis.
- The anterior contour of the chin.
- The outline of the inferior dental canal.
- The crypt of the developing third permanent molars from the time of mineralization of the crown until root formation begins.

6.11 Cephalometric errors

As mentioned previously, cephalometric analysis has limitations and should only be used as a supplement to the clinical assessment. Cephalometric errors can be subdivided as follows: those arising from projection errors, difficulties in identifying landmarks, and subsequent errors in measurements.

6.11.1 Projection errors

A cephalometric radiograph is a slightly enlarged, two-dimensional representation of a three-dimensional (3D) patient; hence, some projection errors are unavoidable. Angular measurements are generally preferred to linear measurements.

6.11.2 Landmark identification

Accurate identification of cephalometric points is often difficult particularly if the radiograph is of poor quality. As described in Section 6.5, some points are more difficult to locate than others, for example, Porion is particularly problematic. Where reference planes are constructed between two points, the errors inherent in determining them are compounded.

6.11.3 Measurement errors

All analyses relate cephalometric points and planes to each other so any errors of landmark identification are multiplied. In addition, operator mistakes may contribute to measurement error.

6.12 3D cephalometric analysis

Cone beam computed tomography (CBCT) is becoming more widely available and as a result, interest in 3D cephalometry is increasing. The potential benefits of 3D views are apparent; more accurate representation of the craniofacial structures, more detailed morphology for diagnosis, and scope for growth monitoring and treatment planning in all three planes. Identification of cephalometric landmarks and measurement using these points is generally accurate; however, there is not currently a standardized method for performing 3D cephalometric analysis. To date, the most common use for 3D cephalometry is orthognathic treatment planning (see Chapter 21, Section 21.10.1), particularly for those patients with facial asymmetry. For extensive discussion around 3D cephalometry, the reader is referred to the publications cited in the section on 'Principal sources and further reading'.

Key point

Cephalometric assessment is an adjunct to clinical assessment and findings from cephalometric analysis should be interpreted with consideration of clinical findings. The aim of orthodontic treatment is to improve the patient's appearance, not to move them nearer to a cephalometric norm.

Principal sources and further reading

Björk, A. (2010). Guide to superimposition of profile radiographs by "The Structural Method". http://www.angle-society.com/case/guide.pdf
A comprehensive guide for undertaking cephalometric superimpositions.

Björk, A. and Skieller, V. (1977). Growth of the maxilla in three dimensions as revealed radiographically by the implant method. *British Journal of Orthodontics*, 4, 53–64. [DOI: 10.1179/bjo.4.2.53] [PubMed: 273440]

Björk, A. and Skieller, V. (1983). Normal and abnormal growth of the mandible. A synthesis of longitudinal cephalometric implant studies over a period of 25 years. *European Journal of Orthodontics*, **5**, 1–46. [DOI: 10.1093/ejo/5.1.1] [PubMed: 6572593]
Two historic papers that used metal implants to examine facial growth.

Drage, N., Carmichael, F., and Brown, J. (2010). Radiation protection: protection of patients undergoing cone beam computed tomography examinations. *Dental Update*, **37**, 542–8. [DOI: 10.12968/denu.2010.37.8.542] [PubMed: 21137846].
Much of the content on radiation protection is relevant to any radiograph.

Ferguson, J. W., Evans, R. I. W., and Cheng, L. H. H. (1992). Diagnostic accuracy and observer performance in the diagnosis of abnormalities in the anterior maxilla: a comparison of panoramic with intra-oral radiography. *British Dental Journal*, **173**, 265–71. [DOI: 10.1038/sj.bdj.4808024] [PubMed: 1449856].

Gaddam, R., Shashikumar, H. C., Lokesh, N. K., Suma, T., Arya, S., and Swetha, G. S. (2015). Assessment of image distortion from head rotation in lateral cephalometry. *Journal of International Oral Health*, **7**, 35–40. [PubMed: 26124597]
An illustration of the effect of positioning errors on linear and angular measurements.

Houston, W. J. B. (1979). The current status of facial growth prediction. *British Journal of Orthodontics*, **6**, 11–17. [PubMed: 396940].

Houston, W. J. B. (1986). Sources of error in measurements from cephalometric radiographs. *European Journal of Orthodontics*, **8**, 149–51. [DOI: 10.1093/ejo/8.3.149] [PubMed: 3464438]

Isaacson, K. G., Thom, A. R., Horner, K., and Whaites, E. (2015). *Guidelines for the Use of Radiographs in Clinical Orthodontics* (4th edn). London: British Orthodontic Society.
An excellent publication that explains the legislative background to taking radiographs and the need to justify every exposure. It contains several helpful flow charts to assist in deciding whether or not to take a radiograph.

Jacobson, A. and Jacobson R. L. (2006). *Radiographic Cephalometry: From Basics to 3-D imaging* (2nd edn). Chicago, IL: Quintessence Publishing, USA.
An authoritative book. This second edition includes a comprehensive description of many methods for analysis, a CD-ROM with practical information for tracing a cephalometric manually and digitally, and detailed description of digital and 3D imaging methods.

Kamoon, A., Dermaut, L., and Verbeek, R. (2001). The clinical significance of error measurement in the interpretation of treatment results. *European Journal of Orthodontics*, **23**, 569–78. [DOI: 10.1093/ejo/23.5.569] [PubMed: 11668876].
An interesting paper which puts into context cephalometric errors in the interpretation of small reported treatment changes.

McNamara, J. A. (1984). A method of cephalometric evaluation. *American Journal of Orthodontics*, **86**, 449–69. [DOI: 10.1016/S0002-9416(84)90352-X] [PubMed: 6594933]
The original paper describing nasion perpendicular.

Millet, D. and Gravely, J. F. (1991). The assessment of antero-posterior dental base relationships. *British Journal of Orthodontics*, **18**, 285–97. [DOI: 10.1179/bjo.18.4.285] [PubMed: 1782187]
An interesting discussion around the reliability and validity of the Eastman conversion, Ballard's and Wits analysis.

Sedentexct Project (2011). *Radiation Protection: Cone Beam CT for Dental and Maxillofacial Radiology (Evidence Based Guidelines)*. Luxembourg: European Commission. http://www.sedentexct.eu/files/radiation-protection_172.pdf
An important and authoritative document that comprises detailed guidelines prepared by a systematic review of the current available evidence.

References for this chapter can also be found at: **www.oup.com/uk/orthodontics5e**. Where possible, these are presented as active links that direct you to the electronic version of the work, to help facilitate onward study. If you are a subscriber to that work (either individually or through an institution), and depending on your level of access, you may be able to peruse an abstract or the full article if available.

7
Treatment planning

S. J. Littlewood

7.1 Introduction

Treatment planning is the most complex area in orthodontics. In order to formulate an appropriate treatment plan the clinician needs to be competent in history taking, examination of the patient, and collection of appropriate records. The clinician also needs to have an understanding of growth and development, facial and dental aesthetics, occlusion, the aetiology of malocclusion, different orthodontic appliances and mechanics, the physiology of tooth movement, the risks and benefits of treatment, retention, and relapse. This chapter must therefore be read in conjunction with other relevant chapters. The aim of this chapter is to offer a logical approach to treatment planning.

7.2 General objectives of orthodontic treatment

When planning treatment, the following areas need to be considered:

● Aesthetics
● Oral health
● Function
● Stability.

Ideally, orthodontic treatment should ensure a good aesthetic result, both facially and dentally; it should not compromise dental health; it should promote good function; and it should produce as stable a result as possible. Treatment should never compromise dental health or function, but occasionally, it may not be possible to produce a treatment plan that creates ideal aesthetics and the most stable result. In these cases, a compromise may need to be reached and this must be discussed with the patient as part of the consent process, explaining the limited treatment objectives (see Section 7.8).

7.3 Forming an orthodontic problem list

By following a logical process, the clinician can draw up a problem list that will help to provide the information needed to form the treatment plan. This process is shown in Fig. 7.1.

The history, examination, and collection of appropriate records are required to identify the problems in any case. This list of problems helps to formulate a diagnosis. Problems can be divided into pathological problems and developmental problems. Pathological problems are problems related to disease, such as caries and periodontal disease, and need to be addressed before any orthodontic treatment is undertaken. Developmental problems are those factors related to the malocclusion and make up the orthodontic problem list. In order to make this problem list more understandable, it can be classified into six sections:

1. The patient's concerns
2. Facial and smile aesthetics
3. Alignment and symmetry within each arch
4. Skeletal and dental relationships in the transverse plane
5. Skeletal and dental relationships in the anteroposterior plane
6. Skeletal and dental relationships in the vertical plane.

7.3.1 The patient's concerns

The patient's role in orthodontic treatment success is vital. The following areas need to be considered:

● Patient's concerns
● Patient's expectations
● Patient's motivation.

A patient will only be satisfied if those aspects of their malocclusion which trouble them are addressed. An appropriate history should reveal which features they are unhappy with and importantly, the result they are hoping for, or expect, at the end of treatment. Where possible, the clinician should formulate a plan that addresses the patient's area of complaint. However, occasionally the patient's perception of their problem or expectations may be unrealistic. The role of the orthodontist is then to counsel the patient carefully to explain what can or cannot be achieved. If the patient's expectations are unrealistic, then treatment should not be undertaken. It is also often helpful for the orthodontist to explain to the patient the parts of the

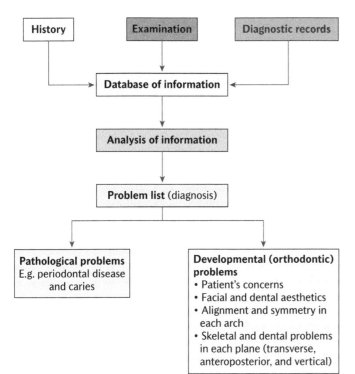

Fig. 7.1 Dividing the problem list into pathological and developmental problems.

occlusion which are normal and that are therefore not going to be changed.

Undergoing orthodontics requires a great deal of active participation and cooperation from the patient. No matter how skilful the orthodontist, treatment will not succeed unless the patient is sufficiently motivated to cooperate with all aspects of their orthodontic care. If the patient is not sufficiently motivated, then treatment should not be undertaken.

7.3.2 Facial and smile aesthetics

Straight teeth do not necessarily create a good smile and appropriate facial aesthetics. The position of the teeth within the face, and the effects of tooth movements on the overlying soft tissues of the lips, need to be considered. This is a complex area for a number of reasons.

The perception of facial aesthetics is affected by personal and cultural factors and also by fashions and trends. There has been a recent trend towards more protrusive profiles, with proclination of both the upper and lower dentitions to produce more lip support. Advocates suggest that this treatment approach leads to increased lip protrusion and can produce a more youthful appearance, but it does come with some potential risks. Firstly, proclination of incisors may move the teeth into areas of increased instability, with a tendency for the lips and cheeks to push the teeth back and cause relapse. In addition, excess expansion and proclination may lead to teeth perforating the buccal plate, causing bony dehiscences and possibly compromising future periodontal health. It is also important for patients to understand that excessive protrusion of the dentition can produce an unaesthetic result.

The effect of tooth movement on the overlying soft tissues is unpredictable. It is untrue to suggest that extracting teeth and retroclining the upper incisors will automatically compromise the facial aesthetics. However, care must be taken in cases where excessive retroclination of the upper labial segment is being considered, to avoid flattening of the facial profile. This would be particularly contraindicated in patients with an increased nasolabial angle, large nose, and retrognathic mandible (Fig. 7.2).

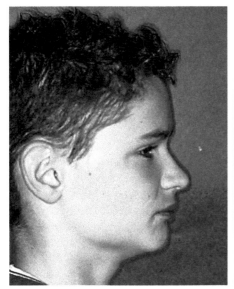
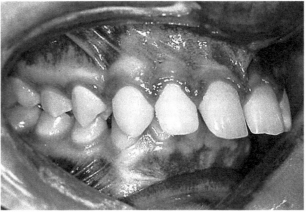

Fig. 7.2 Consideration of facial aesthetics in orthodontic treatment planning. Patient OP presents with a markedly increased overjet of 12 mm. Although the patient complained about the prominent upper teeth, a large proportion of the problem is the retrognathic mandible. Simply retracting the upper labial segment would reduce the overjet, but this would have an unfavourable effect on the facial profile. The soft tissue response to dental movement is unpredictable, but in this case, with such a large dental movement required and the retrognathic mandible, reducing the overjet by reduction of the incisors alone would unfavourably flatten the facial profile. The full treatment of this case is shown in Chapter 19.

Smile aesthetics are discussed in Chapter 5, Section 5.4.4.

Many aspects of facial or smile aesthetics cannot be influenced by orthodontics alone. This needs to be discussed with the patient, and if appropriate, surgical and restorative options may need to be considered.

7.3.3 Alignment and symmetry in each arch

The amount of crowding or spacing in each arch needs to be assessed, as well as the inclination of the upper and lower incisors and any tooth size discrepancies identified. This will play a major role in assessing the amount of space required to treat the case. The process of determining the amount of space required is called 'space analysis' (see Section 7.8). The shape and symmetry within each arch is also noted.

7.3.4 Skeletal and dental relationships in all three dimensions

Chapter 5 emphasized the importance of assessing the patient in all three dimensions (transverse, anteroposterior, and vertical). The aim is to describe the occlusion, distinguishing between the dental and skeletal factors contributing to the malocclusion in each plane. Generally, it is easier to correct malocclusions that are due to dental problems alone—if there are underlying skeletal problems, these are often more difficult to treat. The approaches to treating patients with skeletal problems are discussed in Section 7.5.

7.4 Aims of orthodontic treatment

The orthodontic problem list provides a logical summary of the information collected during the history, examination, and taking of diagnostic records. The next stage is to work through the orthodontic problem list deciding which problems will be addressed and which will be accepted. Any pathological problems need to be addressed. With the developmental problems, it may be helpful to put them in priority order, ensuring that the patient's main complaints are addressed. While it is ideal to be able to address every problem in the list, this may not always be possible, particularly with adults. By producing a prioritized problem list, it ensures that any compromises are acceptable to both the patient and the orthodontist.

This prioritized list of problems can then form the basis of the aims of treatment. Once the aims have been decided, possible solutions can be considered, which will lead to the formulation of the final definitive treatment plan (Fig. 7.3).

There is often more than one treatment plan possible for each patient. The clinician must discuss the realistic options available to the patient, explaining the risks and benefits of each approach, including the effects of no treatment at all. This forms the basis of valid consent (see Section 7.8).

7.5 Skeletal problems and treatment planning

There are three options for treating malocclusions with underlying skeletal problems:

- Orthodontic camouflage
- Growth modification
- Combined orthodontic and surgical approach.

7.5.1 Orthodontic camouflage

Treatment with orthodontic camouflage means that the skeletal discrepancy is accepted, but the labial teeth are moved into a Class I relationship. The smaller the skeletal contribution to the malocclusion, the more likely that orthodontic camouflage will be possible. It is easier to camouflage anteroposterior skeletal problems than vertical problems, which in turn are easier to camouflage than transverse problems.

7.5.2 Growth modification

This type of treatment is also known as dentofacial orthopaedics and is only possible in growing patients. By use of certain orthodontic appliances, minor changes can be made to the skeletal pattern. Most growth modification is used to correct anteroposterior discrepancies as it is

harder to make changes in the vertical dimension and even more difficult to alter transverse skeletal discrepancies.

There is increasing evidence that any growth modification that does occur is usually minimal. In most cases, growth modification is used for treatment of Class II malocclusions using headgear (see Chapters 9 and 15) or functional appliances (see Chapter 19). It can also be used for the early treatment of patients with a Class III skeletal pattern with a retrognathic maxilla, using a protraction facemask (see Chapter 11).

7.5.3 Combined orthodontic and orthognathic surgical treatment

This involves surgical correction of the jaw discrepancy in combination with orthodontics, to position the dentition to produce optimum dental and facial aesthetics. This is undertaken on patients who are fully grown. This may be indicated for patients with severe skeletal or very severe dento-alveolar problems, who are beyond the scope of orthodontics alone. It is also sometimes indicated if the patient is too old for growth modification, and orthodontic camouflage would produce a compromised facial result. Combined orthodontics and orthognathic surgical treatment is discussed further in Chapter 22.

7.6 Basic principles in orthodontic treatment planning

Once the aims of treatment have been established, treatment planning can begin. The basic principles are discussed below.

7.6.1 Oral health

The first part of any orthodontic treatment plan is to establish and maintain good oral health. While definitive restorations, such as crowns and bridges, may be placed after alignment of the teeth, all active disease must be fully treated before beginning any orthodontic treatment.

7.6.2 The lower arch

Traditionally, treatment planning has been based around the lower labial segment. Once the position of the lower labial segment is determined, the rest of the occlusion can be planned around this. In most cases it is advisable to maintain the current position of the lower labial segment. This is because the lower labial segment is positioned in an area of relative stability between the tongue lingually, and the lips and cheeks labially and buccally. Any excessive movement of the lower labial segment would increase the risk of relapse. Treatment planning around the lower incisor position is less rigidly adhered to in contemporary orthodontic treatment planning, due to the increasing emphasis on facial and soft tissue aesthetics, in addition to occlusal goals (see Box 7.1).

Exceptions do exist when the lower labial segment can be either proclined or retroclined. Here are some examples of where it may be appropriate to procline the lower incisors:

- Cases presenting with mild lower incisor crowding.
- Treatment of deep overbites, particularly in Class II division 2 cases (see Chapter 10, Section 10.3).
- Patients who had a digit-sucking habit (where the lower incisors have been held back from their natural position by the habit).
- To prevent unfavourable profile changes in reduction of large overjets when surgery is not indicated or declined.

The lower incisors can also be retroclined to camouflage a Class III malocclusion, or in the treatment of bimaxillary dental proclination.

If the anteroposterior position and inclination of lower incisors are moved excessively this may compromise stability. The patient must be aware of this and implications for retention discussed.

7.6.3 The upper arch

The upper arch should be positioned within the face to provide the best facial and dental aesthetic result, within the confines of the existing skeletal and soft tissue environment. The secret to achieving a Class I incisor relationship is to get the canines into a Class I relationship. It is helpful to anticipate the position of the lower canine once the lower

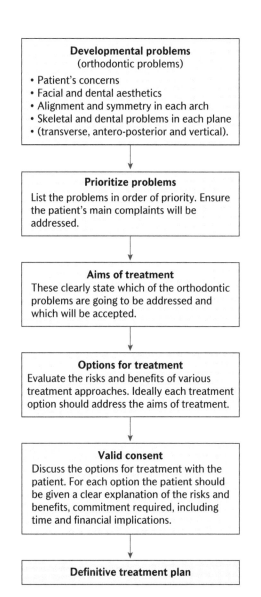

Developmental problems
(orthodontic problems)

- Patient's concerns
- Facial and dental aesthetics
- Alignment and symmetry in each arch
- Skeletal and dental problems in each plane
- (transverse, antero-posterior and vertical).

↓

Prioritize problems
List the problems in order of priority. Ensure the patient's main complaints will be addressed.

↓

Aims of treatment
These clearly state which of the orthodontic problems are going to be addressed and which will be accepted.

↓

Options for treatment
Evaluate the risks and benefits of various treatment approaches. Ideally each treatment option should address the aims of treatment.

↓

Valid consent
Discuss the options for treatment with the patient. For each option the patient should be given a clear explanation of the risks and benefits, commitment required, including time and financial implications.

↓

Definitive treatment plan

Fig. 7.3 Turning the problem list into a definitive treatment plan.

Box 7.1 How upper incisor position influences contemporary treatment planning

The objectives of any orthodontic treatment are optimal aesthetics, oral health, function, and stability. Traditional orthodontic planning was focused on planning around the lower arch by maintaining its initial position to increase stability. However, with greater awareness of facial and smile aesthetics, it has become apparent that this traditional approach may place the upper incisors in a less than ideal aesthetic position in some cases. If the lower arch can be maintained in its current position without compromising aesthetics, then this is the best approach. However, in some cases the stability of the lower arch may need to be compromised to allow better positioning of the upper incisors and hence maximize the aesthetic result. The implications for stability of this approach would then need to be discussed with the patient.

labial segment has been aligned and positioned appropriately. It is then possible to mentally reposition the maxillary canine so that it is in a Class I relationship with the lower canine. This gives the clinician an idea of how much space will be required and how far the upper canine will need to be moved. This will also give an indication of the type of movement and therefore type of appliance required, as well as providing information about anchorage requirements.

7.6.4 Buccal segments

Although the aim is usually to obtain a Class I canine relationship, it is not necessary to always have a Class I molar relationship. If teeth are extracted in the upper arch, but not in the lower, the molars will be in a Class II relationship. Conversely, if teeth are extracted in the lower arch but not in the upper, the molars will be in a Class III relationship. Whether extractions are needed or not will depend upon the space requirement in each arch. Typically, extractions are more likely to be needed in the upper arch in Class II cases, to allow retraction of the upper labial segment to camouflage the underlying skeletal pattern. However, in Class III cases treated orthodontically, extractions are more likely in the lower arch to allow retroclination of the lower labial segment. Factors affecting the need for and choice of extractions are described in the section on creating space (see Section 7.7.1).

7.6.5 Anchorage

Anchorage planning is about resisting unwanted tooth movement. Whenever teeth are moved, there is always an equal and opposite reaction. This means that when teeth are moved there is often a side effect of unwanted tooth movement of other teeth in the arch. When planning a case, it is therefore important to decide how to limit the movement of teeth that do not need to move. It is vital that anchorage is understood

and planned correctly for a treatment plan to work. Anchorage is one of the most difficult areas in orthodontics and is covered in more detail in Chapter 15.

7.6.6 Treatment mechanics

Once the aims of treatment are clear, in many cases the final result could be achieved using different types of appliances and treatment mechanics. When there is a lack of high-quality evidence to support the choice of a particular type of appliance, the choice of treatment mechanics is often determined by the clinician's expertise and experience with different techniques. The clinician should utilize mechanics that produce the desired result in the most efficient and predictable way, while avoiding any risks or undesirable side effects and minimizing the compliance required from the patient.

It is important to mention that the aims of the treatment should be determined first, and then the appropriate appliances and treatment mechanics chosen to deliver these aims. The appliance system and the treatment mechanics should not be used to determine the treatment aims.

7.6.7 Retention

At the end of orthodontic treatment almost every case needs to be retained to prevent relapse back towards the original malocclusion. It is vital that retention must be considered, planned for, and discussed at the beginning of treatment. Wearing retainers requires commitment from the patient and they should be made aware of the need for these retainers before treatment begins (see Chapter 16). Patients who are unwilling or unable to commit to safe long-term wearing of retainers may not be suitable for treatment.

7.7 Space analysis

Space analysis is a process that allows an estimation of the space required in each arch to fulfil the treatment aims. Although not an exact science, it does allow a disciplined approach to diagnosis and treatment planning, particularly for the more inexperienced clinician. It can also help to determine whether the treatment aims are feasible, as well as assisting with the planning of treatment mechanics and anchorage control.

Space planning is carried out in two phases: the first phase is to determine the space required and the second calculates the amount of space that will be created during treatment. This includes creating space for any planned prostheses.

It must be stressed that space analysis can act only as a guide, albeit a useful one, as many aspects of orthodontics cannot be accurately predicted, such as growth, the individual patient's biological response, and patient compliance. It should be used in conjunction with other information collated from the history, examination, and records. It does, however, aid a disciplined approach to treatment planning, particularly for the more inexperienced clinician, or in complex cases. Before undertaking a space analysis, the aims of the treatment should be determined as this will affect the amount of space required or created.

An example of space analysis used in the treatment planning of a clinical case is shown at the end of this chapter (see Section 7.10).

7.7.1 Calculating the space requirements

Space is required to correct the following:

- Crowding.
- Incisor anteroposterior change (usually aiming to achieve a normal overjet of 2 mm).
- Levelling of occlusal curves (flattening the curve of Spee).
- Arch contraction (expansion will create space).
- Correction of upper incisor angulation (mesiodistal tip).
- Correction of upper incisor inclination (torque).

The space requirements to correct incisor angulation and inclination are usually minimal and will not be discussed further here (see section on 'Principal sources and further reading' for more details). However, the other aspects are briefly discussed below.

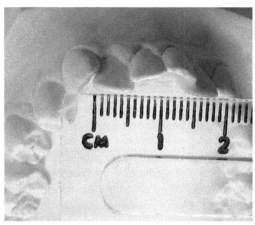 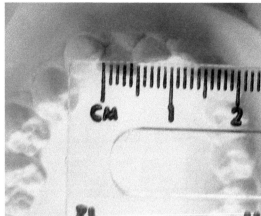

Fig. 7.4 Assessment of crowding. These photographs show the method of assessing the degree of crowding by measuring the width of the misaligned tooth compared with the amount of available space in the arch. In this example, the first photograph shows that the width of the tooth is 6 mm, and the second photograph shows that the amount of space available in the arch for this tooth is 4 mm. This suggests crowding of 2 mm for this tooth. This process is repeated for all the misaligned teeth in the arch to give the total extent of crowding. If two adjacent teeth are displaced, then assessment of crowding can be undertaken by measuring the mesiodistal width of each tooth and determining the combined space available. If digital models are used, software is available to aid efficient calculation of crowding.

Crowding

The amount of crowding present can be calculated by measuring the mesiodistal widths of any misaligned teeth in relation to the available space in the arch (Fig. 7.4).

The amount of crowding present is often classified as:

- mild (<4 mm)
- moderate (4–8 mm)
- severe (>8 mm).

Incisor anteroposterior change

It is often necessary to alter the anteroposterior position of the upper incisors, particularly when reducing an overjet. If incisors are retracted, this requires space; if incisors are proclined, then space is created. The aim is to create an overjet of 2 mm at the end of treatment. Every millimetre of incisor retraction requires 2 mm of space in the dental arch. Conversely, for every millimetre of incisor proclination 2 mm of space are created in the arch: this is helpful in estimating the proclination of incisors that will occur when crowded cases are treated on a non-extraction basis.

For example, if a patient presented with an overjet of 6 mm and the incisors needed to be retracted to create a normal overjet of 2 mm,

then this would require space. Every millimetre of retraction requires 2 mm of space. So, to reduce the overjet by 4 mm would require 8 mm of space.

Levelling occlusal curves

Where there is no occlusal stop, the lower incisors may over-erupt. This may result in an occlusal curve which runs from the molars to the incisors and is known as a curve of Spee as seen in Fig. 7.5. The amount of space required to level an increased curve of Spee is controversial, as it is affected by a number of factors, such as the shape of the archform and tooth shape. However, as a guide, Table 7.1 gives an estimation of the space required. The depth of curve is assessed from the premolar cusps to a flat plane joining the distal cusps of first permanent molars and incisors (Fig. 7.5).

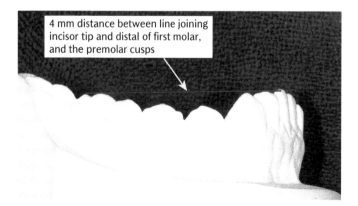

4 mm distance between line joining incisor tip and distal of first molar, and the premolar cusps

Table 7.1 Approximate space requirement to flatten a curve of Spee

Depth of curve (mm)	Space requirement (mm)
3 or less	1
4	1.5
5 or more	2

Fig. 7.5 Assessment of the space requirement for flattening the curve of Spee. It has been decided that the curve of Spee should be flattened in this case, which requires space. The depth of the curve is 4 mm, which requires 1.5 mm of space.

7.7.2 Creating space

The amount of space that will be created during treatment can also be assessed. The aim is to balance the space required with the space created. Space can be created by one or more of the following:

- Extractions
- Distal movement of molars
- Interproximal reduction
- Expansion
- Proclination of incisors
- A combination of any or all of the above.

7.7.3 Extractions

Before planning the extraction of any permanent teeth, it is essential to ensure that all remaining teeth are present and developing appropriately. The following are factors which affect the choice of teeth for extraction:

- Prognosis
- Position
- Amount of space required and where
- Incisor relationship
- Anchorage requirements
- Appliances to be used (if any)
- Patient's profile and the aims of treatment.

Choosing the appropriate teeth for extraction is a complex decision and requires understanding of all aspects of orthodontic treatment.

Incisors

Incisors are rarely the first choice for extraction due to the risk of compromising aesthetics. It can also be difficult to fit four incisors in one arch against three incisors in the opposing arch. However, indications do exist for a lower incisor extraction:

- Incisor has poor prognosis or compromised periodontal support.
- Buccal segments are Class I, but there is moderate lower incisor crowding.
- Adult patient who has a mild Class III skeletal pattern with well-aligned buccal segments.

Fixed appliances are often required to align the teeth following extraction of an incisor and a bonded retainer may be required to maintain the correction.

Management of missing or enforced extraction of upper incisors is discussed in greater detail in Chapter 8.

Canines

Canines form the cornerstone of the arch and are important both aesthetically and functionally (providing canine guidance in lateral movements). However, if severely displaced or ectopic, they may need to be extracted. A reasonable contact between the lateral incisor and first premolar is possible, particularly in the upper arch, but rarely occurs

without the use of fixed appliances. If a canine is missing, the occlusion must also be checked to ensure that there are no unwanted displacing contacts, caused by a lack of canine guidance.

First premolars

These are often the teeth of choice to extract when the space requirement is moderate to severe. Also, extraction of a first premolar in either arch usually gives the best chance of spontaneous alignment. This is particularly true in the lower arch where, provided the lower canine is mesially inclined, spontaneous alignment of the lower labial segment may occur. This spontaneous improvement is most rapid in the first 6 months after the extraction. In the upper arch, the first premolars usually erupt before the upper canines, so the chances of spontaneous improvement in the position of this tooth can be achieved if the first premolar is extracted just before the canine emerges. A space maintainer may be required to keep the space open for the upper canine.

Typically, when using fixed appliances, 40–60% of a first premolar extraction space will be available for the benefit of the labial segment without anchorage reinforcement. The reason why there is some loss of the space available from the extractions is due to mesial movement of the posterior teeth.

Second premolars

Indications for extraction of second premolars include:

- mild to moderate space requirement (3–8 mm space required)
- space closure by forward movement of the molars, rather than retraction of the labial segments is indicated
- severe displacement of the second premolar of a poor prognosis second molar.

Extraction of the second premolars is preferable to first premolars when there is a mild to moderate space requirement. This is because the anchorage balance is altered, favouring space closure by forward movement of the molars. Hence, only an estimated 25–50% of the space created by a second premolar extraction is available to allow labial segment alignment. Fixed appliances are often required to ensure good contact between the first molar and first premolar, particularly in the lower arch.

Early loss of the second deciduous molars often results in crowding of the second premolars palatally in the upper and lingually in the lower. In the upper arch, extraction of the displaced second premolar on eruption may be indicated. Conversely, in the lower arch, extraction of the first premolars is usually easier and, in most cases, uprighting of the second premolars occurs spontaneously following relief of crowding.

First permanent molars

Extraction of first permanent molars often makes orthodontic treatment more difficult and prolonged. However, their extraction may need to be considered if they have a poor long-term prognosis (see Chapter 5, Fig. 5.18). Extraction of first permanent molars is discussed in greater detail in Chapter 3, Section 3.3.8.

Second permanent molars

Extraction of second permanent molars has been suggested in the following cases:

- To facilitate distal movement of upper buccal segments.
- Relief of mild lower premolar crowding.
- Provision of additional space for the third permanent molars, thus avoiding the likelihood of their impaction.

Extraction of the upper second molar will not provide relief of crowding in the premolar or labial segments, due to mesial drift. Relief of mild crowding in the lower premolar region may be possible, as well as providing additional space for eruption of the third permanent molar. The eruption of the third permanent molars is never guaranteed, but the chances can be improved by the correct timing of extraction of the second molar. The following features should ideally be present (Fig. 7.6):

- Angle between the third permanent molar tooth germ and the long axis of the second molar is 10–30°.

- Crypt of developing third molar overlaps the root of the second molar.
- The third permanent molar is developed to the bifurcation.

Even if these criteria are satisfied, eruption of the lower third molar into occlusion cannot be guaranteed, and it should be made clear to the patient that a course of fixed appliance treatment to upright or align the third molar may be necessary.

Third permanent molars

In the past, early extraction of these teeth has been advocated to prevent lower labial segment crowding. However, it is much more likely that late lower incisor crowding is caused by subtle growth and soft tissue changes that continue to occur throughout life (Chapter 16). It is not acceptable to extract third molars purely on the grounds of preventing crowding of the lower labial segment (see Chapter 8, Section 8.2.1).

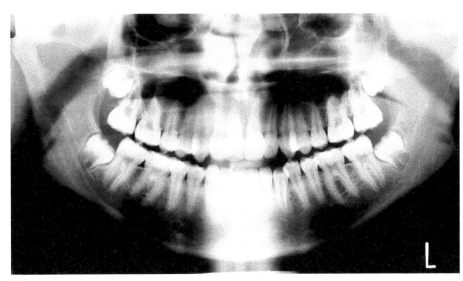

(a)

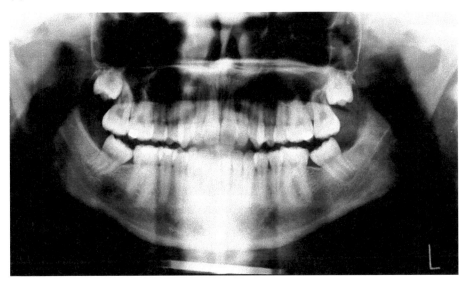

(b)

Fig. 7.6 Example of a case where second permanent molars were extracted. Patient with mild lower arch crowding who had both lower second molars removed in an attempt to treat mild crowding in the lower premolar region. (a) A dental panoramic tomograph (DPT) radiograph prior to extraction of both lower second molars (the upper second molars were not extracted because of concerns over the prognosis for the upper first molars); (b) A DPT radiograph 2 years after the extractions showing eruption of both lower third molars.

7.7.4 Distal movement of molars

Distal movement of molars in the upper arch is possible. This movement can be achieved with headgear or by use of fixed appliances attached to skeletal anchorage in the form of temporary anchorage devices or plates (see Chapter 15). Extra-oral traction using headgear will usually produce up to 2–3 mm per side (creating 4–6 mm space in total). Distalization with clear plastic aligners has also been attempted.

Distal movement of molars tends to be used when there is a mild space requirement where extractions may produce too much space. It can also be used in addition to extractions when there is a very high space requirement.

Examples of clinical situations when it may be used include:

- class I incisor relationship with mild crowding in the upper arch
- class II division 1 incisor relationship with minimally increased overjet and molar relationship of less than half a unit Class II
- where extraction of first premolars does not give sufficient space to complete alignment
- where unilateral loss of a deciduous molar has resulted in mesial drift of the first permanent molar.

7.7.5 Interproximal reduction of enamel

Interproximal reduction ('IPR') of enamel or 'stripping' is the removal of a small amount of enamel on the mesial and distal aspect of teeth and is sometimes known as reproximation. In addition to creating space, the process has been advocated for improving the shape and contact points of teeth, and possibly enhancing stability at the end of treatment. On the anterior teeth, approximately 0.5 mm can be removed on each tooth

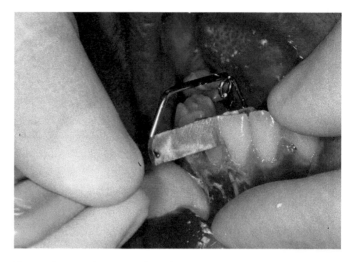

Fig. 7.7 Interproximal reduction using abrasive strips.

(0.25 mm mesial and distal) without compromising the health of the teeth. Slightly more can safely be removed on posterior teeth. Enamel can be carefully removed with a hand-held abrasive strip (Fig. 7.7) or with discs or burs (air-rotor stripping). The abrasive strip can be used in conjunction with pumice mixed with acid etch, to provide a smoother surface finish.

It is felt that interproximal reduction can create an additional 3–6 mm of space in each arch. There is potential for damage to both the teeth and the periodontium unless undertaken carefully. It is important that teeth are reasonably aligned before starting the procedure, and it may be helpful to open up between teeth, either by separators or fixed appliances, before the enamel reduction begins (Fig. 7.8).

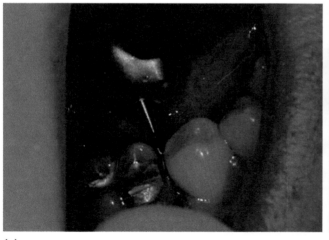

(a)

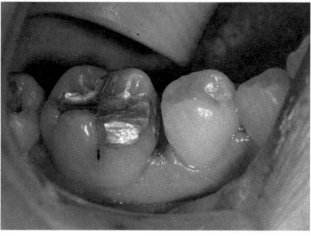

(b)

Fig. 7.8 Air-rotor stripping (ARS). This technique aims to remove interproximal enamel, predominantly in the buccal segments. (a) A small protective wire lies under the contact point to protect the gingival soft tissues. The teeth are already reasonably well aligned and access space has previously been created by use of a separator. The enamel is carefully removed with an air-rotor from the mesial aspect of the first permanent molar and distal aspect of the second premolar. In this case, amalgam is also removed from the mesial side of the first permanent molar. (b) The space has been created and the tooth carefully re-contoured to ensure a good contact point.

7.7.6 Expansion

Space can be created by expanding the upper arch laterally—approximately 0.5 mm is created for every 1 mm of posterior arch expansion. Expansion should be undertaken within the limits of the underlying alveolar bone support, otherwise there is a danger of moving the tooth out of the bone, causing areas of bony dehiscence and compromising the periodontal support.

Expansion of the lower arch may be indicated if a lingual crossbite of the lower premolars and/or molars exists. Any significant expansion in the lower arch, particularly the lower intercanine width, is likely to be unstable.

7.7.7 Proclination of incisors

Space can be created by proclining incisors, but this will be dictated by the aims of the treatment. Each millimetre of incisor advancement creates approximately 2 mm of space within the dental arch.

7.8 Valid consent and the orthodontic treatment plan

7.8.1 Shared decision-making

For some malocclusions there is more than one treatment option, including the option of no treatment. In these situations, the clinical team need to work with the patient and family to determine the best option based on the clinical presentation and the patient's values and preferences. The choice to have no treatment requires that the patient understands and accepts their malocclusion and any associated dental health risks.

Shared decision-making is the collaborative process whereby patients, families, and the clinical team work together to choose the most appropriate treatment. This approach acknowledges that both the orthodontist and the patient have an important role in reaching the best decision about treatment. The orthodontist is an expert in diagnosis of malocclusion who can explain the treatment options, by applying research and clinical evidence, and can help the patient understand this information. The patient knows the daily impact of their malocclusion, their expectations from treatment, their values and preferences for treatment, and their willingness and ability to cope with treatment. Shared decision-making is required at any treatment point where there is more than one option to consider. Where research evidence and clinical experience fail to identify a 'best' treatment, it is essential that patient values and preferences are used to guide decision-making and treatment selection. Supporting patients to be actively involved in treatment choice has been shown to improve satisfaction, adherence, and treatment outcome.

7.8.2 Valid consent in orthodontics

For consent to be valid, it must be voluntary and informed and the patient giving consent must have the capacity to make that decision. Informed consent in orthodontics means the patient is given information to help them to understand the:

- malocclusion
- proposed treatment and alternatives
- commitment required
- duration of treatment
- cost implications.

Treatment alternatives, which must always include no treatment as an option, must be clearly explained, with the risks and benefits of each

approach carefully discussed. Patient consent was changed in 2015 following the Montgomery case in the UK (see 'Principal sources and further reading'). It is no longer sufficient for the clinician to tell the patient the average risks that they feel are important—the emphasis is now on the clinician to find out what the patient wants to know, as well as telling them what you think they should know, so that the consent process is tailored to that particular patient.

Patients who are 16 years or older are presumed to have competence to give consent for themselves. Many orthodontic patients are younger than this, but provided that they fully understand the process, they can give consent. If a competent child consents to treatment, a parent cannot override this decision—this is known as 'Gillick competence'. However, it is preferable to have full parental support for the treatment if possible. If the converse occurs—the parent wants the treatment, but the child does not—then it is best not to proceed. Orthodontic treatment requires a great deal of compliance, and unless the patient is totally committed, it is best to delay until such time as they are.

It is advisable to obtain a written consent for the treatment. A copy should be given to the patient with clear details of the aims of the treatment, risks, and benefits, types of appliances to be used, details of any teeth to be extracted, commitment required, likely duration of treatment, any financial implications, as well as long-term retention requirements. When estimating treatment time, it is always better to slightly overestimate the likely treatment duration ('under-promise and over-deliver'). If the treatment is completed quicker than first promised, the patient will be pleased. However, if the treatment takes longer, the patient may lose interest, resulting in compliance problems.

As well as providing a written record of the aims of the treatment and the treatment plan, it is useful to give the patient a summary of exactly what is expected from them. This involves not only information about good oral hygiene, appropriate diet, and regular attendance, but also any specific requirements relevant to their case, such as headgear wear, turning expansion screws and elastic wear, and any risks that are particularly important to that particular patient. A fully prepared and committed patient is more likely to result in more successful orthodontic treatment.

It is also important to remember that consent is an ongoing process, not a one-off procedure before treatment, so the patient should be kept informed throughout the treatment. This is particularly important in orthodontics as there is often a variation in treatment response among patients, so the treatment plan may need to be reassessed and discussed with the patient.

7.8.3 Limited treatment orthodontics

'Limited treatment orthodontics' or 'LTO' is the term given to compromise orthodontic treatment where there are limited objectives, rather than trying to correct every aspect of the malocclusion. It is more common in adults, where the aim is to try and address the patient's main concerns, without attempting to provide the ideal result. It has also been referred to as 'short-term orthodontics', a name given to try and reflect the shorter treatment time (rather than the limited stability of the result). It has received more attention recently with an increase in adult patients looking to improve the aesthetics of their smile, typically the front six teeth (sometimes referred to as the 'social six'), without resorting to the expense and increased treatment time often associated with more comprehensive treatment.

To consent a patient for limited treatment orthodontics, the orthodontist must ensure the patient understands the limited aims and objectives of treatment, and in particular any compromises that will result. It is certainly acceptable to try and address the cosmetic concerns of adult patients, using limited treatment objectives. However, it is key that all the alternative restorative and comprehensive orthodontic options are fully discussed with the patient, and the patient understands any compromises that will result. It is not acceptable to undertake orthodontic treatment whose long-term consequences could compromise oral health, cause tooth wear, lead to temporomandibular complications, or damage dental restorations.

7.9 Conclusions

This chapter has discussed how the information collected during the history, examination, and collection of records can be used to develop a problem list for each patient. Any pathological problems are treated initially and then the developmental or orthodontic problems can be addressed. The orthodontic problems are divided up into the patient's concerns, facial and smile aesthetics, the alignment and symmetry of each arch, and occlusal problems transversely, anteroposteriorly, and vertically. The skeletal and dental components making up the occlusal problems are identified. Any skeletal problems that are present can be treated by orthodontic camouflage, growth modification, or combined orthodontic and orthognathic surgery treatment.

Once the prioritized problem list is formed, a list of aims can be drawn up, deciding which of the problems will be addressed and which will be accepted. Throughout the planning process, the clinician must consider aesthetics, function, health, and stability. Different treatment options should then be considered to address the treatment aims.

Space analysis involves assessment of the space required and methods of creating this space, and although not an exact science, may help the less experienced orthodontist provide a disciplined approach to diagnosis and treatment planning. It may also help the clinician to assess whether the treatment aims are feasible, and also helps in planning the type of mechanics and anchorage control that are required to treat the case.

The final stage, before formulating the definitive treatment plan, is to discuss the options with the patient using a shared decision-making process. This should lead to valid consent, so the patient is fully aware of their orthodontic problems, how these can be addressed, the risks and benefits of the treatment options, cost implications, the commitment they will need to give, and the likely duration of treatment.

The complete treatment planning process is illustrated in the case discussed in Fig. 7.9.

Key points about treatment planning

- The information gathered from the history, examination, and collection of records is used to form a problem list or diagnosis.
- The problem list is divided into pathological and developmental (orthodontic) problems. Pathological problems are addressed first.
- Any skeletal component of the malocclusion can be treated by one of the following: orthodontic camouflage, growth modification, or a combination of orthodontics and orthognathic surgery.
- By deciding which of the problems will be treated and which accepted, a list of the aims of treatment can be decided upon. Different treatment options can then be considered.
- A space analysis can help provide a disciplined approach to diagnosis and treatment planning, as well as assessing the feasibility of treatment aims, and helping to plan anchorage and treatment mechanics.
- The options for treatment, including no treatment, should be fully discussed with the patient using a shared decision-making process.
- Valid consent should be tailored to each individual patient and is obtained by ensuring the patient understands exactly what the treatment will involve, including the risks and benefits, cost implications, the commitment they will need to give, and the likely duration of the treatment.
- Limited treatment orthodontics is the term given to treatment with more limited treatment objectives and the patient must be fully aware of likely compromises as well as other treatment options.

7.10 Case study: example case to demonstrate treatment planning

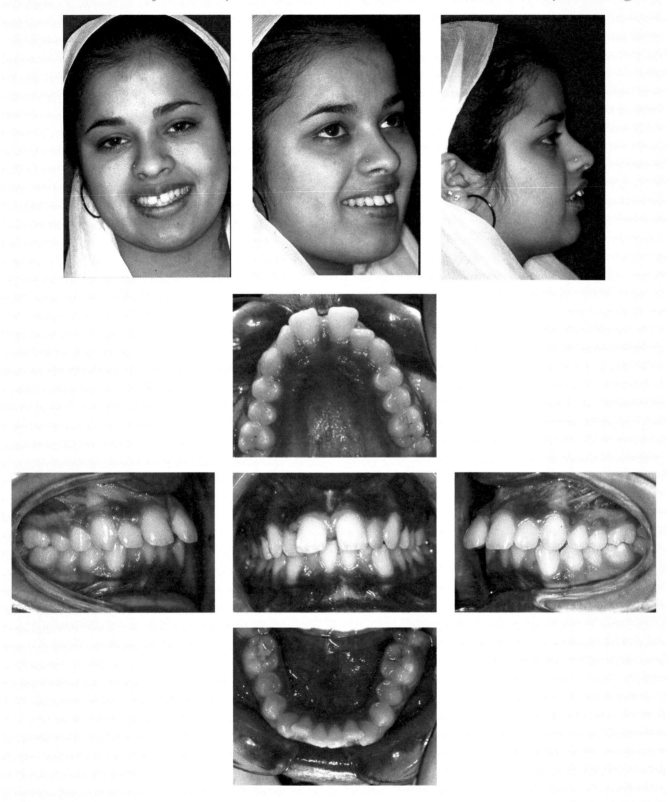

Fig. 7.9 (a) Initial presentation of patient SB. Patient SB presented at age 13 years complaining of prominent upper teeth and a gap between her upper incisors. She was happy to wear fixed appliances and her medical history was clear. She was a regular attendee for dental care and her oral health was good. Radiographs confirmed the presence of third permanent molars, but no pathology. A lateral cephalometric radiograph confirmed a mild Class II skeletal pattern (ANB = 5.5°), normal vertical proportions, proclined upper incisors (117°), and normally inclined lower incisors (92°).

Problem list for SB

Pathological problems

None.

Developmental (orthodontic) problems

Patient's concerns: SB was concerned about prominent upper incisors and a space between the upper incisors. She hoped both these problems would be addressed and was happy to wear orthodontic appliances if required. Her expectations were reasonable and her motivation for treatment was good.

Facial and smile aesthetics: she presented with a slightly everted and protruding upper lip. Her vertical show of incisors on full smile was acceptable (nearly total height of upper incisors). Her mandible was very slightly retrognathic, but acceptable.

Alignment and symmetry in each arch: the lower arch was symmetrical and showed 5 mm of crowding. Her lower labial segment was normally inclined. The upper arch was also symmetrical and overall showed 2 mm of spacing (3 mm diastema and 1 mm crowding of the upper left lateral incisor). The upper incisors were proclined at 117°.

Skeletal and dental problems in transverse plane: there was no skeletal asymmetry. The lower centreline was to the left by 1 mm and the upper centreline was correct. There was no posterior crossbite.

Skeletal and dental problems in anteroposterior plane: the mandible was very slightly retrognathic, but clinically acceptable. There was an increased overjet of 8 mm. The buccal segments were ¼ unit Class II on the left and Class I on the right.

Aims of treatment for SB

The aims of treatment are directly related to the problem list.

Patient's concerns: address the patient's concerns about the prominent upper teeth and upper midline diastema.

Facial and smile aesthetics: accept the slightly retrognathic mandible (in other words, use orthodontic camouflage). Orthodontic treatment effects on the soft tissues are unpredictable, but if the upper incisors have to be retracted this will not have an adverse effect on the facial profile. The vertical position of the incisors can be maintained.

Alignment and symmetry in each arch: relieve the lower crowding, correct the angulation of the upper incisors, and close the residual space in the upper arch.

Skeletal and dental problems in transverse plane: correct the lower centreline.

Skeletal and dental problems in anteroposterior plane: reduce the overjet by retracting the upper labial segment. The anteroposterior position of the lower incisors will be accepted. This is because they have normal inclination, maintaining their

Table 7.2 Space required in each arch to achieve the treatment aims

	Upper (mm)	Lower (mm)
Crowding or spacing	−2	5
Levelling of curve Spee	0	1
AP movement of incisors	12	0
Total	**10**	**6**

position will not compromise facial aesthetics, and the most stable position is their initial position.

Skeletal and dental problems in the vertical plane: reduce the overbite by flattening the lower curve of Spee.

Space analysis for SB

Table 7.2 shows the amount of space required in each arch to achieve the treatment aims. A negative score shows a space gain, a positive score shows a space requirement.

This space analysis shows a larger space requirement in the upper arch, due to the increased overjet. An 8 mm overjet, reduced to a normal overjet of 2 mm, requires 6 mm each side (a total of 12 mm). A curve of Spee of 4 mm in the lower arch requires 1 mm of space for correction.

Now the amount of space required in each arch is known, the methods of creating this space can be considered.

Space creation

The aims of this treatment include achieving an overjet of 2 mm using orthodontic camouflage (i.e. accepting the existing skeletal pattern). Space can be created by extractions, distal movement of molars in the upper arch, enamel stripping, expansion, or proclination of incisors.

In the lower arch, 6 mm of space is required. Expansion of the arch and proclination of the incisors would be unstable, and enamel stripping would not give sufficient space. Extractions are therefore required. Extraction of lower first premolars would provide too much space, so the lower second premolars will be extracted. Each premolar is 7 mm wide, but after anchorage loss (mesial drift of the teeth distal to the second premolars) extraction will provide the appropriate amount of space.

In the upper arch, 10 mm of space requirement is beyond the scope of molar distalization and enamel stripping, and no expansion or incisor proclination is indicated. Therefore, extractions are also required. On this occasion more space is required, so the extraction of first premolars is indicated. Although extraction of first premolars creates a total of 14 mm, part of this is lost to mesial drift. To resist forward movements of the upper molars, anchorage reinforcement will be required. In this case, a palatal arch will help to partially limit the forward movement of the upper first permanent molars.

Definitive treatment plan for SB

1. Palatal arch fitted to upper first molars for anchorage.
2. Extraction of upper first premolars and lower second premolars.
3. Upper and lower fixed appliances.
4. Upper and lower vacuum-formed retainers with a bonded retainer on the palatal of the upper incisors.

(The bonded retainer is indicated in this case due to the risk of relapse of the upper midline diastema. Retention planning is discussed in more detail in Chapter 16.)

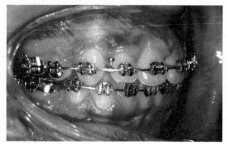 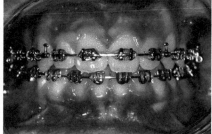 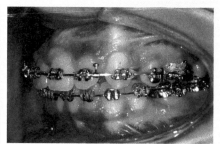

Fig. 7.9 (b) Fixed appliances in place for SB.

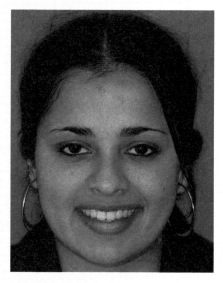 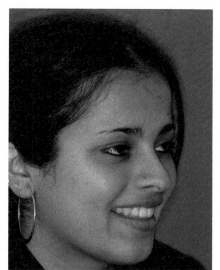 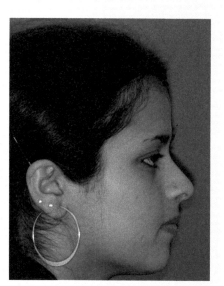

Fig. 7.9 (c) End of treatment extra-oral records for SB.

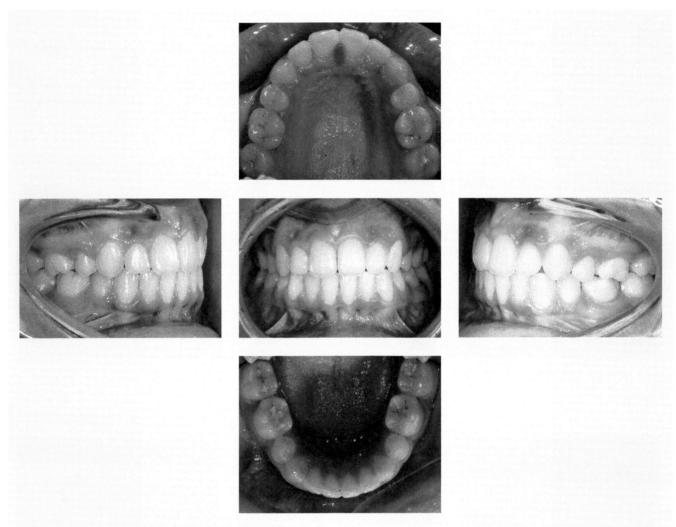

Fig. 7.9 (d) End of treatment intra-oral records for SB.

Principal sources and further reading

Bayliss, C. L. (2017). Informed consent: what's new? *Dental Update*, **44**, 109–13.

Dibiase, A. T. and Sandler, P. J. (2001). Does orthodontics damage faces? *Dental Update*, **28**, 98–102. [DOI: 10.12968/denu.2001.28.2.98] [PubMed: 11819964].
The possible unfavourable effects of orthodontics on the face are debated. Of particular relevance to this chapter is the discussion regarding the unpredictability of the effect of extractions on the facial profile.

Kirshen, R. H., O'Higgins, E. A., and Lee, R. T. (2000). The Royal London Space Planning: an integration of space analysis and treatment planning. Part 1: assessing the space required to meet treatment objectives. Part II:
the effect of other treatment procedures on space. *American Journal of Orthodontics and Dentofacial Orthopedics*, **118**, 448–55, 456–61. [DOI: 10.1067/mod.2000.109031] [PubMed: 11029742] and [DOI: 10.1067/mod.2000.109032] [PubMed: 11029743]
This paper describes one possible approach to space analysis.

Proffit, W. R., Fields, H. R., and Sarver, D. M. (2018). *Contemporary Orthodontics* (6th edn). St. Louis, MO: Mosby.
Section II on orthodontic diagnosis and treatment planning provides more detailed information on the development of a problem list as part of the treatment planning process.

8

Class I

Benjamin R. K. Lewis

Chapter contents

A Class I incisor relationship is defined by the British Standards Institute Incisor Classification as follows: 'the lower incisor edges occlude with or lie immediately below the cingulum plateau of the upper central incisors'. Therefore, Class I malocclusions include those where the anteroposterior occlusal relationship is normal but there is a discrepancy either within the arches, resulting in spacing, crowding, or dental impactions, and/or within the transverse or vertical relationship between the arches.

8.1 Aetiology

8.1.1 Skeletal

In Class I malocclusions, the skeletal pattern is usually Class I, but it can also be Class II or Class III with the inclination of the incisors compensating for the underlying skeletal discrepancy (Fig. 8.1). Marked transverse skeletal discrepancies between the arches are more commonly associated with Class II or Class III occlusions, but milder transverse discrepancies are often seen in Class I cases. Increased vertical skeletal proportions and an anterior open bite can also occur where the anteroposterior incisor relationship is Class I.

8.1.2 Soft tissues

In most Class I cases, the soft tissue environment is favourable and is not an aetiological factor. The major exception to this is bimaxillary proclination, where the upper and lower incisors are proclined. This may be racial in origin, but can also occur because of lack of lip tonicity, which results in the incisors being moulded forwards under tongue pressure, and has implications for planning retention.

8.1.3 Dental factors

Dental factors are the main aetiological influences in Class I malocclusions. The most common are tooth/arch size discrepancies, leading to crowding or, less frequently, spacing.

The size of the teeth is genetically determined and so, to a great extent, is the size of the jaws. Environmental factors can also contribute to crowding or spacing. For example, premature loss of a deciduous tooth can lead to a localization of any pre-existing crowding and possible deviation of centre lines.

Local factors also include displaced or impacted teeth, and anomalies in the size, number, and form of the teeth. These factors can also be found in association with Class II or Class III malocclusions.

8.2 Crowding

Crowding occurs where there is a discrepancy between the size of the teeth and the size of the arches. Approximately 60% of Caucasian children exhibit crowding to some degree. The elective extraction of teeth is one method of alleviating crowding. In a crowded arch, the loss of a permanent or deciduous tooth will result in the remaining teeth tilting

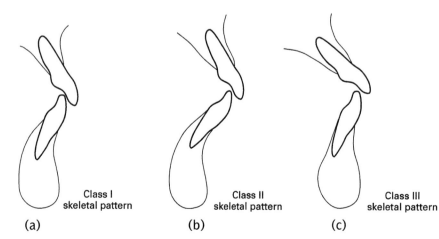

(a) Class I skeletal pattern

(b) Class II skeletal pattern

(c) Class III skeletal pattern

Fig. 8.1 (a) Class I incisor relationship on Class I skeletal pattern; (b) Class I incisor relationship on a Class II skeletal pattern with proclination of the lower incisors; (c) Class I incisor relationship on a Class III skeletal pattern with proclination of the upper incisors and retroclination of the lower incisors.

or drifting into the space created. This tendency is greatest when the adjacent teeth are erupting.

When planning extractions for the management of crowding, the following should be considered:

- The position, presence, and prognosis of the remaining permanent teeth.
- The degree of crowding, which is usually calculated in millimetres.
- The patient's malocclusion and any orthodontic treatment planned, including anchorage requirements (see Chapter 15).
- The patient's age and the likelihood of the crowding increasing or reducing with growth.
- The patient's profile.

These aspects of treatment planning are considered in more detail in Chapter 7.

After relief of crowding, a degree of natural spontaneous movement will take place. In general, this is greater under the following conditions:

- In a growing child.
- If the extractions are carried out just prior to eruption of the adjacent teeth.
- Where the adjacent teeth are favourably positioned to upright if space is made available. For example, considerable improvement will often occur in a crowded lower labial segment provided that the mandibular canines are mesially inclined and can tip distally into the space created.
- Where there are no occlusal interferences with the anticipated tooth movement.

Most spontaneous improvement occurs in the first 6 months after the extractions have been undertaken. If alignment is not complete after 1 year, then further improvement will require active tooth movement with appliances. Fig. 8.2 shows a case which was treated by extraction of all four first premolars without the utilization of orthodontic appliances, and Fig. 8.3 shows a patient whose management required extraction of first molars and the use of fixed appliances. For most patients, the relief of crowding will be an integral part of their overall active orthodontic treatment plan (see Chapter 7).

8.2.1 Late lower incisor crowding

In most individuals, the intercanine width increases up to around 12–13 years of age, and this is followed by a very gradual reduction throughout adult life, with the rate of decrease most noticeable during the mid to late teens. This reduction in intercanine width results in an increase of any pre-existing lower labial crowding, or the emergence of crowding in arches which were previously well aligned or even spaced in the early teens. Therefore, to some extent, lower incisor crowding can be considered as a natural consequence of the ageing process.

The aetiology of late lower incisor crowding is recognized as being multifactorial. The following have all been proposed as being influential in the development of this phenomenon:

- Forward growth of the mandible (either horizontally or manifesting as a growth rotation—see Chapter 4, Section 4.6) when maxillary growth has slowed, together with soft tissue pressures, results in a reduction in lower arch perimeter and labial segment crowding.

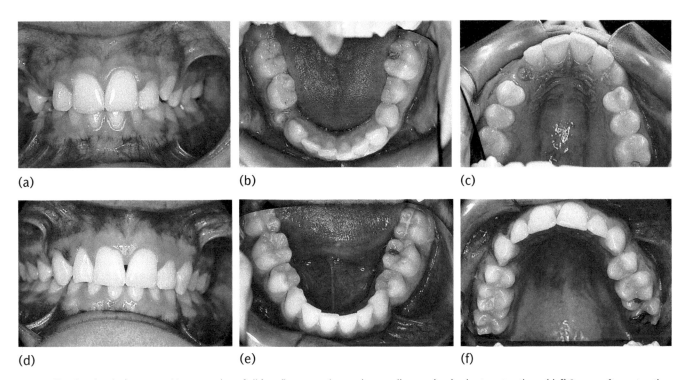

(a) (b) (c)

(d) (e) (f)

Fig. 8.2 Class I malocclusion treated by extraction of all four first premolars and no appliances: (a–c) prior to extractions; (d–f) 3 years after extractions.

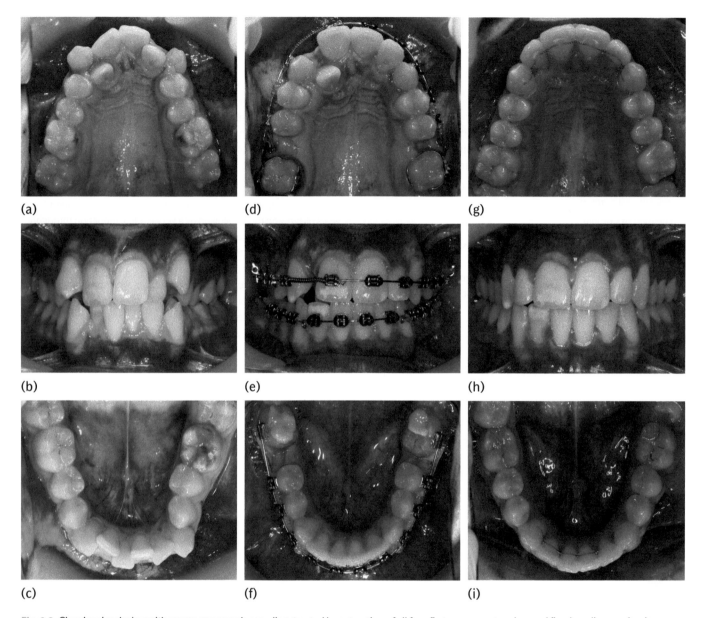

Fig. 8.3 Class I malocclusion with severe upper arch crowding, treated by extraction of all four first permanent molars and fixed appliances: (a–c) pre-treatment; (d–f) during treatment; (g–i) at the end of treatment.

- Soft tissue maturation changing the forces on the incisors.

- Mesial migration of the posterior teeth due to forces from the transseptal fibres and/or from the anterior component of the forces of occlusion.

- The presence of a third molar prevents the pressure which is developed anteriorly (due to either mandibular growth or soft tissue pressures) from being dissipated distally around the arch, that is, the third molar plays a passive role.

- Alteration of the original archform with orthodontic treatment. It is generally accepted that the original lower incisor position and archform should be maintained during orthodontic treatment,

as the original position is likely to be the most stable, because it lies in the zone of balance between the opposing soft tissue forces.

The removal of symptomless lower third molars has been advocated in the past in order to prevent lower labial segment crowding. However, analysis of the evidence indicates that the third permanent molar has a statistically weak association with late lower incisor crowding and that this crowding can still occur in patients with congenitally absent third molars.

Current opinion is that prophylactic removal of lower third molars to prevent lower labial segment crowding cannot be justified—particularly given the associated morbidity with this procedure.

8.3 Spacing

Gencralized spacing is rare and is usually due to either hypodontia or small teeth in well-developed arches. Orthodontic management of generalized spacing is frequently difficult as there is a tendency for the spaces to reopen unless permanently retained. In milder cases, it may be wiser to encourage the patient to either accept the spacing or just to gather the anterior teeth together, which can be more easily maintained with bonded retainers, and accept the posterior spacing. Alternatively, if the teeth are narrower than average, acid-etch composite additions or porcelain veneers can be used to widen them and thus improve aesthetics and the crowns' height-to-width ratios. In severe cases of hypodontia, a combined orthodontic–restorative approach to localize space for the provision of prostheses, or implants, may be required (see Fig. 8.4 and Chapter 23, Section 23.7).

Localized spacing may be due to hypodontia; traumatic loss of a tooth; or because extraction was indicated due to displacement, morphology, or pathology.

8.3.1 Median diastema

A median diastema is a space between the central incisors, which is more common in the upper arch (Fig. 8.5). A diastema is a normal physiological stage in the early mixed dentition when the fraenal attachment

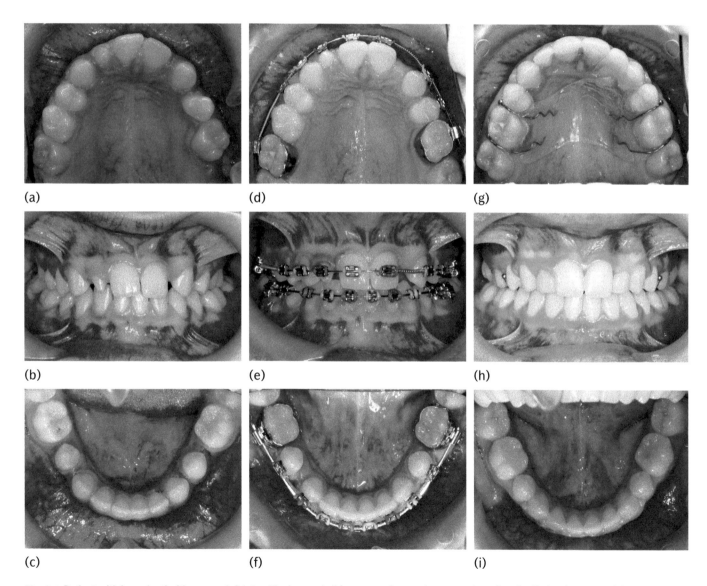

(a)

(b)

(c)

(d)

(e)

(f)

(g)

(h)

(i)

Fig. 8.4 Patient with hypodontia (the upper left lateral incisor and all four second premolars were absent) and a diminutive upper right lateral incisor with associated spacing. Treated with fixed appliances to close the space from the missing premolars, correct the upper centre line, and localize space for prosthetic replacement of upper left lateral incisor and build-up of the diminutive upper right lateral incisor: (a–c) pre-treatment; (d–f) mid-treatment showing fixed appliances; (g–i) completed orthodontic treatment and prior to definitive restorative treatment.

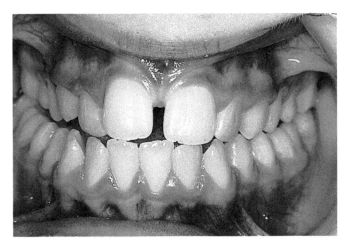

Fig. 8.5 Upper midline diastema with low frenal attachment.

passes between the upper central incisors to attach to the incisive papilla. In normal development, as the lateral incisors and canines erupt, this gap closes and the fraenal attachment migrates labially to the attached mucosa. If the upper arch is spaced or the lateral incisors are diminutive or absent, there is less pressure forcing the upper central incisors together and the diastema may persist. Rarely, the fraenal attachment appears to prevent the central incisors from moving together. In these cases, blanching of the incisive papilla can be observed if tension is applied to the fraenum, and on radiographic examination a V-shaped notch of the interdental bone can be seen between the incisors, indicating the attachment of the fraenum (see Chapter 3, Fig. 3.26). The aetiology and management of median diastema is considered in Chapter 3, Section 3.3.9.

8.4 Early loss of first permanent molars

Decisions about the best options for the management of first permanent molars of poor prognosis in the developing dentition can be a challenging and frequent dilemma in general dental practice. The fact that the first molars erupt at around 6–7 years of age, sometimes unnoticed by the child or their parents, puts them at an increased risk of caries. In addition, because the crowns of these teeth are forming from birth to 3 years of age, they have a greater susceptibility to a range of enamel defects. The pooled prevalence of molar–incisor hypomineralization (MIH) globally has been reported to be 14.2% with even distribution between the sexes. The aetiology of MIH is unknown, however, it is suspected that it is multifactorial and there is some evidence that it is associated with early childhood illnesses, especially fever. The management of first permanent molars of poor prognosis will be determined by many factors including age, associated malocclusion, suitability for future restorative and orthodontic treatment, and the need for a general anaesthetic.

The timing of the first molar extraction and the need to extract the contralateral tooth within the same arch (balancing extraction) and/or the first molar in the opposing arch (compensating extraction) are usually the most fundamental orthodontic-related decisions that need to be made. The response of second molar eruption to the early loss of the adjacent first molar is subject to individual variation. However, it is believed that to achieve the optimum erupted position of the developing second molar without orthodontic appliances, the best time to extract a mandibular first permanent molar is between 8 and 10 years old and prior to the eruption of the second molar. It is suggested that the

calcification of the bifurcation of the mandibular second molar marks the best time to extract the first molar. The timing of upper first molar extractions is usually less critical as the developing second molar has a natural tendency to migrate mesially and erupt into a reasonable position. If a lower first molar is to be extracted, then consideration should be given to extracting the opposing upper first molar to prevent it from over-erupting and creating occlusal interferences. Lower first molars are unlikely to over-erupt therefore when extracting an upper first molar of poor prognosis, the routine extraction of a sound opposing lower first molar is not recommended. Balancing extractions of sound first permanent molars are not usually indicated as the effect of unilateral extractions on the centre line is usually minimal.

The patient's malocclusion will have a bearing on the timing of extraction. The best spontaneous result will be achieved in Class I cases with minimal crowding. If the patient has more moderate crowding, then extraction of the first molars could address the buccal crowding but will have little spontaneous benefit on anterior crowding. In these circumstances, the first molars could be maintained and extracted once the second molars have erupted as part of coordinated orthodontic treatment. In Class II cases, maxillary first molars could be retained as they have the potential to be used for aiding the overjet reduction. Class III cases are more challenging and a specialist opinion is often advisable.

If there is doubt about the best option, especially for patents with a skeletal discrepancy or moderate to severe crowding, then the opinion of an orthodontic specialist should be considered.

8.5 Displaced teeth

Teeth can be displaced for a variety of reasons including the following:

- Abnormal position of the tooth germ: canines (see Chapter 14) and second premolars are the most commonly affected teeth. Management depends upon the degree of displacement. If this is

mild, extraction of the associated primary tooth plus space maintenance, if indicated, may result in an improvement in position. Alternatively, exposure and the application of orthodontic traction may be used to bring the mildly displaced tooth into the arch. If the

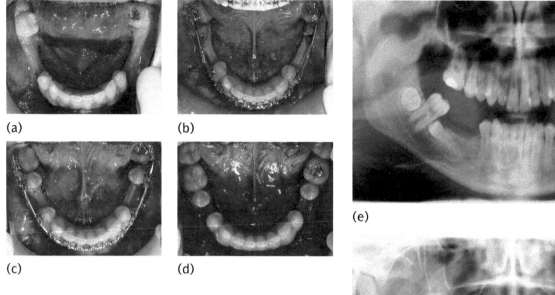

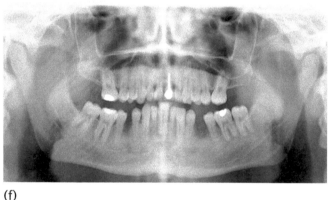

(e)

(f)

Fig. 8.6 (a–f) Severely displaced mandibular second premolars. This was due to the excess space and lack of guidance, following the premature loss of mandibular first permanent molars and the second deciduous molars. Due to the limited alternative restorative options, these teeth were surgically exposed and orthodontically aligned. Full space closure was not possible due to the lack of alveolar bone development as a result of the severity of the original displacement.

displacement is severe, extraction of the affected tooth may be necessary. Very occasionally, orthodontic traction to very displaced teeth can be attempted if the alternative options are limited. However, in these circumstances, the patient must be made fully aware of the potential limitations of treatment and the alternatives, should treatment not be successful (Fig. 8.6).

- Crowding: lack of space for a permanent tooth to erupt within the arch can lead to or contribute to displacement. Those teeth that erupt last in a segment, for example, upper lateral incisors, upper canines (Fig. 8.7), second premolars, and third molars, are most commonly affected. Management involves relief of crowding, followed by active tooth movement where necessary. However, if the displacement is severe, it may be prudent to extract the displaced tooth.

- Prolonged retention of a deciduous predecessor: extraction of the retained primary tooth should be carried out as soon as possible provided that the permanent successor is not severely displaced.

- Secondary to the presence of a supernumerary tooth or teeth (see Chapter 3): management involves extraction of the supernumerary followed by tooth alignment, usually with fixed appliances. Displacements due to supernumeraries have a tendency to relapse, therefore prolonged retention is required.

- Caused by a habit (see Chapter 9).

- Secondary to pathology, for example, a dentigerous cyst.

8.6 Vertical discrepancies

Variations in the vertical dimension can occur in association with any anteroposterior skeletal relationship. Increased vertical skeletal proportions are discussed in Chapter 9 in relation to Class II division 1, in

Chapter 11 in relation to Class III, and in Chapter 12 with respect to anterior open bites.

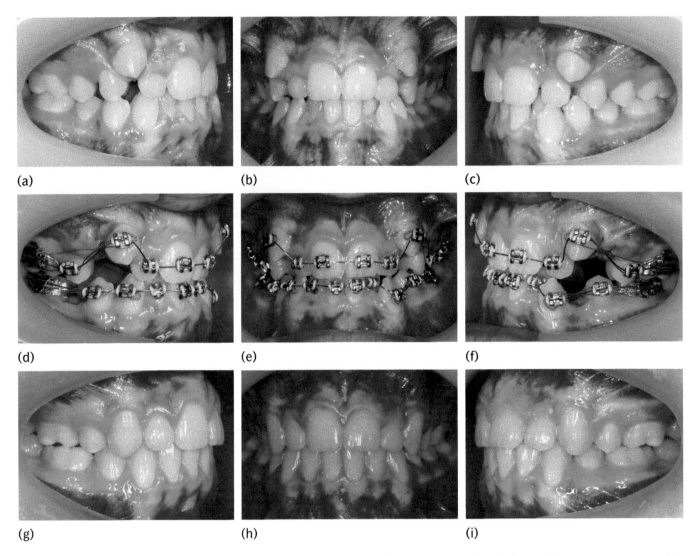

(a)   (b)   (c)

(d)   (e)   (f)

(g)   (h)   (i)

Fig. 8.7 Class I malocclusion with severe upper arch and moderate lower arch crowding. In crowded arches, the last teeth in a segment to erupt, in this case the upper canines, are the most likely to be short of space. (a–c) Initial presentation; (d–f) with fixed appliances *in situ*; (g–i) post treatment.

8.7 Transverse discrepancies

A transverse discrepancy between the arches results in a cross-bite and can occur in association with Class I, Class II, and Class III malocclusions. Classification and management of crossbites is discussed in Chapter 13.

8.8 Bimaxillary proclination

As the name suggests, bimaxillary proclination is the term used to describe occlusions where both the upper and lower incisors are proclined. Bimaxillary proclination is seen more commonly in some racial groups (e.g. Afro-Caribbean), and this needs to be borne in mind during assessment (including cephalometric analysis) and treatment planning.

When bimaxillary proclination occurs in a Class I malocclusion, the overjet is usually increased because of the angulation of the incisors (Fig. 8.8). Management is difficult because both upper and lower incisors need to be retroclined to reduce the overjet. Retroclination of the lower labial segment will encroach on tongue space and therefore has a high likelihood of relapse following removal of the appliances.

For these reasons, treatment of bimaxillary proclination should be approached with caution and consideration should be given to accepting the incisor relationship. If the lips are incompetent, but have a good muscle tone and are likely to achieve a lip-to-lip seal if the incisors are retracted, the chances of a stable result are increased. However, the patient should still be warned that the prognosis for stability is guarded. Where bimaxillary proclination is associated with competent lips, or with grossly incompetent lips which are unlikely to retain the corrected incisor position, permanent retention is advisable.

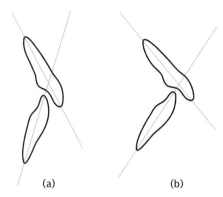

Fig. 8.8 (a) Class I incisor relationship with normal axial inclination (inter-incisal angle is 137°); (b) Class I incisor relationship with bimaxillary inclination showing increased overjet (inter-incisal angle is 107°).

8.9 Trauma

Dental trauma is a common event with approximately 11% of patients being affected prior to the commencement of any orthodontic treatment at 12 years of age. Boys are affected to a greater extent than girls and the incidence of incisor trauma almost doubles in individuals with overjets in excess of 9 mm, especially if the lips are incompetent, which is often the case in this group. With this knowledge, some clinicians favour early orthodontic intervention with the aim to reduce this risk of trauma. The evidence regarding the benefits of early treatment is conflicting. A recent systematic review suggested that early treatment with a functional appliance reduced the incidence of new trauma from 29% to 20% but that ten patients had to be treated to prevent one episode of trauma. This reduction in risk has to be balanced by the significantly extended treatment time of two-phase treatment compare to a one-phase treatment in adolescence, with the associated loss of patient enthusiasm and cooperation as well as the increased cost.

Due to the high incidence of trauma, all orthodontic patients should be questioned about, and examined for, past episodes of trauma. The history should include details of the event, the extent of the injury and any treatment provided, as well as any long-term complications. Any teeth which have, or are suspected to have, suffered from trauma should be assessed with long-cone periapical radiographs and a thorough clinical examination including the tooth colour, mobility, tenderness to percussion, and tenderness of the associated soft tissues along with sensibility tests.

Teeth which have undergone an episode of trauma should be monitored prior to commencing any orthodontic treatment. The period of observation will depend on the severity and occlusal consequences of the trauma. A minimum of 3 months should be allowed for crown fractures, concussion, subluxation, extrusion, and mild lateral luxation. Whereas at least 6 months, and ideally 12 months, should pass before orthodontic movement is undertaken on teeth which have suffered a lateral luxation involving a moderate to severe displacement, intrusion, and avulsion with reimplantation. The clinician should be constantly aware of the possibility of ankylosis. If a tooth becomes non-vital then root canal therapy should be undertaken, with monitoring to ensure the treatment has been successful, prior to commencement of orthodontic treatment. The evidence would suggest that orthodontic treatment on previously traumatized teeth, whether or not they have undergone root canal therapy, is not more likely to cause root resorption, unless there was pre-existing evidence of root shortening due to the episode of trauma itself.

If the dental trauma results in severely displaced tooth positions which interfere with the occlusion, then they can be manually repositioned in the immediate aftermath of the incident. If this is not possible, then consideration can be given to orthodontic repositioning using very light forces. However, this must be undertaken in the knowledge of the potential increased risk of worsening any destructive inflammation present, resulting in ankylosis. Intrusion injuries can be left to spontaneously re-erupt (for patients under 17 years old), or be surgically repositioned or orthodontically extruded. There is some evidence which indicates that, for intrusive luxation in teeth with incomplete root formation, allowing spontaneous re-eruption is the option of first choice. This is because it is associated with the best chance of maintaining vitality and avoiding marginal bone defects, ankylosis, and resorption. In cases where the apex formation has completed, then allowing spontaneous re-eruption can be undertaken when the degree of intrusion has been less than 3 mm. If no improvement occurs within 2–4 weeks, then orthodontic or surgical repositioning should be considered before ankylosis can develop.

Individuals who have suffered dental trauma may benefit from a multidisciplinary approach. Fig. 8.9 demonstrates a patient who suffered severe dental trauma following a collapse. The presentation for dental intervention was delayed due to the required medical investigations which took priority. He suffered intrusion of the upper incisors and canines with associated loss of vitality. The maxillary left lateral incisor and canine were ankylosed on presentation with the canine subsequently requiring removal. A good outcome was achieved through closely coordinated management involving his general dental practitioner, orthodontist, endodontist, restorative dentist, and maxillofacial surgeon.

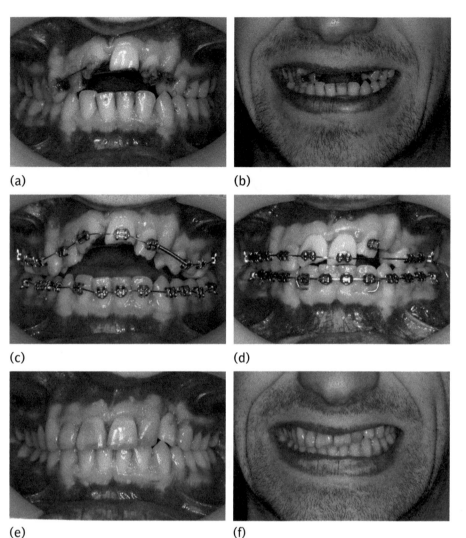

(a)

(b)

(c)

(d)

(e)

(f)

Fig. 8.9 Dental trauma resulting in the intrusion of the maxillary anterior teeth with delayed presentation. (a, b) Initial presentation; (c, d) during orthodontic treatment; (e, f) after treatment with a resin retained bridge to replace the maxillary left canine and composite restorations on the incisors. The slight upper centre-line discrepancy could not be corrected due to the ankylosed maxillary left lateral incisor.

8.9.1 Management following traumatic loss of an incisor

It is important that these cases are managed in close conjunction with all the specialties involved and that prior to the removal of the orthodontic appliances, the patient should be seen by the restorative/surgical specialist, to ensure that the final tooth positions are optimal for any restorative treatment which is planned.

Following traumatic loss of an incisor, a number of options may be considered, including orthodontic space closure; autotransplantation, along with restorative camouflage; or restorative replacement involving the provision of a removable prosthesis, fixed prosthesis, or implant retained prosthesis. The various options can be simulated with a diagnostic (Kesling) set-up which allows the feasibility of different treatment options to be assessed in advance of any active treatment. This diagnostic set-up can be carried out using duplicate models where the teeth to be moved are cut off the model and repositioned in the desired place using wax with any prosthetic units inserted (Fig. 8.10). This allows any number of options to be tested providing an opportunity to evaluate, in detail, the amount and nature of any orthodontic and restorative treatment required by a particular option. This exercise is often helpful in describing the potential outcome of different options to the patient.

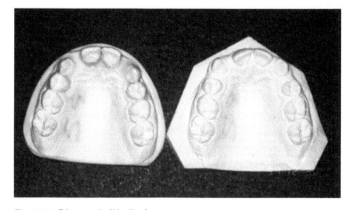

Fig. 8.10 Diagnostic (Kesling) set-up.

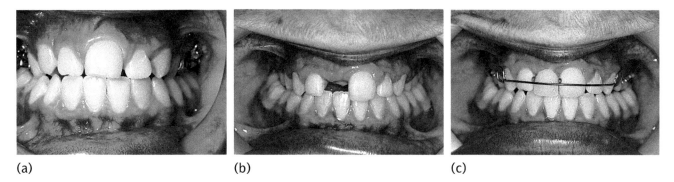

(a)   (b)   (c)

Fig. 8.11 (a) Patient with early traumatic loss of 1/ and partial space closure. Space for prosthetic replacement of 1/ was gained using a fixed appliance. (b) Result on completion of active treatment. (c) Retainer with prosthetic tooth to replace 1/ (NB stops were placed mesial to both 2/ and /1 to help prevent relapse).

After assessment of the above factors, a provisional plan can be discussed with the patient. It is often possible to draw up more than one option and these should all be discussed thoroughly, along with the relative advantages and disadvantages, and the long-term maintenance and associated costs of any prosthetic replacements.

In the immediate post-orthodontic phase of treatment, any prosthetic teeth are usually attached to the orthodontic retainer (see Figs 8.11 and 18.12) to maintain aesthetics while the gingival architecture is settling prior to any definitive restorative intervention.

Implants are becoming more widely available but for most patients may still be relatively expensive and can only be placed when vertical facial development has slowed to adult levels. When planning space opening for placement of an implant, it is wise to bear in mind the results of a recent study which showed that in growing patients 11% of orthodontically repositioned roots relapsed (also see Box 8.1).

Autotransplantation

This is the surgical repositioning of a tooth into a surgically created socket within the same patient. In recent years, the success rate of

Box 8.1 **Requirements for the placement of an implant to replace a missing upper incisor**

- Growth rate slowed to adult levels.
- Adequate bone height.
- Adequate bone width.
- Adequate space between roots of adjacent teeth.
- Adequate space for crown between adjacent crowns and occlusally.

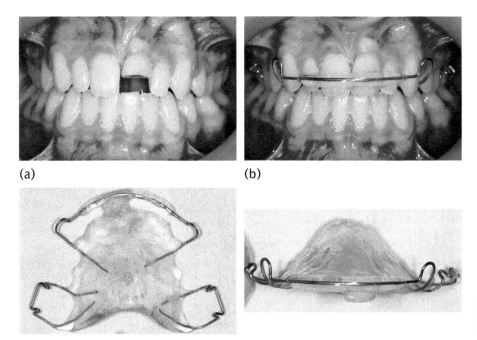

(a)   (b)

(c)   (d)

Fig. 8.12 (a) A traumatically fractured incisor which has been extruded to allow future build-up. (b–d) A modified Hawley retainer to camouflage the fractured tooth.

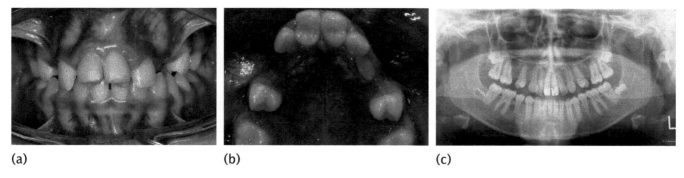

(a)   (b)   (c)

Fig. 8.13 This patient lost both upper central incisors due to trauma. Both upper second premolars were transplanted to replace the missing incisors. The facial surfaces have been modified with composite to improve the appearance. Permanent aesthetic modifications were deferred until orthodontic treatment had been completed and growth had slowed to adult levels. Reproduced with the kind permission of Nadine Houghton.

this procedure has improved in tandem with the understanding of the underlying biology. Autotransplantation has a number of advantages over other methods of tooth replacement:

- Biological replacement: avoids the need for a prosthesis—although the tooth will usually require restorative modification to camouflage its underlying morphology.
- Maintains and can create alveolar bone.
- Has a natural periodontal membrane, normal proprioception, and better gingival contour.
- Can erupt in synchrony with adjacent teeth.
- Can be moved orthodontically once healing is complete.
- Suitable for a growing patient.

However, there are also disadvantages:

- Only feasible if there is a suitable tooth which is planned for extraction.
- Increased burden of care plus a general anaesthetic may be required for the procedure.
- Requires skilled surgical technique.
- Transplanted tooth may undergo resorption and/or ankylosis.

It is now appreciated that the timing of the transplant in terms of the root development of the tooth to be transplanted and a careful

> **Box 8.2 Criteria for successful autotransplantation**
>
> - Root development of tooth to be transplanted: ⅔ to ¾ complete.
> - Sufficient space in arch and occlusally to accommodate transplanted tooth.
> - Careful preparation of donor site to ensure good root to bone adaptation.
> - Careful surgical technique to avoid damage to root surface of transplanted tooth.
> - Transplanted teeth positioned at same level as donor site and splinted for 7–10 days.

surgical technique are important (Box 8.2). When these are satisfied, success rates of the order of 85–90% have been reported by a number of studies. If a patient has premolar crowding, then the teeth of choice for transplanting are the lower premolars or upper second premolars, because of their single root form (Fig. 8.13). Third molars are useful teeth for transplantation, but are usually too bulky for use in the labial segments.

Transplanted teeth should be held in place with a physiological splint for 7–10 days ensuring there is no occlusal contact. A tooth with a closed apex can be used, but root canal treatment should be instituted 7–10 days after transplantation.

Key points

- Class I incisor relationships can occur in association with any skeletal relationship (anteroposterior, vertical, transverse).
- With the exception of bimaxillary proclination, Class I incisor relationships are usually associated with a favourable soft tissue environment.
- Following severe dental trauma, the best outcome requires an interdisciplinary approach.

Relevant Cochrane review

Belmonte F. M., Macedo, C. R., Day, P. F., Saconato, H., and Fernandes Moça Trevisani, V. (2013). Interventions for treating traumatised permanent front teeth: luxated (dislodged) teeth. *Cochrane Database of Systematic Reviews*, Issue 4. Art. No.: CD006203. DOI: 10.1002/14651858.CD006203.pub2. https://www.cochranelibrary.com/cdsr/doi/10.1002/14651858.CD006203.pub2/full
Unfortunately, no studies could be included within this review due to the poor nature of the evidence currently available.

Principal sources and further reading

Bishara, S. E. (1999). Third molars: a dilemma! Or is it? *American Journal of Orthodontics and Dentofacial Orthopedics*, **115**, 628–33. [DOI: 10.1016/S0889-5406(99)70287-8] [PubMed: 10358244]

Cobourne, M. T., Williams, A., and Harrison, M. (2014). *A Guideline for the Extraction of First Permanent Molars in Children (Update of the 2009 Guidelines)*. London: Royal College of Surgeons of England.

Costa, L. A., Ribeiro, C. C., Cantanhede, L. M., Santiago Júnior, J. F., de Mendonça, M. R., and Pereira, A. L. (2017). Treatments for intrusive luxation in permanent teeth: a systematic review and meta-analysis. *International journal of Oral and Maxillofacial Surgery*, **46**, 214–29. [DOI: 10.1016/j.ijom.2016.08.021] [PubMed: 27649968]
A review of the current literature in this area, which suggests the degree of root formation and the severity of intrusion are key influences on the outcome of these cases. The authors highlight the need for higher-quality investigations to be undertaken.

Day, P. F., Kindelan, S. A., Spencer, J. R., Kindelan, J. D., and Duggal, M. S. (2008). Dental trauma: part 2. Managing poor prognosis anterior teeth – treatment options for the subsequent space in a growing patient. *Journal of Orthodontics*, **35**, 143–55. [DOI: 10.1179/146531207225022590] [PubMed: 18809778]
An excellent review of the treatment options for the traumatic loss of an incisor in a growing patient.

Dental Trauma Guide (DTG): http://www.dentaltraumaguide.org
The definitive guide to the management of dental injuries.

Harradine, N. W. T., Pearson, M. H., and Toth, B. (1998). The effect of extraction of third molars on late lower incisor crowding: a randomised controlled trial. *British Journal of Orthodontics*, **25**, 117–22. [DOI: 10.1093/ortho/25.2.117] [PubMed: 9668994].
This excellent study is essential reading.

International Association of Dental Traumatology: http://www.iadt-dental-trauma.org

Kindelan, S. A., Day, P. F., Kindelan, J. D., Spencer, J. R., and Duggal, M. S. (2008). Dental trauma: an overview of its influence on the management of orthodontic treatment. Part 1. *Journal of Orthodontics*, **35**, 68–78. [DOI: 10.1179/146531207225022482] [PubMed: 18525070]
An excellent summary of the impact of dental trauma on orthodontic management.

Little, R. M., Reidel, R. A., and Artun, J. (1981). An evaluation of changes in mandibular anterior alignment from 10–20 years postretention. *American Journal of Orthodontics and Dentofacial Orthopedics*, **93**, 423–8. [PubMed: 3163221]
Classic paper. The authors found that lower labial segment crowding tends to increase even following extractions and appliance therapy.

Mittal, M., Murray, A. M., and Sandler, J. (2011). Maxillary labial frenectomy: indications and technique. *Dental Update*, **38**, 159–62. [DOI: 10.12968/denu.2011.38.3.159] [PubMed: 21667829].

National Institute for Health and Care Excellence (2000). *Guidance on the Extraction of Wisdom Teeth*. London: NICE. https://www.nice.org.uk/guidance/ta1

Shashua, D. and Artun, J. (1999). Relapse after orthodontic correction of maxillary median diastema: a follow-up evaluation of consecutive cases. *The Angle Orthodontist*, **69**, 257–63. [DOI: 10.1043/0003-3219(1999)069<0257:RAOCOM>2.3.CO;2] [PubMed: 10371432].

Thiruvenkatachari, B., Harrison, J., Worthington, H., and O'Brien, K. (2015). Early orthodontic treatment for class II malocclusions reduced the chance of incisal trauma: results of a Cochrane systemic review. *American Journal of Orthodontics and Dentofacial Orthopedics*, **148**, 47–59. [DOI: 10.1016/j.ajodo.2015.01.030] [PubMed: 26124027]

Waldon, K., Barber, S. K., Spencer, R. J., and Duggal, M. S. (2012). Indications for the use of auto-transplantation of teeth in the child and adolescent. *European Archives of Paediatric Dentistry*, **13**, 210–16. [DOI: 10.1007/BF03262872] [PubMed: 22883361]
This paper demonstrated the indications for the use of the autotransplantation techniques with seven clinical examples.

References for this chapter can also be found at: **www.oup.com/uk/orthodontics5e**. Where possible, these are presented as active links which direct you to the electronic version of the work, to help facilitate onward study. If you are a subscriber to that work (either individually or through an institution), and depending on your level of access, you may be able to peruse an abstract or the full article if available.

9

Class II division 1

S. J. Littlewood

Chapter contents

The British Standards classification defines a Class II division 1 incisor relationship as follows: 'the lower incisor edges lie posterior to the cingulum plateau of the upper incisors, there is an increase in overjet and the upper central incisors are usually proclined'. In a Caucasian population, the incidence of Class II division 1 incisor relationship is approximately 15–20%.

Class II division 1 malocclusions are the commonest type of malocclusions treated in the Western world and therefore many aspects are covered in more detail in other chapters. The aims of this chapter are to discuss the aetiology and presentation of Class II division 1 malocclusions, and provide a broad overview on the objectives of treatment and factors affecting treatment planning in these cases. Where appropriate, the reader will be referred to the relevant chapter elsewhere in the book for more details.

9.1 Aetiology

9.1.1 Skeletal pattern

A Class II division 1 incisor relationship is usually associated with a Class II skeletal pattern, commonly due to a retrognathic mandible (Fig. 9.1). More rarely, it is possible for patients with a Class II division 1 incisor relationship to have a Class I (or even a Class III) skeletal pattern. This can occur when the upper incisors are proclined and/or the lower incisors are retroclined, either by the soft tissues (see Section 9.1.2) or a habit (see Section 9.1.3). The increased overjet could also be due to a buccally displaced or crowded upper incisor.

A Class II division 1 incisor relationship is found in association with a range of vertical skeletal patterns and asymmetries. As a general rule, the more significant the underlying skeletal discrepancy in any plane, the more difficult it is to treat.

9.1.2 Soft tissues

The tongue, lips, and cheeks can be aetiological factors in a Class II division 1 malocclusion. The influence of the soft tissues on a Class II division 1 malocclusion is mainly mediated by the skeletal pattern, both anteroposteriorly and vertically. However, the resting position of the patient's soft tissues and their functional activity can also be important.

In a Class II division 1 malocclusion, the lips are often incompetent due to the prominence of the upper incisors and/or the underlying skeletal pattern. If the lips are incompetent, a patient can try to achieve an anterior oral seal in a number of different ways. How this anterior oral seal is achieved will affect the presentation of the Class II division 1 incisor relationship. The following are different methods of achieving an anterior seal:

- Circumoral muscular activity to achieve a lip-to-lip seal (Fig. 9.2).
- The mandible is postured forwards to allow the lips to meet at rest.
- The lower lip is drawn up behind the upper incisors (Fig. 9.3).
- The tongue is placed forwards between the incisors to contact the lower lip, often contributing to the development of an incomplete overbite.
- A combination of these.

Where the patient can achieve lip-to-lip contact by circumoral muscle activity or the mandible is postured forwards, the influence of the soft tissues is often to moderate the effect of the underlying skeletal pattern by dento-alveolar compensation. The action of achieving lip-to-lip contact will tend to mould the upper incisors back, reducing the overjet.

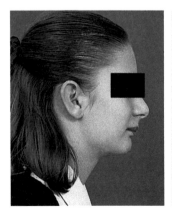
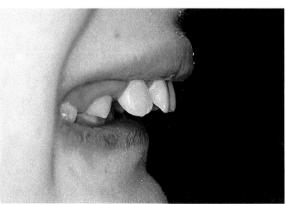

Fig. 9.1 A Class II division 1 incisor relationship on a Class II skeletal pattern with a retrognathic mandible.

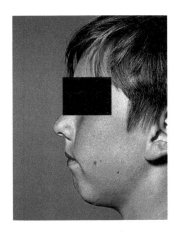

Fig. 9.2 Marked circumoral muscular activity is visible as this patient attempts to achieve an anterior oral seal by a lip-to-lip seal.

If lip-to-lip contact is not possible, which is more likely as the skeletal pattern becomes more severe, the lower lip functions by being drawn up behind the upper incisors (Fig. 9.4). The effect of this is to retrocline the lower labial segment and/or procline the upper incisors, resulting in an incisor relationship that is more severe than the underlying skeletal pattern.

If the tongue habitually comes forward to contact the lower lip, proclination of the lower incisors may occur, helping to compensate for the underlying skeletal pattern. This type of soft tissue behaviour is often associated with increased vertical skeletal proportions and/or grossly incompetent lips, or a habit which has resulted in an increase in overjet and an anterior open bite. In practice, it is often difficult to determine

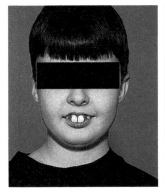
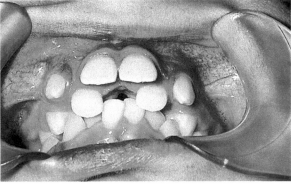

Fig. 9.3 In this patient with a Class II division 1 malocclusion, the lower lip lies behind the upper central incisors which have been proclined, and in front of the lateral incisors which have been retroclined as a result.

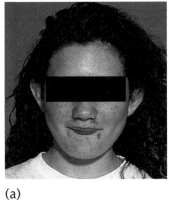
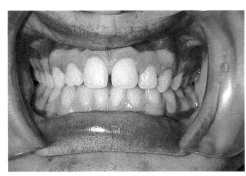
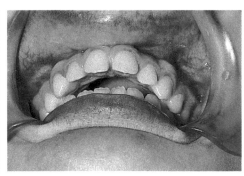

(a) (b) (c)

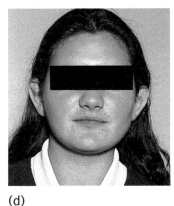
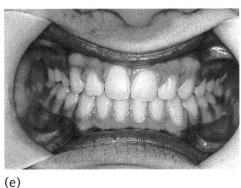

(d) (e)

Fig. 9.4 A Class II division 1 malocclusion due mainly to retroclination of the lower labial segment by an active lower lip. This patient achieved an anterior oral seal by contact between the tongue and the lower lip. (a–c) Prior to treatment; (d, e) post treatment.

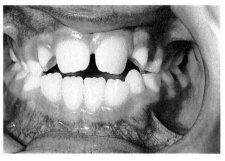 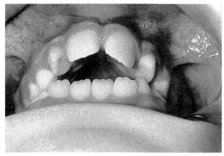

(a)   (b)

Fig. 9.5 The effects of a persistent digit-sucking habit on the occlusion: the upper incisors have been proclined and the lower incisors retroclined.

the degree to which this is adaptive tongue behaviour, or whether a rarer endogenous tongue thrust exists (see Chapter 12, Section 12.2.2).

Infrequently, a Class II division 1 incisor relationship occurs as a result of retroclination of the lower incisors by a very active lower lip sometimes referred to as 'strap-like' (Fig. 9.4).

9.1.3 Dental factors

A Class II division 1 incisor relationship may occur as a result of crowding. Due to the shortage of space, the upper incisors may be displaced labially leading to an increased overjet. It is also possible to have an increased overjet as a result of an ectopic incisor that has developed labially. Treatment of the increased overjet in these situations is aimed at creating space to relieve the crowding and/or bringing the ectopic tooth back into the line of the arch.

9.1.4 Habits

(See also Chapter 12, Section 12.2.3.)

An increased overjet can be the result of a persistent digit-sucking habit. A prolonged force on the teeth from the digit lasting several hours a day is sufficient to move teeth. The severity of the effects produced will depend upon the duration and the intensity, but the following are commonly associated with a determined habit (Fig. 9.5):

- Proclination of the upper incisors.
- Retroclination of the lower labial segment.

- An incomplete overbite or a localized anterior open bite.
- Narrowing of the upper arch thought to be mediated by the tongue taking up a lower position in the mouth (so it no longer balances the inward pressure from the cheeks) and also the negative pressure generated during sucking of the digit.

The effects may be asymmetric if a single finger or thumb is sucked (Fig. 9.6).

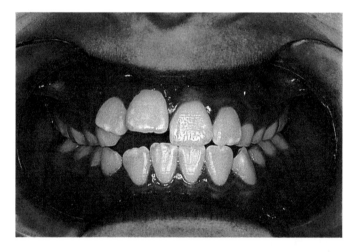

Fig. 9.6 An asymmetrical increase in overjet in a patient with a habit of sucking one finger on the right hand.

9.2 Objectives of treating Class II division 1 malocclusions

Like all orthodontic cases, the following areas need to be considered:

- Aesthetics
- Oral health
- Function
- Stability.

9.2.1 Aesthetics

As discussed in Chapter 7, Section 7.3.2, in order to achieve a good aesthetic result, it is important to consider the patient's facial and smile aesthetics. Simply reducing an overjet, without considering the position

of the teeth within the face and relation to the lips, will not necessarily produce an aesthetic result. It is important to determine the aetiology of the Class II division 1 malocclusion, and identify where the abnormalities lie (see Chapter 5). For example, the case study in Chapter 19, Fig. 19.1 shows a patient who has a markedly increased overjet, and this is partly due to proclined incisors, but is also as a result of a retrognathic mandible, so treatment was planned to address both of these aetiological factors.

9.2.2 Oral health

One major objective for treating Class II division 1 malocclusions is to reduce the risk of traumatic injuries. The risk of injury is more than doubled in individuals with an overjet greater than 3 mm, and the risk of injury increases with overjet size and lip incompetence.

An increased overjet and increased vertical proportions can sometimes lead to grossly incompetent lips which are habitually apart at rest. This can result in drying of the gingivae, exacerbating any pre-existing gingivitis. Reducing the overjet to improve lip incompetence may help reduce this drying effect.

9.2.3 Function

Although aesthetics and health issues may be more common reasons for treating a Class II division 1 malocclusion, it is important to aim for a functional result that allows the patient to incise foods normally.

9.2.4 Stability

The soft tissues are the major determinant of stability following overjet reduction. Ideally, at the end of overjet reduction the lower lip should lie on the labial incisal one-third of the upper incisors and the patient should be able to achieve a competent lip seal. For example, the patient shown in Chapter 19, Fig. 19.1, has an increased overjet on a Class II skeletal pattern with the lower lip functioning behind the upper incisors. However, following treatment with a functional appliance and fixed appliances the overjet has been reduced, and the lower lip lies passively at rest over the lower third of the upper incisors, increasing the chances of stability. In contrast, the patient shown in Fig. 9.7 has a Class II skeletal pattern with increased vertical skeletal proportions and

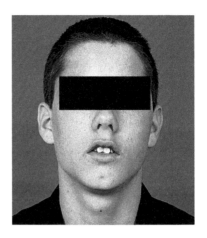

Fig. 9.7 Class II division 1 malocclusion with a poor prognosis for the stability of overjet reduction due to the markedly incompetent lips and increased vertical proportions. Prolonged retention would be advisable.

markedly incompetent lips. In this case, overjet reduction is unlikely to be stable as, following retraction, the upper labial segment would not be controlled by the lower lip.

If it is not possible to get the upper incisors under the control of the lower lip at the end of orthodontic treatment, additional fixed retention may be indicated, or in some cases surgical input may be required.

9.3 Treatment planning for Class II division 1 malocclusions

A full history, examination, and special tests will have identified a list of problems, including the increased overjet and any associated Class II skeletal discrepancy. From this, a list of aims can be produced, identifying which problems will be addressed and which will be accepted. Once the aims are established, possible solutions can be considered. Of particular relevance to treatment planning for Class II division 1 malocclusions are:

• aetiology

• age of the patient

• any underlying skeletal problems

• anchorage

• retention.

9.3.1 Aetiology

It is important to identify the aetiology of the increased overjet, as this will determine the appropriate treatment plan. If there is an underlying skeletal aetiology then a decision needs to be made whether to accept the underlying skeletal component and move the teeth into a Class I relationship (orthodontic camouflage, see Chapter 7, Fig. 7.9), to try to modify the skeletal component (growth modification, see Chapter 19, Fig. 19.1), or to use a combined orthodontics and surgical approach (orthognathic surgery, see Chapter 22, Fig. 22.3).

If there is a soft tissue cause to the malocclusion, then the treatment plan should aim to place the teeth in such a position that the lips will meet passively in a competent position at rest.

Addressing underlying dental causes of an increased overjet are usually simpler, as this typically involves relieving crowding and/or aligning irregular teeth.

If habits are contributing to this type of malocclusion it is vital that the habit is broken before any treatment begins, as the pressures from the digit are likely to inhibit the corrective forces of any orthodontic appliances, and certainly would significantly increase the risk of any relapse.

9.3.2 Age

The patient's age is important as it will determine whether there will be any further significant facial growth. This is important for two reasons:

• Future growth—favourable or unfavourable?

• Utilizing favourable growth for treatment.

In the 'average' growing child, forward growth of the mandible occurs during the pubertal growth spurt and the early teens. This is advantageous in the management of Class II malocclusions. However, correction of the incisor relationship in a child with increased vertical skeletal proportions and a backward-opening rotational pattern of growth has a poorer prognosis. This is because the anteroposterior discrepancy will worsen with growth, and in addition an increase in the lower face height may reduce the likelihood of lip competence at the end of treatment.

In a growing patient, growth modification may be used to correct underlying Class II skeletal problems, and it is also makes it easier to treat other possible aspects of the malocclusion, such as a deep overbite.

9.3.3 Skeletal problems

Patients with an underlying skeletal discrepancy (usually Class II), can be treated by:

- orthodontic camouflage
- growth modification
- a combined orthodontic and surgical approach.

Orthodontic camouflage can be used to treat Class II division 1, by moving the teeth into a Class I relationship, but accepting the underlying skeletal discrepancy. This is usually more likely when the skeletal contribution to the malocclusion is small and may involve allowing the lower incisors to come forwards, or retracting the upper incisors, or both. Retracting the upper incisors sometimes requires space to be created to move the incisors into. This space can be created by removing tooth tissue, using extractions (see Chapter 7, Section 7.7.3) or interproximal reduction of enamel. Space can also be created by applying distalizing forces to the upper molars with headgear (see Chapter 15, Section 15.5) or from temporary anchorage devices (see Chapter 15, Section 15.4.8).

Growth modification is possible in growing patients. This can be undertaken with headgear (see Chapter 15, Section 15.5) or functional appliances (see Chapter 19). It is likely that any skeletal changes are minimal and that the majority of changes are dento-alveolar, however these orthodontic appliances often offer an efficient way to correct the more severe Class II division 1 malocclusions. One particularly controversial area of growth modification treatment of Class II division 1

malocclusions with functional appliances is the timing of treatment: should it be early (typically before the age of 10 years in the mixed dentition) or in the late mixed dentition? The best research evidence available would suggest that starting treatment earlier takes longer, requires more compliance from patients, and does not result in a better final result, either occlusally or skeletally. Early treatment is however indicated to reduce the risk of incisal trauma or when a patient is being teased or bullied about their Class II division 1 malocclusion. Further details are available in Chapter 19, Section 19.5.

Combined orthodontic and orthognathic surgery treatment is usually reserved for adults with more severe skeletal discrepancies that are beyond the scope of orthodontics alone or where orthodontic camouflage would produce a compromised facial result. Combined orthodontic and orthognathic surgery treatment is discussed further in Chapter 22.

9.3.4 Anchorage

Anchorage is the resistance to unwanted tooth movement. Whenever teeth are moved, there is always an equal and opposite force that may cause unwanted tooth movement elsewhere in the mouth. Anchorage is needed to minimize this unwanted tooth movement. In the treatment of Class II division 1 malocclusions, there is often a challenge in keeping the upper posterior teeth still while retracting the upper labial segment to reduce an overjet. Planning, applying, and monitoring anchorage is discussed in detail in Chapter 15.

9.3.5 Retention

Retention is a vital part of any orthodontic treatment plan. Of particular relevance to retaining the result of corrected Class II division 1 malocclusions is to ensure the upper incisors are under control of the lower lip at the end of treatment, to help minimize relapse of the overjet. Retention is discussed in more detail in Chapter 16.

Key points

- Class II division 1 malocclusions are commonly associated with an underlying Class II skeletal pattern with a retrusive mandible.
- When treating Class II division 1 malocclusions, it is important to identify the aetiology, which can be skeletal, due to soft tissues, dental factors, or habits.
- For cases with an underlying Class II skeletal pattern, the options are growth modification, camouflage, or surgery.
- Growth modification can only be undertaken in growing patients.
- Stability of treated Class II division 1 malocclusions is improved if the upper incisors are under the control of the lower lip at the end of treatment.

Relevant Cochrane review

Batista, K. B., Thiruvenkatachari, B., Harrison, J. E., and O'Brien, K. D. (2018). Orthodontic treatment for prominent upper front teeth (Class II malocclusion) in children. *Cochrane Database of Systematic Reviews*, Issue 3, Art. No.: CD003452. DOI: 10.1002/14651858.CD003452.pub4 https://www.cochranelibrary.com/cdsr/doi/10.1002/14651858.CD003452.pub4/full This systematic review discusses the evidence behind the treatment of patients with increased overjets, and includes summaries of the best quality studies using functional appliances.

Principal sources and further reading

Nguyen, Q. V., Bezemer, P. D., Habets, L., and Prahl-Andersen, B. (1999). A systematic review of the relationship between overjet size and traumatic dental injuries. *European Journal of Orthodontics*, **21**, 503–15. [DOI: 10.1093/ejo/21.5.503] [PubMed: 10565091]

Petti, S. (2015). Over two hundred million injuries to anterior teeth attributable to large overjet: a meta-analysis. *Dental Traumatology*, **31**, 1–8. [DOI: 10.1111/edt.12126] [PubMed: 25263806]
These two papers discuss the increased risk of trauma to the incisors of patients with increased overjets.

References for this chapter can also be found at: **www.oup.com/uk/orthodontics5e**. Where possible, these are presented as active links which direct you to the electronic version of the work, to help facilitate onward study. If you are a subscriber to that work (either individually or through an institution), and depending on your level of access, you may be able to peruse an abstract or the full article if available.

10

Class II division 2

S. K. Barber

Chapter contents

Class II division 2 incisor relationship is defined by the British Standards Institute classification as an occlusion where the lower incisor edges occlude posterior to the cingulum plateau of the upper incisors and the upper central incisors are retroclined (Fig. 10.1). The overjet may be normal or increased. The prevalence of this malocclusion in a Caucasian population is approximately 10%.

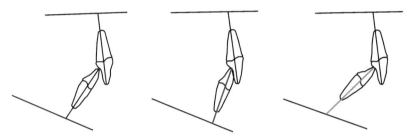

Fig. 10.1 Class II division 2 malocclusion: the lower incisor edges occlude posterior to the cingulum plateau of the upper incisors and the upper central incisors are retroclined. The lower incisors may be normal inclination (black), retroclined (blue), or proclined (green).

10.1 Aetiology

The majority of Class II division 2 malocclusions arise from a number of interrelated skeletal, soft tissue, and dental factors (Table 10.1).

10.1.1 Skeletal pattern

Class II division 2 malocclusion is commonly associated with a mild Class II anteroposterior skeletal pattern, but may also occur in association with a Class I or even a Class III dental base relationship. Where the skeletal pattern is more markedly Class II, the upper incisors usually lie outside the control of the lower lip resulting in a Class II division 1 relationship, but where the lower lip line is high relative to the upper incisors, a Class II division 2 malocclusion can result.

The vertical skeletal dimension is important in the aetiology of Class II division 2 malocclusions. Typically, the lower anterior face height (LAFH) and the Frankfort–mandibular plane angle (FMPA) and maxillary–mandibular plane angle (MMPA) are reduced as a result of a forward (anticlockwise) rotational pattern of growth (see Chapter 4). A reduced LAFH occurring in conjunction with a Class II jaw relationship usually results in the absence of an occlusal stop to the lower incisors. This has the effect of increasing the overbite through further eruption of the incisors (Fig. 10.2).

10.1.2 Soft tissues

The position and activity of the lips and the activity of the masticatory muscles have both been suggested as aetiological factors in Class II division 2 malocclusions. The influence of the lips in Class II division 2 malocclusions is usually mediated by the skeletal pattern. If the lower facial height is reduced, the lower lip line will effectively be higher relative to the crown of the upper incisors (more than the normal one-third coverage). A high lower lip line will tend to retrocline the upper incisors (Fig. 10.3). In some cases, the upper lateral incisors, which have a shorter crown length, will escape the action of the lower lip. In these cases, the central incisors are retroclined while the lateral incisors are

Table 10.1 Common aetiological factors in Class II division 2 malocclusion

Skeletal	Class II anteroposterior skeletal base relationship
	Vertical anterior proportion is often reduced
Soft tissue	High lower lip line can retrocline the maxillary incisors
	Highly active lips can cause bimaxillary dental retrusion
	Increased masticatory muscle tone is associated with reduced facial proportion
Dental	Lack of occlusal stop resulting in increased overbite
	Abnormal crown–root is a possible aetiological factor for increased inter-incisor angle

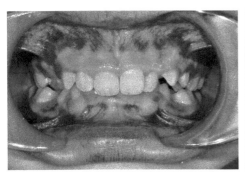
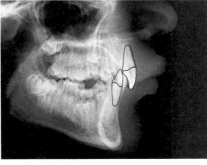

Fig. 10.2 Lack of an occlusal stop allowed the incisors to continue erupting, leading to a significantly increased overbite.

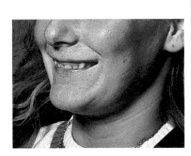
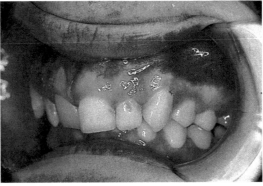

Fig. 10.3 Class II division 2 malocclusion with retroclination of all the upper incisors due to a high lower lip line, which is evident in the view of the patient smiling.

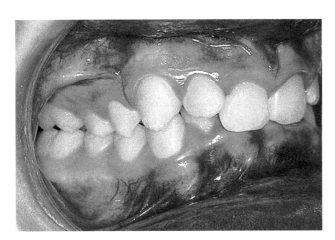

Fig. 10.4 Typical Class II division 2 malocclusion with retroclination of the upper central incisors. The lateral incisors, which are shorter, escape the effect of the lower lip and lie at an average inclination and are slightly mesiolabially rotated as a result of crowding.

average inclination or proclined, commonly with mesiobuccal rotation due to crowding (Fig. 10.4). Class II division 2 incisor relationships may also result from bimaxillary retroclination caused by active muscular lips (Fig. 10.5), irrespective of the skeletal pattern.

Increased masticatory muscle force has been associated with anticlockwise rotational growth patterns and reduced vertical facial proportions. The cause-effect relationship is unclear and it is possible that altered muscular activity is a result of the underlying skeletal pattern or that it contributes to the development of the skeletal pattern. The potentially increased muscular force is an important consideration during treatment planning and management, particularly in non-growing patients, as this may pose challenges for correction of the deep bite.

10.1.3 Dental factors

The increased overbite seen in Class II division 2 malocclusion arises from the lack of effective occlusal stop to limit eruption of the lower

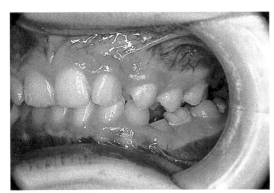
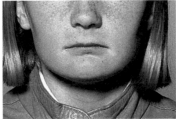

Fig. 10.5 Patient with bimaxillary retroclination due to the action of the lips.

incisors. This results in their continued eruption and an increased inter-incisial angle. This effect may be secondary to a Class II skeletal pattern or a result of retroclination of the incisors by the action of the lips. In some cases the increased inter-incisal angle arises from an abnormal crown-root angulation in the central incisors (Fig. 10.6). However, it has not been established whether the acute crown–root angulation causes the incisor relationship or is itself a result of root development arising from deflection of the crown of the tooth relative to the root after eruption by a high lower lip line.

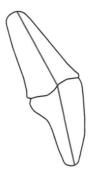

Fig. 10.6 Altered root crown angulation in the maxillary incisors has been suggested as an aetiological factor in Class II division 2 incisal relationship.

10.2 Common features of Class II division 2 malocclusion

10.2.1 Extra-oral features

Typically, Class II division 2 malocclusions are associated with a mild Class II skeletal pattern with reduced vertical proportions. A forward rotational pattern of growth tends to result in the mandible becoming more prognathic and this can be helpful in camouflaging the underlying anteroposterior discrepancy. Reduced LAFH and forward rotation of the mandible commonly results in a more pronounced labio-mental fold (Fig. 10.7).

10.2.2 Occlusal features

The skeletal, soft tissue and dental aetiological factors in Class II division 2 malocclusion result in a number of typical occlusal features (Box 10.1).

Classically, in Class II division 2 malocclusions the upper central incisors are retroclined and the lateral incisors are at average angulation or proclined, depending upon their vertical position relative to the lower lip. Crowding is commonly seen in conjunction with a Class II division 2 incisor relationship as any existing shortage of space is exacerbated by the retroclination of the upper central incisors, resulting in the incisors

being positioned in an arc of smaller circumference. This usually manifests as a lack of space for the upper lateral incisors, which typically rotate mesiolabially out of the arch (Fig. 10.4). Lower arch crowding is similarly exacerbated by retroclination of the lower labial segment, in cases where the lower labial segment has become 'trapped' behind the upper labial segment by an increased overbite (Fig. 10.8). The sagittal curvature of the occlusal plane, known as the curve of Spee, is commonly increased in Class II division 2 malocclusions.

In mild Class II skeletal patterns, the lower incisors occlude with the upper incisors, but in patients with a more severe skeletal discrepancy, the overbite may be complete to the palatal mucosa. In a small proportion of Class II division 2 incisor relationships, a 'traumatic' overbite may occur, where the lower incisors cause ulceration of the palatal tissues, or retroclination of the upper incisors causes stripping of the labial gingivae of the lower incisors (Fig. 10.9).

Another feature associated with a more severe underlying Class II skeletal pattern is lingual crossbite of the first and occasionally the second premolars (Fig. 10.10). This may be a consequence of the relative positions and widths of the arches and/or trapping of the lower labial segment within a retroclined upper labial segment.

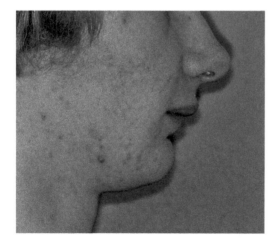

Fig. 10.7 Deep labiomental fold is typical of a forward (anticlockwise) rotational growth pattern, often seen with Class II division 2 malocclusions.

Box 10.1 Common occlusal features in Class II division 2 malocclusion

- Retroclined central maxillary incisors, which are often overerupted.
- Normal, proclined, or retroclined maxillary lateral incisors—lateral incisors are often rotated due to crowding.
- Retroclined mandibular incisors due to 'trapping' behind maxillary incisors.
- Crowding—this can be exacerbated by retroclined incisors.
- Increased overbite.
- Increased curve of Spee.
- Lingual crossbite in premolar region.
- Buccal segment relationship is commonly Class II.

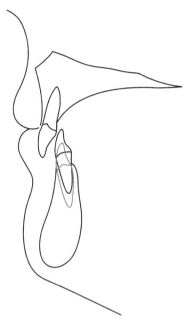

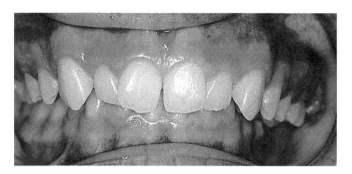

Fig. 10.10 Particularly severe lingual crossbite of the entire left buccal segment due to a Class II skeletal pattern resulting in wider portion of upper arch occluding with narrower section of lower arch.

Fig. 10.8 'Trapping' of the lower incisor teeth behind the cingulum of the upper incisors in a Class II division 2 malocclusion. Note the space created labial to the lower incisor crown by reduction of the overbite (blue line) within the soft tissue environment.

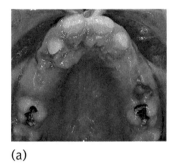

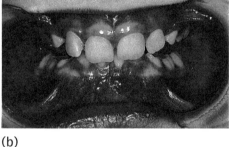

(a)   (b)

Fig. 10.9 'Traumatic overbite' caused by Class II division 2 incisor relationship. (a) Ulceration of the palatal mucosa of 1/1 caused by the occlusion of the lower incisor edges. (b) Stripping of the labial gingivae of the lower incisors caused by the severely retroclined upper incisors.

10.3 Aims of treatment

Class II division 2 malocclusion is one of the most challenging occlusal anomalies to manage due to the underlying aetiological skeletal and soft tissue factors. A recent Cochrane review was unable to find any high-quality evidence to advocate any treatment approach over another and much of the evidence around treatment effectiveness comes from case series, clinical experience, and expert opinion.

Stable correction of a Class II division 2 incisor relationship has two key components to prevent re-eruption of the incisors after treatment (Fig. 10.11):

1. Correction of the inter-incisal angle.
2. Reduction of the increased overbite.

These treatment objectives can be addressed simultaneously along with other aspects of the malocclusion but are discussed separately here for clarity.

Class II division 2 malocclusions are often associated with an underlying Class II skeletal discrepancy and the decision whether to correct or camouflage the anteroposterior discrepancy will depend on the desired final incisor position relative to the face and upper lip. Similarly, the vertical component of the malocclusion will determine the preferred treatment mechanics for correcting the overbite.

10.3.1 Correction of inter-incisal angle

If re-eruption of the incisors and an increase in overbite is to be resisted, the inter-incisal angle needs to be reduced, preferably close to 135°, to create an effective occlusal stop. It has been suggested that stability is increased if, at the end of treatment, an edge–centroid relationship is achieved (Fig. 10.12), where the lower incisor edge lies

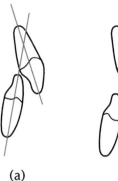
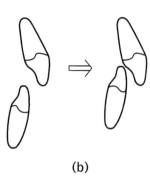

(a)   (b)

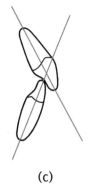

(c)

Fig. 10.11 If a Class II division 2 incisor relationship is to be corrected, not only the overbite but also the inter-incisal angle must be reduced to prevent re-eruption of the incisors after treatment: (a) Class II division 2 incisor relationship; (b) reduction of the overbite alone will not be stable as the incisors will re-erupt following removal of appliances; (c) reduction of the inter-incisal angle in conjunction with reduction of the overbite has a greater chance of stability.

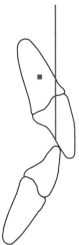

Fig. 10.12 Edge–centroid relationship: the midpoint of the maxillary incisor root axis (centroid) lies palatal to the lower incisor incisal edge.

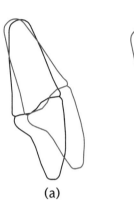

(a)   (b)

Fig. 10.13 Correction of the upper incisor inclination can be achieved in two ways: (a) proclination of the incisor crown while the root position is maintained; (b) palatal torque of the incisor root while the crown position is maintained.

0–2 mm anterior to the midpoint of the root axis of the upper incisors, known as the centroid.

Incisor inclination can be corrected by movement of the crown, root, or both (Fig. 10.13). As a result, there are a number of possible approaches to reducing the inter-incisal angle. The preferred treatment approach will depend upon the aetiology of the malocclusion, the presence and degree of crowding, the extra-oral profile and subsequent preferred incisor position, and the patient's age and wishes.

Inter-incisal correction can be achieved through one or a combination of the following approaches (Fig. 10.14):

- Torquing the incisor roots palatally/lingually.

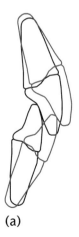
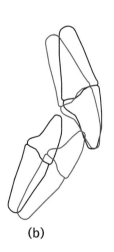
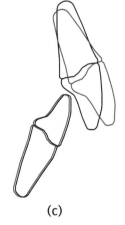

(a)   (b)   (c)

Fig. 10.14 Effect of correcting the inclination of the incisors. Black lines = pre-treatment; red lines = treatment effect. (a) Proclination of both upper and lower incisors corrects the inter-incisal angle and reduces the overbite (e.g. in cases with bimaxillary retrusion). (b) Correction of overjet and overbite by proclination of the lower labial segment and torque of the upper incisor (e.g. in a more severe Class II malocclusion). (c) Proclination of the upper incisors without alteration of the lower incisor position usually leads to an increased overjet. This malocclusion can then be treated as a Class II division 1 malocclusion.

- Proclination of the lower labial segment.
- Proclination of the upper labial segment, then managing as a Class II division 1 malocclusion.

Torquing the incisor roots

Fixed appliances can be used to torque the incisor roots palatally or lingually while maintaining the crown position. Theoretically, if the incisor crown position is unchanged, treatment will have little effect on lip support and facial profile. Torquing incisor apices is dependent upon the presence of sufficient cortical bone palatally/lingually and places a considerable strain on anchorage. This type of movement is also more likely to result in resorption of the root apices than other types of tooth movement. Palatal and lingual incisor root torque requires space in the arch due to the palatal/lingual shift in the contact points of the teeth, leading to a reduction in the arc circumference and a relative reduction in the arch length.

Proclination of incisors

An alternative method for correcting the incisor angulation involves proclination of the teeth. This moves the crown of the tooth labially while maintaining the root position, resulting in space gain by increasing the arc circumference. The relative proclination or torque of upper and/or lower incisors will determine the final incisor relationship.

Proclination of the lower incisors may gain space for alignment and assist overjet and overbite reduction; however, excessive movement of the lower labial segment increases the risk of relapse, bony dehiscence through the labial bone, and gingival recession (see Chapter 1, Section 1.6). Lower incisor proclination is discussed in more detail in Section 10.4.2.

In the upper arch, proclination of the incisors will convert the incisal relationship into a Class II division 1 malocclusion, usually with an increased overjet. In cases where lip support is reduced, labial movement of the upper incisors may be desirable. Where proclination of the upper labial segment results in an increased overjet, management for correcting the anteroposterior inter-arch discrepancy to achieve a Class I incisor relationship follows the same principles as a Class II division 1 malocclusion (see Chapter 9).

10.3.2 Reduction of overbite

The levelling phase of treatment aims to correct the overbite and the increased curve of Spee associated with Class II division 2 malocclusion. A number of approaches can be used to correct the overbite:

- Intrusion of incisors
- Eruption of molars
- Extrusion of molars
- Proclination of incisors.

Due to the difficulty in creating isolated effects with orthodontic appliances, it is likely that, in reality, any mechanics will result in a combination of these tooth movements to varying degrees. The decision whether anterior or posterior vertical tooth movement is preferred depends on the amount of incisor and gingival show at rest and smiling and the LAFH. Considerations for proclination of incisors are

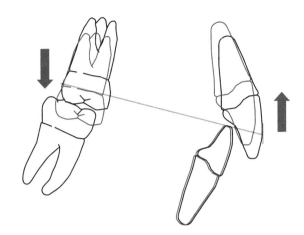

Fig. 10.15 Incisor intrusion with fixed appliance with a continuous archwire will lead to some molar extrusion.

discussed in Section 10.4.2. Levelling the curve of Spee requires space (see Chapter 7, Section 7.7.1) and may result in proclination of the lower labial segment unless there is space in the arch.

Incisor intrusion

True intrusion of the incisors is difficult to achieve with fixed appliances alone, as the mechanics tend to pit intrusion of the incisors against extrusion of the buccal segment teeth (Fig. 10.15). It is easier to move molars occlusally than to intrude the incisors into bone and consequently, the former tends to predominate. In practice, relative intrusion is achieved, where the incisors are held while vertical growth of the face occurs with additional extrusion of the molars. Where there is a step in the occlusion, arches such as the utility arch can be used (Fig. 10.16). This bypasses the canines and premolars to enable levelling of the labial segment and reduction of overbite by intrusion of the incisors, although some molar extrusion does occur.

Molar extrusion alongside incisor intrusion may be acceptable, or even desirable, for example, in cases with reduced vertical proportions. However, in those with normal or increased facial proportions, it

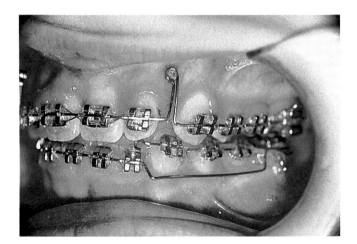

Fig. 10.16 Lower utility arch for overbite reduction. Note the difference in level between the lower incisor brackets and the buccal segment teeth.

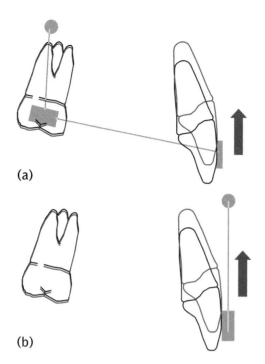

(a)

(b)

Fig. 10.17 Altering the anchorage balance to increase incisor intrusion with minimal molar extrusion: (a) increasing posterior anchorage by including more teeth in the anchor unit or using posterior skeletal anchorage; (b) providing a stable force for application of intrusive force, such as anterior skeletal anchorage.

may be undesirable to have molar movement and methods may be used to alter the anchorage balance and increase true incisor intrusion (Fig. 10.17). Posterior anchorage can be increased to limit reciprocal molar extrusion during incisor extrusion. The two most common methods to increase posterior anchorage are increasing the number of molars included in anchorage unit, for example, bonding the second molars, and use of skeletal anchorage ligated to the fixed appliance in the molar region to restrict molar movement. Alternatively, skeletal anchorage in the incisor region allows direct application of intrusive forces to the upper labial segment with minimal effect on the molars. However, care must be taken not to apply excessive intrusive force, as this increases the risk of root resorption (see Section 4.10). Temporary anchorage devices (TADs) are the most common method for gaining skeletal anchorage and can be used in conjunction with fixed or removable appliances (see Chapter 15, Section 15.4.8).

10.4 Treatment methods

The decision to embark on orthodontic treatment should be based on a thorough risk–benefit analysis. In milder Class II division 2 cases, where the overbite is only slightly increased, the arches are not significantly crowded, and the aesthetics acceptable, it may be preferable to accept the malocclusion (Fig. 10.19).

Where treatment is indicated, the overall malocclusion will determine the treatment objectives. Treatment modalities for Class II division

Eruption of the molars

Eruption of the buccal segment will aid levelling of the curve of Spee and overbite reduction but this is limited to growing patients. Methods can be used to encourage molar eruption while simultaneously limiting further eruption of the incisors (Fig. 10.18). This is most commonly achieved with an upper removable appliance that incorporates a flat anterior bite-plane (FABP) or a functional appliance that frees the occlusion of the posterior teeth, such as a medium opening activator (see Chapter 19, Section 19.7.3). If worn conscientiously, these appliances result in rapid reduction of the overbite.

Eruption of the molars to correct the overbite results in an increase in the vertical dimension. This must be judged to be favourable to the overall facial balance and in addition, the patient must still be growing to enable adaptation and prevent re-intrusion of the molars under the forces of occlusion once the appliance is withdrawn. Resistance to re-intrusion is aided if the treatment creates an effective occlusal stop and reduces the inter-incisal angle.

Extrusion of the molars

As previously described, the major effect of attempting intrusion of the incisors is often extrusion of the molars. This is advantageous in Class II division 2 cases with reduced vertical proportions. Vertical growth is required if the overbite reduction achieved is to be stable and it can be very difficult to extrude the molars in a stable manner in adult patients due to the lack of growth.

10.3.3 Correction of other aspects of malocclusion

When determining the aims of treatment for Class II division 2 malocclusions, it is important to consider all aspects of the malocclusion and how these may be corrected, as this may have implications for the best method for correcting the inter-incisal angle and overbite. Space requirements need to be judged based on crowding, change in incisor inclination, and any anteroposterior, vertical, or transverse discrepancies (see Chapter 7, Section 7.7).

Lingual crossbites often affect the first premolars only and may be inadvertently managed by extraction of the upper first premolars. If extractions are not indicated or if multiple teeth are involved, elimination of the crossbite will commonly involve fixed appliances to achieve a combination of contraction across the affected upper teeth and expansion of the lower premolar width.

2 malocclusion include fixed appliances, functional appliances, and orthognathic treatment (Table 10.2).

10.4.1 Extractions

The decision to extract in Class II division 2 malocclusion cases depends on the overall space requirements to correct all aspects of the

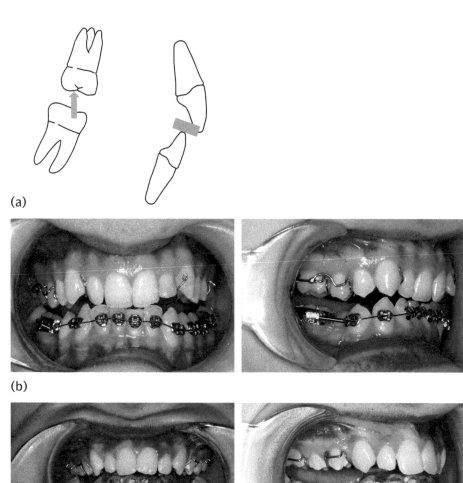

(a)

(b)

(c)

Fig. 10.18 (a) The effect of 'opening the bite'. Further eruption of the incisors is limited while the molars are encouraged to erupt to reduce the overbite. (b) An upper removable appliance with a flat anterior bite plane. The posterior teeth are out of occlusion, providing space for eruption. The levelling effect can be increased by placing a lower fixed appliance. (c) A similar effect can be achieved using a functional appliance that separates the posterior teeth, such as a medium opening activator.

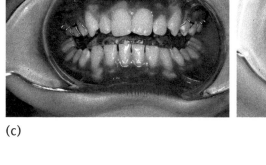

Fig. 10.19 An acceptable mild Class II division 2 incisor relationship.

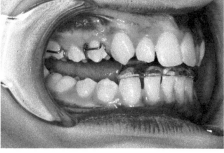

malocclusion and the proposed final position of the incisors based on optimizing facial aesthetics.

In the lower arch, it is preferable to limit any lingual movement of the lower incisors to avoid worsening the overbite. In cases with little space requirement, it may be preferable to accept proclination of the lower incisors rather than risking lower incisor retraction. Clinical experience suggests that space closure occurs less readily in patients with reduced vertical skeletal proportions and, as this is a common feature of Class II division 2 malocclusions, this is often cited as a further reason to avoid lower arch extractions. In cases where lower arch extractions are necessary, treatment mechanics must be planned and executed to ensure space closure without lingual movement of the lower incisors (Fig. 10.20). Most commonly, lower second premolars rather than first premolars are the extraction choice.

In the upper arch, extractions may be required to provide space and anchorage for torquing the incisor roots palatally or for retracting the

Table 10.2 Treatment methods in Class II division 2 malocclusion

Method	Aim
Fixed appliances	Torque incisor roots to correct inter-incisal angle Procline lower incisors to correct inter-incisal angle, reduce overbite, and create space Intrusion of incisors and/or extrusion of molars to reduce overbite
Removable appliance	Flat anterior bite plane—eruption of molars and allow lower incisors to spontaneously procline Use with TADS as a splint to intrude upper labial segment
Headgear	Distalization of buccal segments Extrusion of molars Anchorage
Temporary anchorage device (TAD)	Provide anchorage to support desired tooth movements
Inter-arch elastic traction	Anteroposterior or vertical correction Anchorage
Functional appliance	Modifications to procline upper incisors Anteroposterior inter-arch correction
Orthognathic surgery	Manage severe anteroposterior and vertical skeletal discrepancy

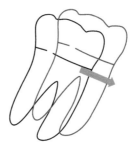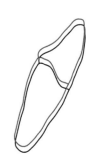

Fig. 10.20 Residual extraction space in the lower arch is ideally closed by protraction of the buccal segments to prevent labial segment retraction and worsening of the overbite.

Reduced buccal alveolar bone and thin gingival biotype are associated with iatrogenic gingival recession, particularly in the presence of poor plaque control. In non-growing patients with an underlying skeletal discrepancy, lower labial segment proclination is often desirable; however, the increased risk of gingival recession may be inhibitory.

10.4.3 Fixed appliances

Fixed appliances can be used to correct the inter-incisal angle and reduce the overbite, as well as correcting other aspects of the malocclusion such as malalignment and crossbites (Fig. 10.21). Fixed appliances can be used alone or in conjunction with other appliances.

Headgear can be used alongside fixed appliances to provide additional anchorage or for distal movement of the buccal segments. A direction of pull below the occlusal plane (cervical pull) is indicated in Class II division 2 malocclusions with reduced vertical facial proportions to aid extrusion of molar and increase face height.

Skeletal anchorage from TADs has increased the scope for correction of more severe Class II division 2 malocclusions with orthodontics alone. TADs can be used with fixed or removable appliances to provide a point for direct application of force or to increase anchorage (see Chapter 15, Section 15.4.8).

10.4.4 Removable appliances

Removable appliances are useful as a stand-alone treatment or as an adjunct to other appliances. In cases where the lower incisors have been trapped behind the upper labial segment by an increased overbite, fitting an upper removable appliance (URA) with FAPB may allow the lower labial segment to procline spontaneously.

URAs can also be used in conjunction with other treatment modalities:

- URA with FABP used with a lower fixed appliance to eliminate interference from the upper incisors while the lower arch is aligned and levelled

- URA with headgear to gain buccal segment correction

- URA with anterior capping with traction to anterior temporary anchorage devices to intrude the labial segment.

labial segment. Care must be taken to determine the desired maxillary incisor crown position relative to the face and upper lip to prevent over-retraction of the upper labial segment. Identifying the proposed incisor position at the outset ensures the treatment plan is feasible, identifies any additional anchorage requirements, and helps to plan mechanics.

10.4.2 Lower incisor proclination

Proclination of the lower incisors is helpful in reducing both overbite and the inter-incisal angle. In general, proclination of the lower labial segment should be considered unstable but it has been argued that in some Class II division 2 malocclusions, the lower labial segment is trapped behind the upper labial segment by the increased overbite. This results in retroclination of the lower incisors and constriction of the lower intercanine width during growth. In these cases, it is suggested that a limited increase in intercanine width and a degree of proclination of the lower labial segment can be stable. In the majority of patients, movement of the lower labial segment labially increases the likelihood of relapse and therefore carefully planned retention is particularly important (see Chapter 16).

If the treatment plan involves proclination of the lower labial segment, it is critical that the lower labial supporting tissues are assessed.

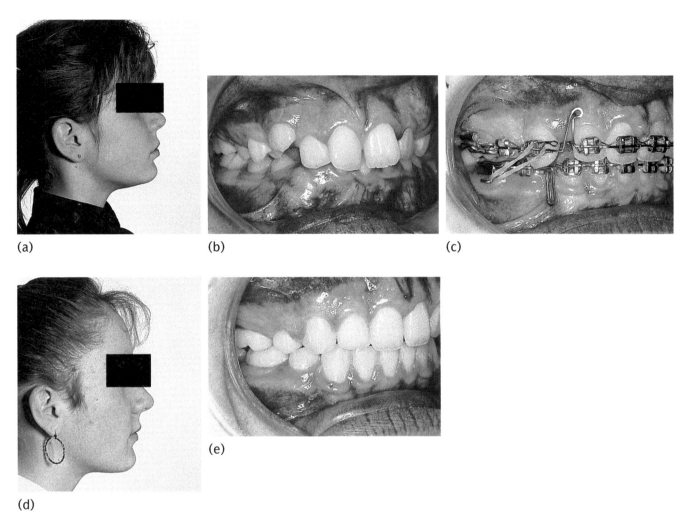

(a)   (b)   (c)

(d)   (e)

Fig. 10.21 (a) A 12-year-old female with a Class II division 2 incisor relationship on a Class I skeletal pattern with crowded and rotated incisors. (b) The second premolars were extracted and fixed appliances were used. (c) At the end of treatment, the deep bite and crowding were corrected and some favourable mandibular growth is also evident (d, e).

10.4.5 Functional appliances

See also Chapter 19, Section 19.6.2.

Functional appliances can be utilized in the correction of Class II division 2 malocclusions in growing patients with a mild to moderate Class II skeletal pattern. Reduction of the inter-incisal angle is achieved mainly by proclination of the upper incisors, although some proclination of the lower labial segment may also occur. In some cases a removable appliance might be used prior to the functional appliance to procline the incisors and expand the upper arch to ensure the correct buccolingual arch relationship at the end of treatment (Fig. 10.22).

Alternatively, to eliminate the need for an additional treatment stage, modifications can be incorporated into some types of functional appliance. Twin-block functional appliances can be designed to incorporate a spring and a midline expansion screw into the upper block to procline the incisors and gain expansion respectively. Alternatively, a sectional-fixed appliance can be placed on the upper

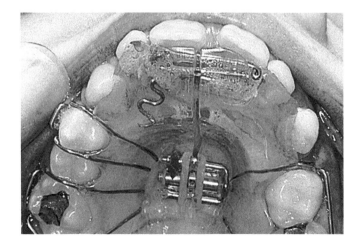

Fig. 10.22 A URA can be used prior to functional appliance treatment to procline the upper incisors and gain upper arch expansion, known as the 'Expansion and Labial Segment Alignment Appliance' (ELSAA).

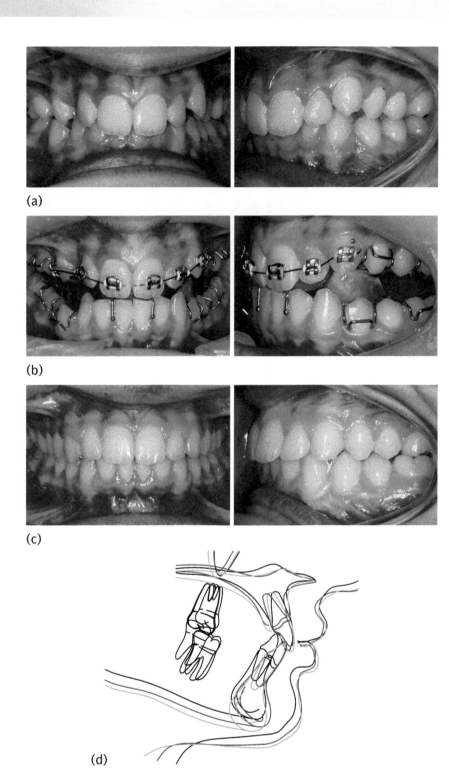

(a)

(b)

(c)

(d)

Fig. 10.23 (a) A Class II division 2 malocclusion. (b) A sectional fixed was used in conjunction with a twin-block appliance to procline the upper labial segment and gain anteroposterior correction. (c) Following this, fixed appliances were used to correct all remaining aspects of the malocclusion. (d) The cephalometric superimposition demonstrates the maxillary incisors have been torqued and the lower incisors proclined to correct the inter-incisal angle, alongside reduction of the overbite (black = pre-treatment, green = post-functional, red = near end of treatment).

labial segment teeth to achieve alignment during the functional phase (Fig. 10.23). After anteroposterior correction with the functional appliance, fixed appliances are nearly always required to detail the occlusion.

10.4.6 Surgery

See Chapter 22.

A stable aesthetic orthodontic correction may not be possible in patients with an unfavourable skeletal pattern anteroposterior or vertical, particularly if growth is complete (Fig. 10.24). In these cases, surgery may be necessary. A phase of pre-surgical orthodontics is required to align the teeth. However, arch levelling is usually not completed as extrusion of the molars is much more easily accomplished after surgery (see Chapter 21, Section 21.8.2).

10.4.7 Retention

In cases where the lower incisors have been proclined, the stability of their position should be assessed. Permanent retention is advised after

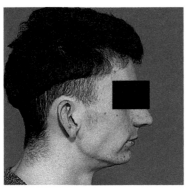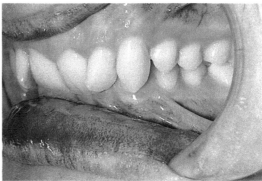

Fig. 10.24 Adult patient with severe Class II division 2 malocclusion on a marked Class II skeletal pattern with reduced vertical proportions. It was decided that a combined orthodontic and orthognathic surgery approach was required to correct this malocclusion.

most orthodontic correction and retention phase is particularly important in Class II division 2 malocclusions, with regard to:

- preventing an increase in overbite
- retaining any de-rotated teeth, for example, the upper lateral incisors

- maintaining alignment of the lower labial segment, particularly if it has been proclined during treatment.

For further details, see Chapter 16.

Key points

- Careful assessment of the aetiological factors contributing to the incisor relationship and the degree to which they can be reduced or eliminated is essential if treatment is to be successful.
- The threshold for extractions in the lower arch is higher than other malocclusions.
- The inter-incisal angle needs to be reduced and an adequate occlusal stop for the lower incisors created to increase the chances of a stable overbite reduction.

Relevant Cochrane review

Millett, D. T., Cunningham, S. J., O'Brien, K. D., Benson, P. E., and de Oliveira, C. M. (2018). Orthodontic treatment for deep bite and retroclined upper front teeth in children. *Cochrane Database of Systematic Reviews*, Issue 2, Art No.: CD005972. DOI: 10.1002/14651858.CD005972.pub4 https://www.cochranelibrary.com/cdsr/doi/10.1002/14651858.CD005972.pub4/full
The authors concluded it was not possible to provide any evidence-based guidance for the management of this malocclusion in children.

Principal sources and further reading

Baccetti, T., Franchi, L., and McNamara, J. (2011). Longitudinal growth changes in subjects with deepbite. *American Journal of Orthodontics and Dentofacial Orthopedics*, **140**, 202–9. [DOI: 10.1016/j.ajodo.2011.04.015] [PubMed: 21803258]
An interesting paper reporting changes in overbite during growth.

Burstone, C. R. (1977). Deep overbite correction by intrusion. *American Journal of Orthodontics*, **72**, 1–22. [DOI: 10.1016/0002-9416(77)90121-X] [PubMed: 267433].
A useful paper for the more experienced orthodontist using fixed appliances.

Dyer, F. M., McKeown, H. F., and Sandler, P. J. (2001). The modified twin block appliance in the treatment of Class II division 2 malocclusions. *Journal of Orthodontics*, **28**, 271–80. [DOI: 10.1093/ortho/28.4.271] [PubMed: 11709592]
Describes the management of two Class II division 2 cases treated with functional and fixed appliances with excellent illustrations.

Houston, W. J. (1989). Incisor edge-centroid relationships and overbite depth. *European Journal of Orthodontics*, **11**, 139–43. [DOI: 10.1093/oxfordjournals.ejo.a035976] [PubMed: 2767146]
The original paper describing edge–centroid and its relationship to overbite.

Lee, R. T. (1999). Arch width and form: a review. *American Journal of Orthodontics and Dentofacial Orthopedics*, **115**, 305–13. [DOI: 10.1016/S0889-5406(99)70334-3] [PubMed: 10066980]
A classic article.

Leighton, B. C. and Adams, C. P. (1986). Incisor inclination in Class II division 2 malocclusions. *European Journal of Orthodontics*, **8**, 98–105. [DOI: 10.1093/ejo/8.2.98] [PubMed: 3459666]
A historically important paper investigating the incisor inclination at stages of tooth development.

Kim, T. W. and Little, R. M. (1999). Post retention assessment of deep overbite correction in Class II division 2 malocclusion. *Angle Orthodontist*, **69**, 175–86. [DOI: 10.1043/0003-3219(1999)069<0175:PAODOC>2.3.CO;2] [PubMed: 10227559]

Lapatki, B. G., Mager, A. S., Sculte-Moenting J., and Jonas, I. E. (2002). The importance of the level of the lip line and resting lip pressure in Class II, Division 2 malocclusion. *Journal of Dental Research*, **85**, 323–8. [DOI: 10.1177/154405910208100507] [PubMed: 12097445]
Evidence to suggest that high pressure from a high lip line is an important aetiological factor in Class II division 2 malocclusion.

Melsen, B. and Allais, D. (2005). Factors of importance for the development of dehiscence during labial movement of mandibular incisors: a retrospective study of adult orthodontic patients. *American Journal of Orthodontics and Dentofacial Orthopedics*, **127**, 552–61. [DOI: 10.1016/j.ajodo.2003.12.026] [PubMed: 15877035]
Although this is a retrospective study, it does have a sample size of 150 adults. The authors concluded that thin gingivae pre-treatment, presence of plaque, and inflammation were useful predictors of gingival recession.

Millett, D. T., Cunningham, S., O'Brien, D., Benson, P., and de Oliveira, C. M. (2012). Treatment and stability of Class II division 2 malocclusion in children and adolescents: a systematic review. *American Journal of Orthodontics and Dentofacial Orthopedics*, **142**, 159–69. [DOI: 10.1016/j.ajodo.2012.03.022] [PubMed: 22858324]
The authors provide guidelines for treatment of Class II division 2 malocclusion but emphasize the lack of good evidence currently available.

Mills, J. R. E. (1973). The problem of overbite in Class II division 2 malocclusion. *British Journal of Orthodontics*, 1, 34-48 [DOI: 10.1179/bjo.1.1.34]
A classic paper describing the aetiology of malocclusion and aims of treatment.

Ng, J., Major, P. W., Heo, G., and Flores-Mir, C. (2005). True incisor intrusion attained during orthodontic treatment: a systematic review and meta-analysis. *American Journal of Orthodontics and Dentofacial Orthopedics*, **128**, 212–19. [DOI: 10.1016/j.ajodo.2004.04.025] [PubMed: 16102407]
The authors found limited true incisor intrusion in non-growing patients.

Selwyn-Barnett, B. J. (1991). Rationale of treatment for class II division 2 malocclusion. *British Journal of Orthodontics*, **18**, 173–81. [DOI: 10.1179/bjo.18.3.173] [PubMed: 1931851]
This paper contains a carefully constructed argument for management of Class II division 2 malocclusion by proclination of the lower labial segment rather than extractions, in order to avoid detrimental effects upon the profile.

 References for this chapter can also be found at: **www.oup.com/uk/orthodontics5e**. Where possible, these are presented as active links that direct you to the electronic version of the work, to help facilitate onward study. If you are a subscriber to that work (either individually or through an institution), and depending on your level of access, you may be able to peruse an abstract or the full article if available.

11
Class III

Benjamin R. K. Lewis

Chapter contents

The British Standards definition of Class III incisor relationship includes those malocclusions where the lower incisor edge occludes anterior to the cingulum plateau of the upper incisors. Class III malocclusions affect around 3% of Caucasians.

11.1 Aetiology

11.1.1 Skeletal pattern

The skeletal relationship is often the most important aetiological factor, with the majority of Class III incisor relationships being associated with an underlying Class III skeletal relationship. Cephalometric studies have shown that, compared with Class I occlusions, Class III malocclusions exhibit the following:

● Increased mandibular length.

● A more anteriorly placed glenoid fossa so that the condylar head is positioned more anteriorly leading to mandibular prognathism.

● Reduced maxillary length.

● A more retruded position of the maxilla leading to maxillary retrognathia.

The first two of these factors are the most influential. Fig. 11.1 shows a patient with a Class III malocclusion with mandibular prognathism and Fig. 11.2 illustrates maxillary retrognathia (maxillary retrusion). To help determine the extent to which the maxilla and mandible are contributing to the facial Class III appearance, the zero meridian can be used. This an imaginary line dropped vertically from the soft tissue nasion and perpendicular to the true horizontal, when the individual is in natural head position. In a Class I skeletal relationship the chin point should lie on the line or slightly behind it (see Chapter 5, Fig. 5.2).

Class III malocclusions occur in association with a range of vertical skeletal proportions, ranging from increased to reduced. A backward, opening rotation pattern of facial growth will tend to result in a reduction of overbite with a longer lower face height but less mandibular forward projection; whereas, a forward rotating pattern of facial growth will lead to a more marked increase in the prominence of the chin.

There is evidence to indicate that Class III skeletal patterns exhibit less maxillary growth and more mandibular growth than Class I skeletal patterns.

11.1.2 Soft tissues

In the majority of Class III malocclusions, the soft tissues do not play a major aetiological role. In fact, the reverse is often the case, with the soft tissues tending to tilt the upper and lower incisors towards each other so that the incisor relationship is often less severe than the underlying skeletal pattern. This dento-alveolar compensation occurs in Class III malocclusions because an anterior oral seal can frequently be achieved by upper to lower lip contact. This has the effect of moulding the upper and lower labial segments towards each other. The main exception

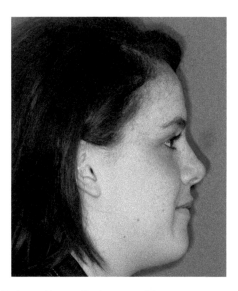

Fig. 11.1 Patient with mandibular prognathism.

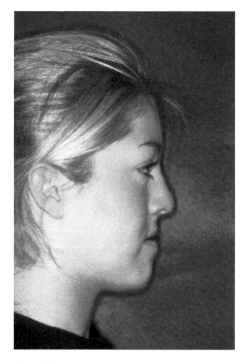

Fig. 11.2 Patient with maxillary retrognathia.

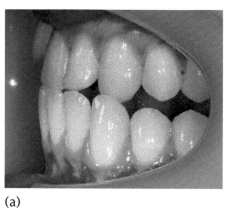
(a)

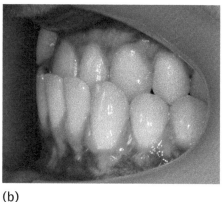
(b)

Fig. 11.3 (a) Initial contact on the incisors in retruded contact position; (b) anterior displacement resulting in a full anterior crossbite in maximum intercuspation.

to this occurs in patients with increased vertical skeletal proportions where the lips are more likely to be incompetent and an anterior oral seal is often accomplished by tongue to lower lip contact, resulting in less dental camouflage being generated.

11.1.3 Dental factors

Class III malocclusions are often associated with a narrow upper arch and a broad lower arch, with the result that crowding is seen more commonly, and to a greater degree, in the upper arch compared with the lower. Frequently, the lower arch is well aligned or even spaced.

11.2 Occlusal features

By definition, Class III malocclusions occur when the lower incisors are positioned more labially relative to the upper incisors. Therefore, an anterior crossbite of one or more of the incisors is a common feature of Class III malocclusions. Generally, the more anterior teeth that are in crossbite, the more severe the underlying skeletal Class III base. As with any crossbite, it is essential to check for a displacement of the mandible on closure from a premature contact into maximal interdigitation (Fig. 11.3). In Class III malocclusions, this can be ascertained by asking the patient to try to achieve an edge-to-edge incisor position. If such a displacement is present, the prognosis for correction of the incisor relationship is more favourable. In the past, it was thought that such a displacement led to overclosure and greater prominence of the mandible, with the condylar head displaced forward. In fact, cephalometric studies suggest that in most cases, although there is a forward displacement of the mandible, to allow disengagement from the premature contact of the incisors, as closure into maximum occlusion occurs, the mandible subsequently moves backwards until the condyles regain their normal position within the glenoid fossa (Fig. 11.4).

Another common feature of Class III malocclusions is buccal crossbite, which can occur for two main reasons. Due to the relationship between the upper and lower jaws, there is a discrepancy in the relative width of the arches, with the lower arch being positioned relatively more anteriorly in Class III malocclusions. In addition, the upper jaw can be intrinsically small both in the anteroposterior and transverse dimensions which will often result in severe crowding of the upper arch (Fig. 11.5).

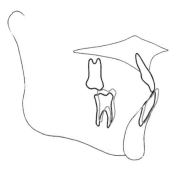

Fig. 11.4 Diagram illustrating the path of closure in a Class III malocclusion from an edge-to-edge incisor relationship into maximal occlusion. Although the mandible is displaced forwards from the initial contact of the incisors to achieve maximal interdigitation, the condylar head is not displaced out of the glenoid fossa.

As mentioned previously, Class III malocclusions often exhibit dentoalveolar compensation with the upper incisors proclined and the lower incisors retroclined, which reduces the severity of the incisor relationship when compared to the underlying skeletal position (Fig. 11.6).

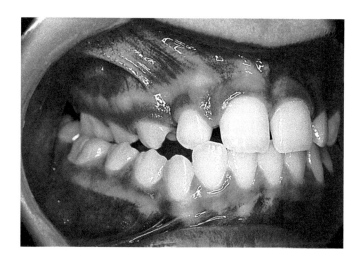

Fig. 11.5 A Class III malocclusion with a narrow crowded upper arch and a broader less crowded lower arch with associated buccal crossbite.

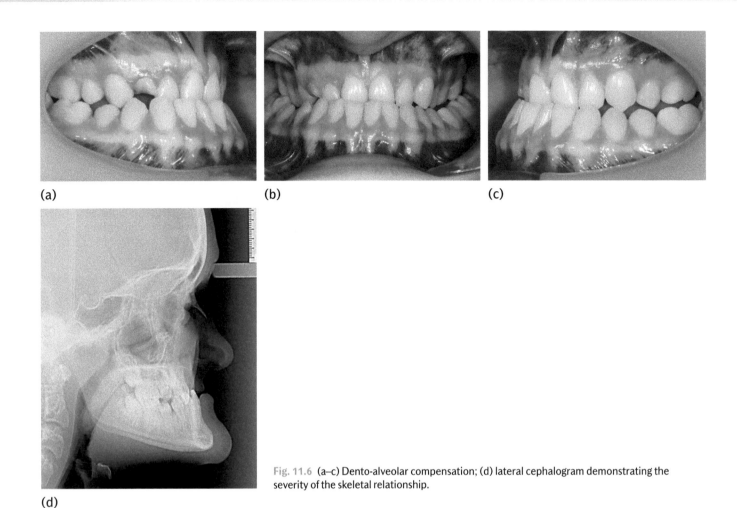

(a) (b) (c)

(d)

Fig. 11.6 (a–c) Dento-alveolar compensation; (d) lateral cephalogram demonstrating the severity of the skeletal relationship.

11.3 Treatment planning in Class III malocclusions

A number of factors should be considered when planning treatment:

The patient's opinion regarding their occlusion and facial appearance must be taken into account, as facial concerns will have a significant bearing on the appropriateness of an orthognathic surgical approach. This subject needs to be approached with some tact.

The severity of the skeletal pattern, in all three planes of space, anteroposteriorly, transversely, and vertically, should be assessed. This is the major determinant of the difficulty and prognosis of orthodontic treatment.

The amount and expected pattern of future growth, both anteroposteriorly and vertically, should be considered. It is important to remember that average growth will tend to result in a worsening of the relationship between the arches as the maxilla completes its growth before the mandible, and a significant deterioration can be anticipated if growth is unfavourable (see Chapter 4, Section 4.5). When evaluating the likely direction and extent of facial growth, the patient's age, sex, facial pattern, and family history of Class III malocclusions should be taken into consideration (see Chapter 4). Children with increased vertical skeletal proportions may continue to exhibit a vertical pattern of growth, which often leads to the increases in mandibular length being split between anteroposterior and

vertical projection, resulting in relatively less mandibular prognathism, but an increased lower face height with reduced incisor overbite. For patients on the borderline between different management regimens, it is wise to err on the side of pessimism (as growth will often prove this to be correct) and a period of monitoring is advisable (Fig. 11.7).

In Class III malocclusions, a normal or increased overbite is an advantage, as sufficient vertical overlap of the upper and lower incisors after treatment is vital for stability.

If the patient can achieve an edge-to-edge incisor contact and then displaces forwards into a reverse overjet, this increases the prognosis for correction of the incisor relationship with orthodontic camouflage.

In general, orthodontic management of Class III malocclusion will aim to increase dento-alveolar compensation. Therefore, if considerable dento-alveolar compensation is already present, trying to increase it further may not be an aesthetic or stable treatment option. Cephalometrically, it has been suggested that, for the majority of patients, an upper incisor angle of 120° to the maxillary plane and a lower incisor angle of 80° to the mandibular plane, are the limits of an acceptable compromise.

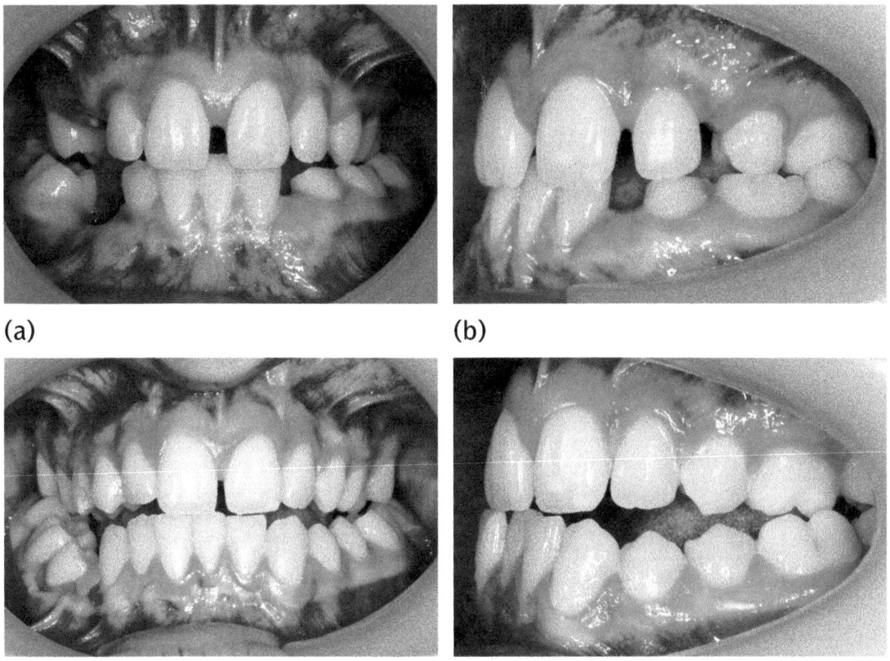

(a)

(b)

(c)

(d)

Fig. 11.7 Worsening of the occlusal relationship in both the anteroposterior and vertical dimensions. (a, b) Initial presentation; (c, d) presentation 4 years later.

The degree of crowding in each arch should be considered. In Class III malocclusions, crowding occurs more frequently, and to a greater degree, in the upper arch than in the lower. Extractions only in the upper arch should be resisted as this will often lead to a worsening of the incisor relationship. Where upper arch extractions are necessary, it is advisable to extract at least as far forwards in the lower arch, to allow maximum opportunity to establish a positive overjet at the end of treatment. Using headgear for distal movement of the upper buccal segments to gain space for alignment is inadvisable in Class III malocclusions as this may have the effect of restraining growth of the maxilla which could worsen the underlying skeletal relationship.

Functional appliances are less widely used in Class III malocclusions because it is difficult for patients to posture posteriorly to achieve an active working bite. However, they can be useful in mild cases in the mixed dentition where a combination of proclination of the upper incisors together with retroclination of the lower incisors is required.

In patients with a severe Class III skeletal pattern and/or reduced overbite, the possibility that a surgical approach may ultimately be

Box 11.1 **Summary of factors to be considered when planning treatment**

- Patient's concerns and motivation towards treatment.
- Severity of skeletal pattern.
- Amount and direction of any future growth.
- Can patient achieve edge-to-edge incisor contact?
- Overbite.
- Amount of dento-alveolar compensation present.
- Degree of crowding.

required must be considered, particularly before any permanent tooth extractions are undertaken (see Chapter 11, Section 11.4.4).

Box 11.1 summarizes those features which need to be considered when planning treatment in Class III patients.

11.4 Treatment options

11.4.1 Accepting the incisor relationship

In mild Class III malocclusions, particularly those cases where the overbite is minimal, it may be preferable to accept the incisor relationship and direct treatment towards achieving arch alignment.

For younger patients, who present with a more severe Class III incisor relationship with upper arch crowding, an initial course of orthodontic treatment may be undertaken to align the upper teeth. This provides

the psycho-social benefits of an improved dental appearance during the early teenage years, while awaiting the completion of facial growth. At this stage, the options may be to accept the residual malocclusion, undergo orthodontic camouflage, or proceed with full comprehensive treatment involving further orthodontic treatment and orthognathic surgery. The most appropriate option would be dependent on the degree of adverse growth and the concerns of the patient.

11.4.2 Early orthopaedic treatment

Orthopaedic correction of Class III malocclusions aims to enhance or encourage maxillary growth and/or restrain or redirect mandibular growth. Although a number of different treatment modalities have been shown to be successful in the short to mid term, given the propensity for unfavourable growth in skeletal Class III, the results of long-term follow-up are awaited with interest.

There is an increasing body of evidence that orthopaedic correction treatment is more likely to be successful if it is carried out prior to the pubertal growth spurt. The techniques in most common usage are as follows:

● Protraction face-mask used to advance the maxilla. The forces applied in this technique are in the region of 400 g per side and a cooperative patient is necessary to achieve the 14 hours per day wear required (Fig. 11.8). A recent multicentre randomized controlled trial in patients under the age of 10 years showed a success rate of 70% in terms of achieving a positive overjet over a follow-up period of 15 months. They reported that by the average age of 15 years, despite

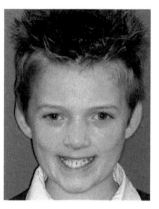
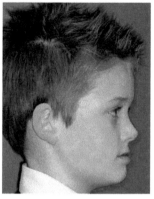
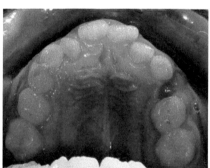
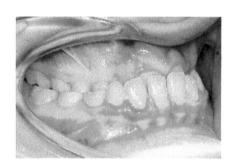
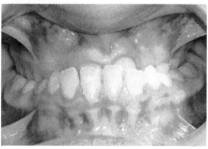
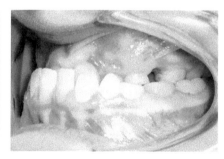
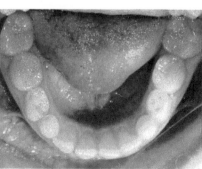

(a–g)

Fig. 11.8 Patient treated by reverse headgear and rapid maxillary expansion. (a–g) pre-treatment; (h–k) showing face mask and rapid maxillary expansion appliance which was cemented in position. Elastic traction was applied from the hooks on the intra-oral appliance adjacent to the first deciduous molars to hooks on the face frame; (l–n) after 10 months of treatment; (o–s) 2 years after completion of treatment showing good stability.

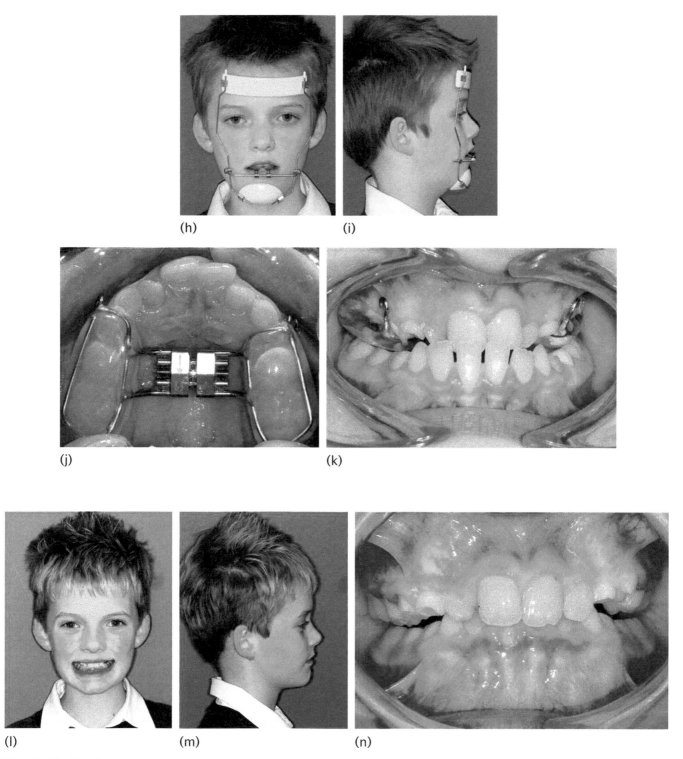

(h)

(i)

(j)

(k)

(l)

(m)

(n)

Fig. 11.8 (*Continued*)

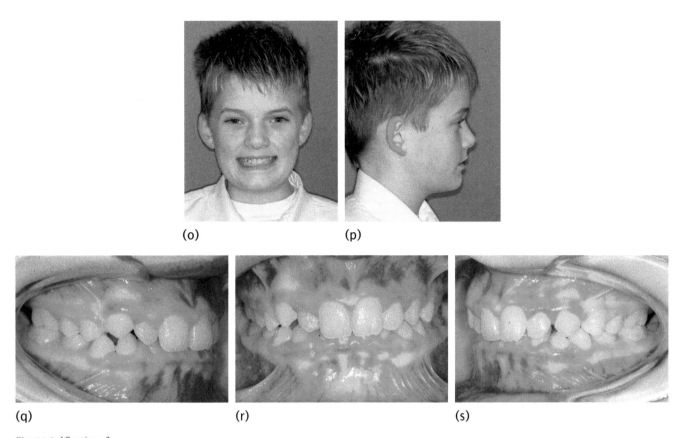

(o)

(p)

(q)

(r)

(s)

Fig. 11.8 (*Continued*)

the initial skeletal benefits not being maintained, 68% of patients still maintained a positive overjet and remarkably only a third of patients who had undergone face-mask treatment had, at this age, a perceived need for orthognathic surgery, compared with two-thirds of the control group. It is hypothesized that this difference in the perceived need for surgery could be due to the maintained clockwise rotation of the maxilla and mandible, along with the increase prevalence of a positive overjet with the associated elimination of the mandibular displacement in the face-mask treatment group. A number of workers advocate the use of rapid maxillary expansion (see Chapter 13, Section 13.4.6) in conjunction with protraction face-mask therapy even if no posterior crossbites are present initially. This is in the belief that the expansion will disrupt the circum-maxillary sutures and enhance the skeletal effects. Although more recent work has suggested that this additional appliance is not essential to success, some trials have indicated that alternative expansion and constriction of the maxilla during the protraction phase may confer an advantage in the short term.

- Bone-anchored maxillary protraction (known as BAMP). Screws or mini-plates are used in the posterior maxilla and anterior mandible for Class III elastics. There is some evidence to show that a greater degree of maxillary advancement is achieved than with face-mask therapy alone, but further research is required in this area.
- A combination of these two techniques—elastics are run between skeletal anchorage in the maxilla and a face mask.

- Chin-cup—this has the effect of rotating the mandible downwards and backwards, reducing the overbite but with no reported orthopaedic change, so is a largely historic technique.

11.4.3 Orthodontic camouflage

Correction of an anterior crossbite in a Class I or mild Class III skeletal pattern can be undertaken in the mixed dentition when the unerupted permanent canines are high above the roots of the upper lateral incisors. This is often achieved with an upper removable appliance which results in tipping of the upper incisors labially to correct the anterior crossbite; this also has the benefit of moving the apices of these teeth palatally and away from the developing canines (Fig. 11.9). This can also be achieved with an upper fixed appliance. Using a fixed appliance may be cheaper and quicker, with less effect on speech than the removable appliance, but patients may complain of more difficulty biting and chewing initially with the fixed appliance. Extraction of the lower deciduous canines at the same time may allow the lower labial segment to move lingually slightly. Early correction of a Class III incisor relationship has the advantage that further forward mandibular growth may be counterbalanced by further dento-alveolar compensation (Fig. 11.10). Later in the mixed dentition when the developing canines drop down into a buccal position relative to the lateral incisor root, there may be a risk of resorption if the incisors are moved labially. In this situation, correction is then best deferred until the permanent canines have erupted.

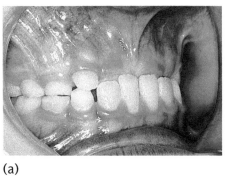 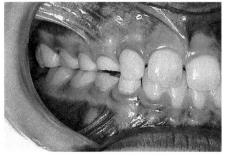

(a) (b)

Fig. 11.9 Mild Class III malocclusion that was treated in the mixed dentition by proclination of the upper labial segment with a removable appliance: (a) prior to treatment; (b) post treatment.

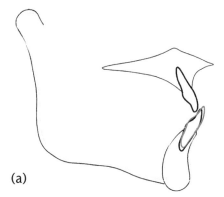

(a)

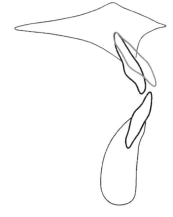

Fig. 11.11 Diagram to show how proclination of the upper incisors results in a reduction of overbite.

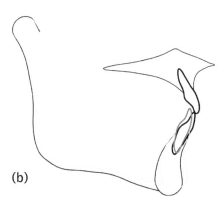

(b)

Fig. 11.10 (a) Forward growth rotation is the most common pattern of mandibular growth. In a Class III malocclusion, this will lead to a worsening of the skeletal pattern and the incisor relationship. (b) If a Class III incisor relationship is corrected in the mixed dentition, dento-alveolar compensation may help to mask the effects of further growth provided that this is not marked.

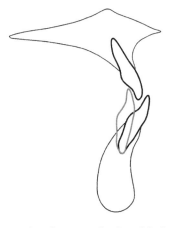

Fig. 11.12 Diagram to show how retroclination of the lower incisors results in an increase of overbite.

Orthodontic correction of a Class III incisor relationship can be achieved by proclination of the upper incisors, retroclination of the lower incisors, or a combination of both. Proclination of the upper incisors reduces the overbite (Fig. 11.11) whereas retroclination of the lower incisors helps to increase overbite (Fig. 11.12). Although the pitfalls of significant movement of the lower labial segment have been emphasized in earlier chapters, in the correction of Class III malocclusions, if the positions of the upper and lower incisors are adjusted within the zone of soft tissue balance

then, provided that there is an adequate overbite and further growth is not unfavourable, the corrected incisor relationship has a good chance of stability. Although functional appliances can be used to advance the upper incisors and retrocline the lower incisors, in practice these tooth movements are accomplished more efficiently with fixed appliances.

Space for relief of crowding in the upper arch can often be gained by expansion of the arch anteriorly to correct the incisor relationship and/or buccolingually to correct buccal segment crossbites. Therefore, it may be prudent to delay permanent extractions until after the crossbite is corrected and the degree of crowding is reassessed (Fig. 11.13). Expansion of the upper arch to correct a crossbite will have the effect of reducing overbite, which is a disadvantage in Class III cases. This reduction in overbite occurs because expansion of the upper arch is achieved primarily by tilting the upper premolars and molars buccally, which results in the palatal cusps of these teeth swinging down and 'propping open' the occlusion (see Fig. 13.11). Therefore, if upper arch expansion is indicated and the overbite is reduced, expansion should be achieved using rectangular archwires with buccal root torque added to try and minimize this sequela.

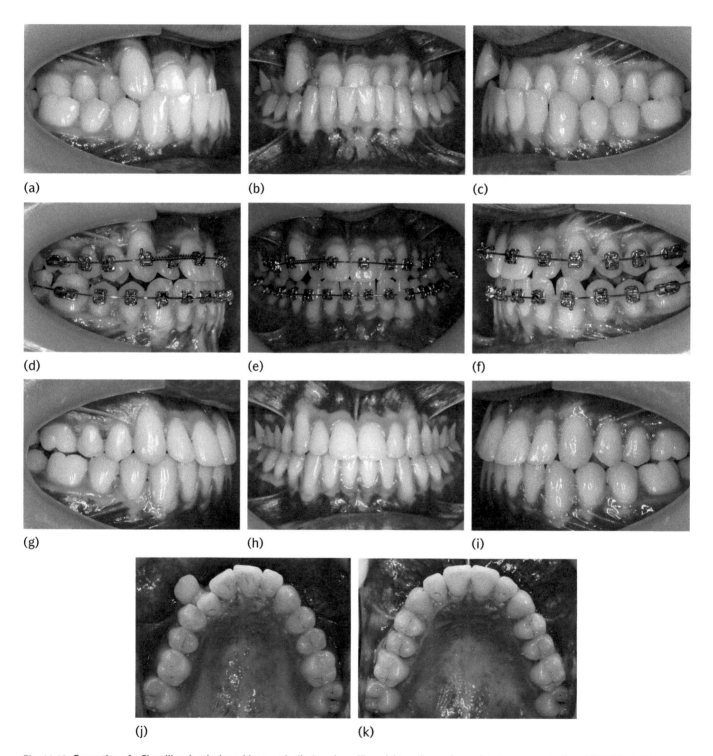

Fig. 11.13 Correction of a Class III malocclusion with severely displaced maxillary right canine and associated upper centreline shift to the right. (a–c) Initial presentation; (d–f) appliances *in situ*; (g–i) completed treatment with arch alignment and correction of the anterior and posterior crossbites; (j, k) before and after maxillary arch alignment.

Space is required in the lower arch for retroclination of the lower labial segment, and therefore extractions may be required unless the arch is naturally spaced. Use of a round archwire in the lower arch and a rectangular arch in the upper arch along with judicious space closure can be used to help correct the incisor relationship (Fig. 11.14).

Intermaxillary Class III elastic traction (see Chapter 15, Section 15.4.6) from the lower labial segment to the upper molars can also be used to help move the upper arch forwards and the lower arch backwards, but care is required to avoid extrusion of the molars which will reduce the overbite.

A patient treated using orthodontic camouflage is shown in Fig. 11.14.

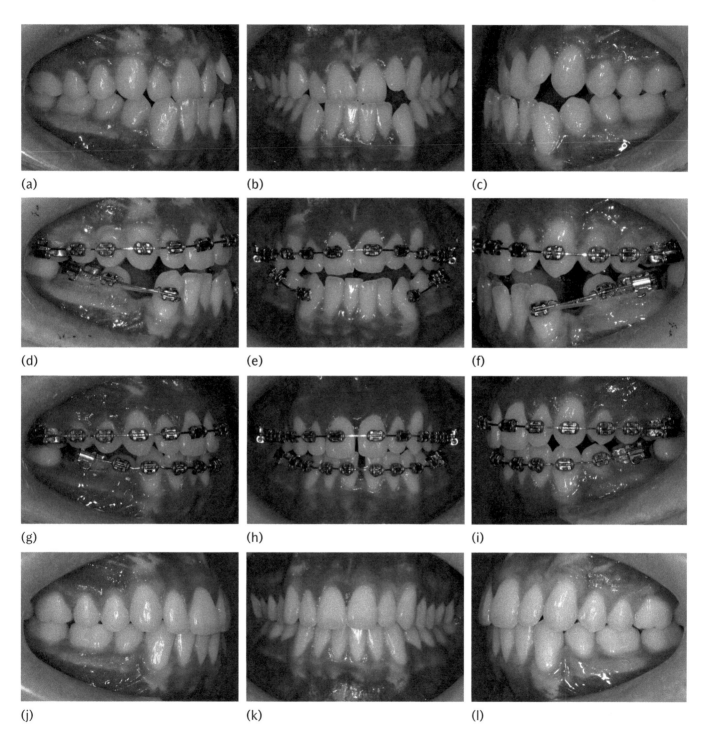

Fig. 11.14 Patient with Class III malocclusion on a Class III skeletal pattern with increased vertical skeletal proportions and crowding. Orthodontic camouflage was the approach used and involved the extraction of the mandibular first premolars and fixed appliances. (a–c) Initial presentation; (d–f) upper fixed appliance and lower sectional appliance to conserve mandibular posterior anchorage; (g–i) upper and lower fixed appliances with round wire in the mandibular arch to help control reverse overjet correction; (j–l) post treatment.

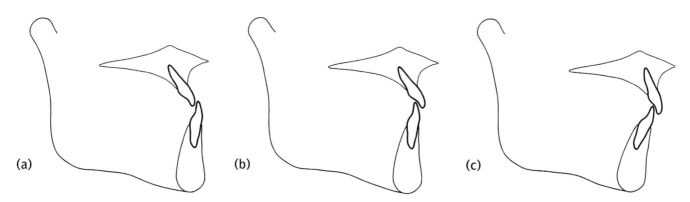

Fig. 11.15 (a) Severe Class III malocclusion with dento-alveolar compensation. (b) Without reduction of the dento-alveolar compensation, surgery to produce a Class I incisor relationship will only achieve a limited correction of the underlying skeletal pattern, thus constraining the overall aesthetic result. (c) Decompensation of the incisors to bring them nearer to their correct axial inclination allows a complete correction of the underlying skeletal pattern.

11.4.4 Surgery

In a proportion of cases, the severity of the skeletal pattern and/or the presence of a reduced overbite or an anterior open bite preclude orthodontics alone, and surgery is necessary to correct the underlying skeletal discrepancy. It is impossible to produce hard and fast guidelines as to when to choose surgery rather than orthodontic camouflage, but it has been suggested that surgery is almost always required if the value for the ANB angle is below −4° and the inclination of the lower incisors to the mandibular plane is less than 80°. However, the cephalometric and clinical findings, in all three planes of space, should be considered in conjunction with the patient's concerns and facial appearance.

For those patients where orthodontic camouflage treatment will be challenging due to the severity of the skeletal pattern and/or a lack of overbite, a surgical approach should be considered before any permanent extractions are carried out, and preferably before any appliance treatment. The reason for this is that management of Class III malocclusions by orthodontics alone involves dento-alveolar compensation of the underlying skeletal pattern. However, in order to achieve a satisfactory occlusal and facial result with a surgical approach, any dento-alveolar compensation must first be removed or reduced (Fig. 11.15). For example, if lower premolars are extracted in an attempt to retract the lower labial segment but this fails and a surgical approach is subsequently necessary, the pre-surgical orthodontic phase will probably involve proclination of the incisors to a more average inclination with reopening of the extraction spaces and possible subsequent restoration. This is a frustrating experience for both patient and operator.

Because the actual surgery needs to be delayed until the growth rate has diminished to adult levels, planning and commencement of a combined orthodontic and orthognathic approach is best delayed until around the age of 16 years. This has the advantage that the patient is of an age when they can make up their own mind as to whether they wish to proceed with a combined approach. As the pre-surgical phase of orthodontic treatment is likely to take 18–24 months, this will allow for any further adverse facial growth to occur prior to surgery at around 18 years old. The patient will then undergo finishing orthodontic treatment for about 6–12 months postoperatively to optimize the occlusal result. An example of a patient treated by a combination of orthodontics and surgery is shown in Fig. 11.16. Surgical approaches to the correction of Class III malocclusions are considered in Chapter 22.

Key points

- Growth is often unfavourable in Class III malocclusions.
- If orthopaedic treatment might be an option then it is important to refer the patient to a specialist before 10 years of age.

Relevant Cochrane review

Watkinson, S., Harrison, J. E., Furness, S., and Worthington, H. V. (2013). Orthodontic treatment for prominent lower front teeth (Class III malocclusion) in children. *Cochrane Database of Systematic Reviews* Issue 9, Art. No.: CD003451. DOI: 10.1002/14651858.CD003451.pub2 https://www.cochranelibrary.com/cdsr/doi/10.1002/14651858.CD003451.pub2/full
This review included seven randomized controlled trials and indicated that there was some evidence that the use of a face mask to correct a Class III incisor relationship was effective on a short-term basis. There was no evidence to show whether the short-term benefits will be maintained when the child is fully matured and the use of rapid maxillary expansion solely as an adjunct to improve the efficacy of face-mask treatment cannot be recommended. The studies were generally of poor quality with further research required.

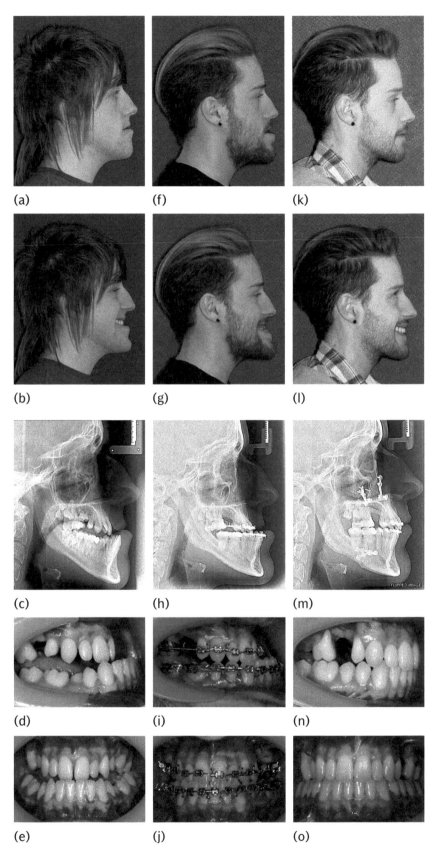

Fig. 11.16 Patient with a severe Class III skeletal pattern, further complicated by developmentally absent maxillary second premolars and grossly infra-occluded deciduous predecessors, treated with a combination of orthodontics and bimaxillary orthognathic surgery: (a–e) initial presentation; (f–j) post-orthodontic decompensation; (k–o) post treatment.

Principal sources and further reading

Baccetti T., Rey, D., Oberti, G., Stahl, F., and McNamara, J. A. (2009). Long-term outcomes of Class III treatment with mandibular cervical headgear followed by fixed appliances. *Angle Orthodontist*, **79**, 828–34. [DOI: 10.2319/111408-580.1] [PubMed: 19705951].
The patients in the treatment group were followed up over 5 years. The favourable dento-skeletal changes seen were maintained.

Battagel, J. M. (1993). The aetiological factors in Class III malocclusion. *European Journal of Orthodontics*, **15**, 347–70. [DOI: 10.1093/ejo/15.5.347] [PubMed: 8223970].

Bryant, P. M. F. (1981). Mandibular rotation and Class III malocclusion. *British Journal of Orthodontics*, **8**, 61–75. [DOI: 10.1179/bjo.8.2.61] [PubMed: 6942886].
This paper is worth reading for the introduction alone, which contains a very good discussion of growth rotations. The study itself looks at the effect of growth rotations and treatment upon Class III malocclusions.

Cevidanes, L., Baccetti, T., Franchi, L., McNamara, J.A., and De Clerk, H. (2010). Comparison of two protocols for maxillary expansion: bone anchors versus face mask with rapid maxillary expansion. *Angle Orthodontist*, **80**, 799–806. [DOI: 10.2319/111709-651.1] [PubMed: 20578848]
An interesting paper.

De Toffol, L., Pavoni, C. Baccetti, T., Franchi, L., and Cozza, P. (2008). Orthopedic treatment outcomes in Class III malocclusion. *Angle Orthodontist*, **78**, 561–73. [DOI: 10.2319/030207-108.1] [PubMed: 18416617]
Unfortunately, like many systematic reviews the available evidence on this topic at the time of this review was not strong.

Fareen, N., Alam, M. K., Khamis, M. F., and Mokhtar, N. (2017). Treatment effects of reverse twin-block and reverse pull fask mask on craniofacial morphology in early and late mixed dentition. *Orthodontics & Craniofacial Research*, **20**, 134–9. [DOI: **10.1111/ocr.12179**] [PubMed: 28440029]
This study indicated that reverse pull fask-mask treatment produced more favourable craniofacial changes than reverse twin-block therapy, especially in the late mixed dentition phase.

Gravely, J. F. (1984). A study of the mandibular closure path in Angle Class III relationship. *British Journal of Orthodontics*, **11**, 85–91. [DOI: 10.1179/bjo.11.2.85] [PubMed: 6587912].
A very readable and clever article which examines the displacement element of Class III malocclusions.

Kerr, W. J. S., Miller, S., and Dawber, J. E. (1992). Class III malocclusion: surgery or orthodontics? *British Journal of Orthodontics*, **19**, 21–4. [DOI: 10.1179/bjo.19.1.21] [PubMed: 1562575].

An interesting study which compares the pre-treatment lateral cephalometric radiographs of two groups of Class III cases treated by either surgery or orthodontics alone. The authors report the thresholds for three cephalometric values which would indicate when surgery is required.

Kim, J. H., Viana, M. A., Graber, T. M., Omerza, F. F., and BeGole, E. A. (1999). The effectiveness of protraction face mask therapy: a meta-analysis. *American Journal of Orthodontics and Dentofacial Orthopedics*, **115**, 675–85. [DOI: 10.1016/S0889-5406(99)70294-5] [PubMed: 10358251]

Mandall, N., DiBiase, A., Littlewood, S., Nute, S., Stivaros, N., McDowall, R., et al. (2010). Is early Class III protraction facemask treatment effective? A randomized, controlled trial: 15-month follow-up. *Journal of Orthodontics*, **37**, 149–61. [DOI: 10.1179/14653121043056] [PubMed: 20805344]
A well-designed multicentre randomized controlled trial. One of the few studies in this area to look at patient-related outcomes, but interestingly found that early treatment did not result in a clinically significant psychosocial benefit.

Mandall, N., Cousley, R., DiBiase, A., Dyer, F., Littlewood, S., Mattick, R., et al. (2016). Early class III protraction facemask treatment reduces the need for orthognathic surgery: a multi-centre, two arm parallel randomized controlled trial. *Journal of Orthodontics*, **43**, 164–75. [DOI: 10.1080/14653125.2016.1201302] [PubMed: 27564126]
An excellent multicentre randomized controlled trial which indicates the potential medium- to long-term benefits of interceptive treatment of Class III malocclusions with protraction facemask to reduce the need for orthognathic surgery in the future.

Vaughan, G. A., Mason, B., Moon, H. B., and Turley, P. K. (2005). The effects of maxillary protraction therapy with or without rapid palatal expansion: a prospective randomized clinical trial. *American Journal of Orthodontic and Dentofacial Orthopedics*, **132**, 467–74. [DOI: 10.1016/j.ajodo.2005.04.030] [PubMed: 16168327]

Wiedel, A. and Bondemark, L. (2015). Fixed versus removable orthodontic appliances to correct anterior crossbite in the mixed dentition – a randomised controlled trial. *European Journal of Orthodontics*, **32**, 123–7. [DOI: 10.1093/ejo/cju005] [PubMed: 25114123]

Woon, S. C. and Thiruvenkatachari, B (2017). Early orthodontic treatment for CIII malocclusion: a systematic review and meta-analysis. *American Journal of Orthodontics and Dentofacial Orthopedics*, **151**, 28–52. [DOI: 10.1016/j.ajodo.2016.07.017] [PubMed: 28024779]

 References for this chapter can also be found at: **www.oup.com/uk/orthodontics5e**. Where possible, these are presented as active links which direct you to the electronic version of the work, to help facilitate onward study. If you are a subscriber to that work (either individually or through an institution), and depending on your level of access, you may be able to peruse an abstract or the full article if available.

12
Anterior open bite and posterior open bite

Benjamin R. K. Lewis

Chapter contents

12.1 Definitions

- **Anterior open bite (AOB):** there is no vertical overlap of the incisors when the buccal segment teeth are in occlusion (Fig. 12.1).
- **Posterior open bite (POB):** when the teeth are in occlusion there is a space between the posterior teeth (Fig. 12.2). This can sometimes be referred to as a lateral open bite (LOB).

- **Incomplete overbite:** the lower incisors do not occlude with the opposing upper incisors or the palatal mucosa when the buccal segment teeth are in occlusion (Fig. 12.3). The overbite may be decreased or increased.

12.2 Aetiology of anterior open bite

In common with other types of malocclusion, both inherited and environmental factors are implicated in the aetiology of an AOB. These factors include the skeletal pattern, soft tissues, habits, trauma, and a localized failure of development. In many cases, the aetiology is multifactorial, and in practice it can be difficult to determine the extent to which each of these potential influences has had as the presenting malocclusions often appear similar (Box 12.1). However, a thorough history and examination, perhaps with a period of observation, may be helpful.

12.2.1 Skeletal pattern

Individuals with a tendency to vertical rather than horizontal facial growth exhibit increased vertical skeletal proportions (see Chapter 4). Where the lower face height is increased, there will be an increased

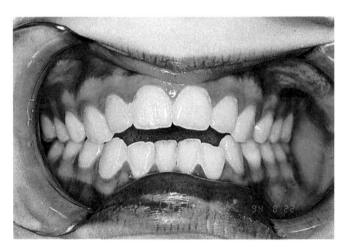

Fig. 12.1 Anterior open bite.

Box 12.1 Prevalence differs between racial groups

- Caucasians: 2–4%.
- Afro-Caribbean: 5–10%.
- Chinese: 1.5–6%.

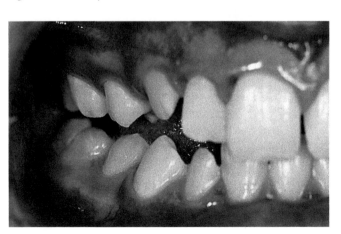

Fig. 12.2 Posterior open bite.

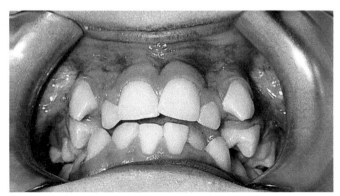

Fig. 12.3 Incomplete overbite.

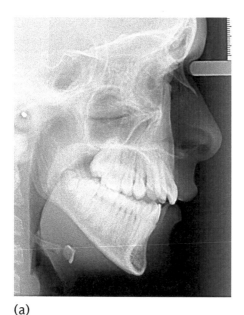

(a)

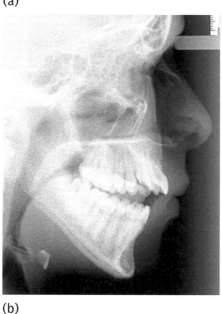

(b)

Fig. 12.4 A patient with increased vertical skeletal proportions and an anterior open bite. (a) Initial presentation; (b) deterioration 2.5 years later due to adverse vertical growth and eruption of second molars.

inter-occlusal distance between the maxilla and mandible. Although the labial segment teeth appear to be able to compensate for this to a limited extent by further eruption, where the inter-occlusal distance exceeds this compensatory ability an AOB will result. If the vertical, downwards, and backwards pattern of growth continues, the AOB will become more marked.

In this group of patients, the AOB is usually symmetrical and in the more severe cases may extend distally around the arch so that only the most posterior molars are in contact when the patient is in maximal interdigitation. The AOB can also deteriorate with the eruption of the second and third molars and vertical growth (Fig. 12.4). The vertical development of the labial segments results in typically extended

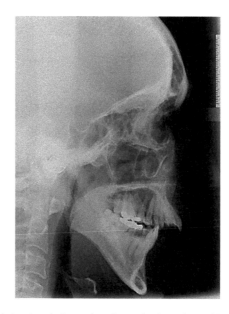

Fig. 12.5 Lateral cephalometric radiograph of a patient with a marked Class II division 1 malocclusion on a Class II skeletal pattern with increased vertical skeletal proportions. Note the thin dento-alveolar processes.

alveolar processes when viewed on a lateral cephalometric radiograph (Fig. 12.5).

AOBs can also be present in individuals as a consequence of damage to the condylar anatomy either due to local problems such as osteoarthritis, necrosis, and trauma, or due to systemic problems involving connective tissue or autoimmune disease, for example, rheumatoid arthritis.

12.2.2 Soft tissue pattern

In order to be able to swallow, it is necessary to create an anterior oral seal. In younger children the lips are often incompetent and a proportion will achieve an anterior seal by positioning their tongue forward between the anterior teeth during swallowing. Individuals with increased vertical skeletal proportions have an increased likelihood of incompetent lips and may continue to achieve an anterior oral seal in this manner even when the soft tissues have matured. This type of swallowing pattern is also seen in patients with an AOB due to a digit-sucking habit (see Section 12.2.3). In these situations, the behaviour of the tongue is adaptive and as such can potentially revert to a conventional swallowing pattern once the AOB has been closed. An endogenous or primary tongue thrust is rare, but it is difficult to distinguish it from an adaptive tongue thrust as the presenting occlusal features are similar. However, it has been suggested that an endogenous tongue thrust is associated with sigmatism (lisping), and in some cases, both the upper and lower incisors are proclined by the action of the tongue.

The facial and masticatory soft tissue environment can also be affected by generalized muscular dysfunctionality as demonstrated in individuals with cerebral palsy and muscular dystrophy. These conditions tend to lead to low tonicity of the facial muscles and uncoordinated movements of the lips and tongue with lip incompetency, which

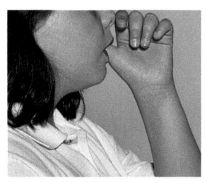
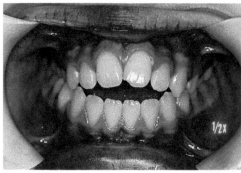

Fig. 12.6 The occlusal effects of a persistent digit-sucking habit. Note the anterior open bite and the unilateral posterior crossbite.

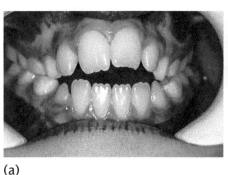
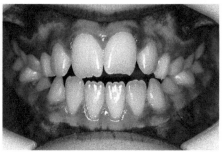

(a)   (b)

Fig. 12.7 A patient aged 10 years with a dummy-sucking habit: (a) at presentation; (b) 4 months after habit stopped.

could explain the increased finding of AOBs and increased vertical proportions in these individuals

12.2.3 Habits

See also Chapter 9, Section 9.1.4

Oral habits are common in young children and the consequences of a habit will depend upon its duration and intensity. If a persistent digit-sucking habit continues into the mixed and permanent dentitions, this can result in an AOB due to restriction of development of the incisors by the finger or thumb (Fig. 12.6). Characteristically, the AOB produced is asymmetrical (unless the patient sucks two fingers) and it is often associated with a posterior crossbite due to constriction of the upper arch which is believed to be caused by cheek pressure and a low tongue position.

After a sucking habit stops the open bite tends to at least partially resolve (Fig. 12.7), although this may take several months. During this period, the tongue may continue to come forward during swallowing to achieve an anterior seal and as a consequence may limit spontaneous AOB correction. In a small proportion of cases, where the habit has continued until growth is complete, the open bite may persist.

12.2.4 Localized failure of development

This is seen in patients with a cleft of the lip and alveolus (see also Chapter 24, Fig. 24.3), although rarely it may occur for no apparent reason.

12.2.5 Mouth breathing

It has been suggested that the open-mouth posture adopted by individuals who habitually mouth breathe, either due to nasal

obstruction or habit, results in overdevelopment of the buccal segment teeth. This leads to an increase in the height of the lower third of the face and consequently a greater incidence of an AOB. In support of this argument, it has been shown that patients referred for tonsillectomy and adenoidectomy had significantly increased lower facial heights compared with controls, and that postoperatively, the disparity between the two groups diminished. However, the differences demonstrated were small. Other workers have shown that children referred to ear, nose, and throat clinics exhibit the same range of malocclusions as the general population, and no relationship has been demonstrated between nasal airway resistance and skeletal pattern in normal individuals.

On balance, it would appear that mouth breathing per se does not play a significant role in the development of AOB in most patients.

12.2.6 Trauma

See also Chapter 8, Section 8.9.

Trauma to the upper anterior teeth can lead to intrusion injuries which can result in an AOB. Traumatically intruded teeth can sometimes have the potential to erupt spontaneously, especially in young patients with incomplete root development. Alternatively, surgical repositioning or an interceptive course of orthodontic treatment can be undertaken to reposition the teeth and gently extrude them back to their original vertical position. If the episode of trauma resulted in avulsion of a permanent tooth/teeth with subsequent reimplantation, then there is a risk of ankylosis occurring. Depending on the age and skeletal maturity of the patient when the ankylosis occurs, then this can result in a marked restriction of the future development of the dento-alveolar complex.

12.3 Management of anterior open bite

Notwithstanding the difficulties faced in determining the aetiology, treatment of an AOB is one of the more challenging aspects of orthodontics. Management of an AOB due purely to a digit-sucking habit can be straightforward, but where the skeletal pattern, growth, and/or soft tissue environment are unfavourable, correction without resorting to orthognathic surgery may not be possible.

In the mixed dentition, a digit-sucking habit that has resulted in an AOB should be gently discouraged. If a child is keen to stop, a removable or bonded appliance can be fitted to act as a reminder. However, if the child derives emotional support from their habit and does not want to stop, forcing them to wear an appliance to discourage it is unlikely to be successful, and even if the habit did stop in the short term, it is very likely that it would recommence on discontinuing the appliance. The simplest type of appliance is a removable plate with a long labial bow for anterior retention and cribs on the first molars. After fitting, the acrylic behind the upper incisors should be trimmed to allow any spontaneous alignment. Once the permanent dentition is established, more active steps can be taken, usually in combination with treatment for other aspects of the malocclusion.

A period of observation may be helpful in the management of children with an AOB which is not associated with a digit-sucking habit (Fig. 12.4). In some cases, an AOB may reduce spontaneously, possibly due to the maturation of the soft tissues and improved lip competence, or favourable growth. Skeletal open bites with increased vertical proportions are often associated with a downward and backward rotation of the mandible with growth. Obviously, if growth is unfavourable, it is better to know this before planning treatment rather than experiencing difficulties once treatment is under way.

There is no evidence to show that correction of AOB improves lisping/speech problems and this is best managed by the involvement of a speech and language therapist after any orthodontic intervention to correct the malocclusion.

The best predictor of stability following correction is the extent of the AOB at the outset. Some advocate active retention, for example, continuing with high-pull headgear if this has been used during treatment. Certainly, there is some evidence to suggest that this can be an advantage when molar intrusion has been achieved using temporary anchorage devices (see Section 12.3.1).

12.3.1 Approaches to the management of anterior open bite

There are three possible approaches to management.

Acceptance of the anterior open bite

In this case, treatment is aimed at relief of any crowding and alignment of the arches. This approach can be considered in the following situations (particularly if the AOB does not present a problem to the patient):

- Mild cases.
- Where the soft tissue environment is not favourable, for example, where the lips are markedly incompetent and/or an endogenous tongue thrust is suspected (Fig. 12.8). Sometimes it is possible to

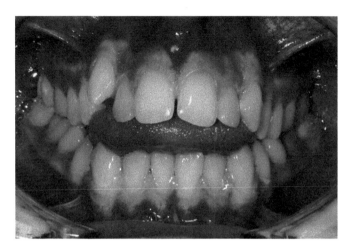

Fig. 12.8 A forward lying tongue at rest rather than just when swallowing which suggests a greater risk of relapse if any intervention was undertaken, unless the tongue position can be retrained using a tongue crib (not shown here).

retrain the tongue position with a tongue crib, encouraging the patient to keep the tongue tip on the anterior palate, rather than between the incisors.
- More severe malocclusions where the patient is not motivated towards surgery.

Orthodontic correction of the anterior open bite

If growth and the soft tissue environment are favourable, an orthodontic solution to address the AOB can be considered. A careful assessment should be carried out, including the anteroposterior and vertical skeletal pattern, the feasibility of the tooth movements required, and the likelihood of post-treatment stability.

Extrusion of the incisors to close an AOB is generally inadvisable as there is a significant risk of vertical relapse once the appliances are removed. The few occasions when incisor extrusion could be considered are in cases where there has been a previous non-intrinsic intrusion force which has been subsequently removed, such as a digit-sucking habit or after an episode of trauma. Rather, treatment should aim to try and intrude the molars, or at least control their vertical development (Box 12.2). This will allow for a mandibular clockwise forward rotation to close the AOB.

Box 12.2 Methods of intruding the molars

- High-pull headgear
- Fixed appliance mechanics
- Buccal capping on a removable/functional appliance
- Repelling magnets
- Temporary anchorage devices (TADs).

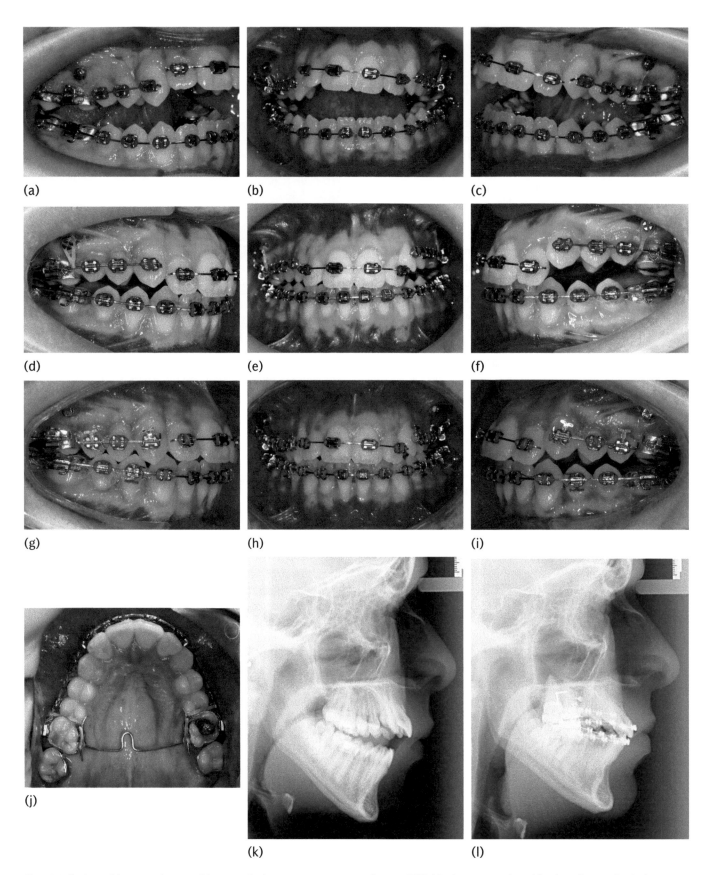

Fig. 12.9 Patient with an anterior open bite treated using temporary screw anchorage (TADs) in the upper arch and fixed appliances: (a–c) placement of TADs buccally and elastic chain to arms on a transpalatal arch (TPA). Note the sectioned wires in the upper arch which allow the upper incisors to act as a reference point to judge the amount of posterior intrusion. If the whole arch is connected there is a risk of extruding the incisors and an anterior rotation of the maxillary plane. (d–f) True intrusion of the buccal segments with a positive overjet established—note the vertical movement of the canines relative to the lateral incisors. (g–i) Following one visit of settling elastics. The buccal wires are sectioned to allow the settling elastics to bring the premolars and canines into occlusion. (j) TPA *in situ* to prevent buccal flaring of the molars when the intrusion elastics are placed. (k, l) Close-up views on the lateral cephalographs before and after intrusion—note the vertical movement of the molar apices.

In the milder malocclusions, the use of high-pull headgear during conventional treatment may suffice. In cases with a more marked AOB associated with a Class II skeletal pattern, a removable appliance or a functional appliance incorporating buccal blocks and high-pull headgear can be used to try to restrain vertical maxillary growth. In order to achieve true growth modification, it is necessary to apply an intrusive force to the maxilla for at least 14–16 hours per day during the pubertal growth spurt, and preferably this would be continued until the growth rate has slowed. This is only achievable with excellent patient cooperation and favourable growth.

Modified functional appliances are also used for Class II malocclusions with increased vertical proportions. A number of designs have been described, but usually they incorporate high-pull headgear and buccal capping (see Chapter 19, Section 19.7).

Successful reduction of AOB has been achieved using fixed appliance mechanics that tip the molar teeth distally. This can be achieved using multi-loop archwires, otherwise known as 'Kim mechanics', or continuous 'rocking-horse' archwires in conjunction with anterior vertical elastics. The rationale is that as the molars tip distally, the posterior vertical dimensions reduce and the vertical elastics prevent the incisors from intruding and allow them to come together as the posterior teeth intrude.

The introduction of skeletal anchorage devices has also expanded the envelope in terms of the severity of AOB that can be treated non-surgically. A greater degree of molar intrusion can be achieved utilizing bone anchorage either with screws (Fig. 12.9) or plates (see Chapter 15, Fig. 15.18). There is a risk of tipping the molars towards the traction force so some advocate using both palatal and buccal implants. Not surprisingly the evidence suggests that relapse following this mode of treatment is greatest in the first year, so active retention is often advocated. This involves continuing with an intrusive force from the skeletal anchorage to the retention appliances. Further work is required to determine if this just offsets the timing of, rather than the extent of, relapse.

In cases with bimaxillary crowding and proclination, relief of crowding with retraction and alignment of the incisors can result in a reduction of an open bite (Fig. 12.10). Stability of this correction is more likely if the lips were incompetent prior to treatment but become competent following retroclination of the incisors.

If it is difficult to ascertain the exact aetiology of an AOB but a primary tongue thrust is suspected, even though these are uncommon, it is wise to err on the side of caution regarding treatment objectives (and extractions) and to warn patients of the possibility of relapse with the re-establishment of an AOB and intra-arch spacing if extractions were undertaken. An alternative is to try and retrain the tongue position with a crib appliance.

Surgery

This option can be considered, once growth has slowed to adult levels, for severe problems with a skeletal aetiology and/or where dental compensation will not give an aesthetic or stable result. In some patients, an AOB is associated with a 'gummy' smile which can be difficult to reduce by orthodontics alone, necessitating a surgical approach. The same principle is utilized as when using temporary anchorage devices. The maxillary posterior teeth are moved up vertically allowing the mandible to auto-rotate and close the AOB (Fig. 12.11). The assessment and management of such cases is discussed in Chapter 22.

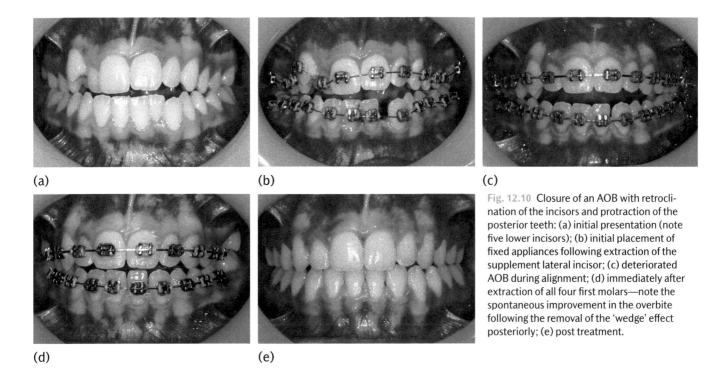

(a)　(b)　(c)

(d)　(e)

Fig. 12.10 Closure of an AOB with retroclination of the incisors and protraction of the posterior teeth: (a) initial presentation (note five lower incisors); (b) initial placement of fixed appliances following extraction of the supplement lateral incisor; (c) deteriorated AOB during alignment; (d) immediately after extraction of all four first molars—note the spontaneous improvement in the overbite following the removal of the 'wedge' effect posteriorly; (e) post treatment.

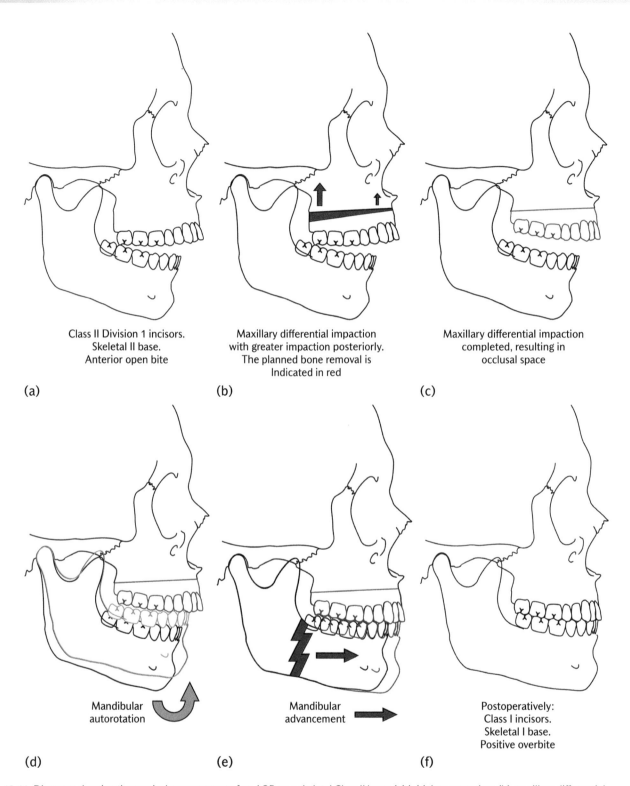

Class II Division 1 incisors.
Skeletal II base.
Anterior open bite

(a)

Maxillary differential impaction
with greater impaction posteriorly.
The planned bone removal is
Indicated in red

(b)

Maxillary differential impaction
completed, resulting in
occlusal space

(c)

Mandibular
autorotation

(d)

Mandibular
advancement

(e)

Postoperatively:
Class I incisors.
Skeletal I base.
Positive overbite

(f)

Fig. 12.11 Diagrams showing the surgical management of an AOB on a skeletal Class II base: (a) initial presentation; (b) maxillary differential impaction where the posterior teeth are lifted up; (c) occlusal space generated by the maxillary differential impaction; (d) mandibular autorotation to close the AOB; (e) mandibular advancement to address the retrognathia; (f) post-surgical correction.

12.3.2 Management of patients with increased vertical skeletal proportions and reduced overbite

The treatment specifics of patients with increased vertical skeletal proportions will obviously be influenced by the other aspects of their malocclusion (see appropriate chapters), but management of the mechanics requires careful planning to try and prevent an iatrogenic deterioration of the vertical excess. The following points should be borne in mind:

- Space closure appears to occur more readily in patients with increased vertical skeletal proportions. This will have an influence on anchorage considerations (see Chapter 15).

- Avoid extruding the molars as this will result in an increase of the lower facial height. If headgear is required, a direction of pull above the occlusal plane is necessary, that is, high-pull headgear. Cervical-pull headgear is contraindicated.

- Upper arch expansion should be undertaken with care. When the upper arch is expanded, the upper molars are tilted buccally which may result in the palatal cusps being tipped downwards (see Chapter 13, Fig. 13.11). If arch expansion is required, this is best achieved in combination with a fixed appliance so that buccal root torque can be used to limit this downward tipping of the palatal cusps.

- Use Class II or Class III intermaxillary traction minimally as this may extrude the molars.

12.4 Posterior open bite

POBs affecting the permanent dentition occur more rarely than an AOB and the aetiology is less well understood. In some cases, an increase in the vertical skeletal proportions is a factor, although this is more commonly associated with an AOB which also extends posteriorly. A LOB is occasionally seen in association with early extraction of first permanent molars (Fig. 12.12), possibly occurring as a result of lateral tongue spread.

12.4.1 Infra-occluded deciduous molars

Infra-occlusion, due to ankylosis, of the deciduous molars, which affects 8–14% of children aged 6 to 11 years, can result in a localized POB (Fig. 12.13) The current evidence suggests that this is best managed with observation as up to 96% of ankylosed deciduous molars, which have a permanent successor developing in a reasonable position, will undergo spontaneous exfoliation within 12 months of their normal range of exfoliation. However, if there is evidence of significant infra-occlusion of the deciduous tooth, ectopic development of the permanent successor, significant tipping of adjacent teeth, and relative spacing or infra-occlusion of the adjacent permanent dentition, then the extraction of the infra-occluded deciduous molar should be considered.

If there is no permanent successor, then the deciduous molar is unlikely to exfoliate naturally within the usual age range. As such, there is an increased risk of ankylosis and subsequent infra-occlusion. These situations are best managed on a case-by-case basis taking into consideration the factors mentioned above as well as the patient's age and the long-term orthodontic and restorative implications of the hypodontia (see Chapter 23).

12.4.2 Eruption disturbances of permanent teeth

A POB can also be seen in cases with eruption disturbances. The two main categories of eruption disorder are primary failure of eruption (PFE) and mechanical failure of eruption (MFE). PFE is a condition which almost exclusively affects molar teeth and affects all teeth distal to the most mesially affected tooth (Fig. 12.14). Although these teeth are not ankylosed they do not respond normally to orthodontic forces and indeed usually become ankylosed if traction is applied.

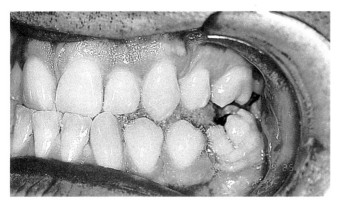

Fig. 12.12 POB in a patient who had all four first permanent molars extracted in the mixed dentition.

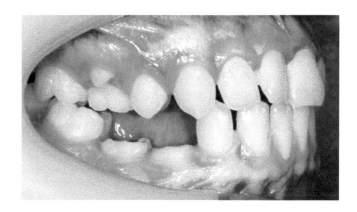

Fig. 12.13 Lateral open bite due to infra-occluded deciduous teeth.

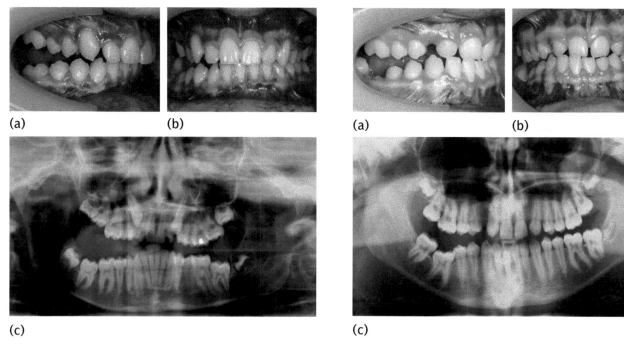

(a) (b)

(c)

Fig. 12.14 (a–c) Primary failure of eruption of the posterior teeth on the right-hand side—note that the open bite increases as you progress further back into the mouth.

(a) (b)

(c)

Fig. 12.15 (a–c) Mechanical failure of eruption of the mandibular right first permanent molar and the appearance on the OPT radiograph—note that the mandibular right second molar has continued to erupt.

PFE has recently been linked to a specific gene in several familial cases. In contrast, MFE is associated with radiographical signs of ankylosis and often affects the first permanent molar with the more distal teeth developing and erupting normally (Fig. 12.15). In both types, the affected teeth may erupt and then cease to keep pace with continued vertical development becoming relatively infra-occluded, or may fail to erupt at all. Extraction is often the only treatment alternative.

12.4.3 Condylar hyperplasia

More rarely, POB can be seen in association with unilateral condylar hyperplasia, which also results in facial asymmetry. If this problem is suspected, a bone scan may be required. If the scan indicates excessive cell division in the condylar head region, a condylectomy alone, or in combination with orthognathic surgery to correct the resultant deformity, may be required.

Key points

- The definitive aetiology of AOBs and POBs can be difficult to confirm as the resulting presentation will often have similar appearances.
- Cessation advice should be given as soon as possible to help stop any oral habits which are thought to contribute to the malocclusion.
- Adverse facial growth can worsen AOB and POB so a period of monitoring can be useful.
- There is generally a higher risk of relapse following treatment for AOB, especially if there is a persistent soft tissue component to the aetiology.

Relevant Cochrane reviews

Lentini-Oliveira, D. A., Carvalho, F. R., Rodrigues, C. G., Ye, Q., Prado, L. B., Prado, G. F., et al. (2014). Orthodontic and orthopaedic treatment for anterior open bite in children. *Cochrane Database of Systematic Reviews*, Issue 9, Art. No.: CD005515. DOI: 10.1002/14651858.CD005515.pub3 https://www.cochranelibrary.com/cdsr/doi/10.1002/14651858.CD005515.pub3/full
Three randomized controlled trials were included in this review; however, due to the quality of the evidence, the authors concluded that recommendations for clinical practice could not be made.

Borrie, F. R. P., Bearn, D. R., Innes, N. P., and Iheozor-Ejiofor, Z. (2015). Interventions for the cessation of non-nutritive sucking habits in children. *Cochrane Database of Systematic Reviews*, Issue 3, Art. No.: CD008694. DOI: 10.1002/14651858.CD008694.pub2 https://www.cochranelibrary.com/cdsr/doi/10.1002/14651858.CD008694.pub2/full
Six trials which looked at the effectiveness of methods to stop digit-sucking habits were included in this review. The authors concluded that there was low-quality evidence that orthodontic appliances (palatal arch and palatal crib) and psychological interventions (including positive and negative reinforcement) are effective at improving sucking cessation in children. There was some evidence that the palatal crib was effective at improving the AOB reduction. The authors felt that further research was required.

Principal sources and further reading

Baek, M. -S., Choi, Y. -J., Yu, H. -S., Lee, K. -L., Kwak, J., and Park, Y. C. (2010). Long-term stability of anterior open-bite treatment by intrusion of maxillary posterior teeth. *American Journal of Orthodontics and Dentofacial Orthopedics*, **138**, 396.e1–396.e9 (Editorial **138**, 396–8). [DOI: 10.1016/j.ajodo.2010.05.006] [PubMed: 20889043]
A short online article with an interesting Q&A section with the lead author and the journal's editor.

Chate, R. A. C. (1994). The burden of proof: a critical review of orthodontic claims made by some general practitioners. *American Journal of Orthodontics and Dentofacial Orthopedics*, **106**, 96–105. [DOI: 10.1016/S0889-5406(94)70026-5] [PubMed: 8017355].
An excellent discussion of the evidence on the postulated and actual effects of mouth breathing upon the dentition, plus much other information. Highly recommended.

Dung, D. J. and Smith, R. J. (1988). Cephalometric and clinical diagnoses of open bite tendency. *American Journal of Orthodontics and Dentofacial Orthopedics*, **94**, 484–90. [DOI: 10.1016/0889-5406(88)90006-6] [PubMed: 3195512]
The authors also look at predictors of successful treatment.

Frazier-Bowers, S. A., Koehler, K. E., Ackerman, J. L., and Proffit, W. R. (2007). Primary failure of eruption: further chacterization of a rare eruption disorder. *American Journal of Orthodontics and Dentofacial Orthopedics*, **131**, 578.e1–11. [DOI: 10.1016/j.ajodo.2006.09.038] [PubMed: 17482073]
An update with clinical and radiographic images from the authors who first described the condition.

Greenlee, G. M., Huang, G. J. Chen, S. S. -H., Chen, J., Koepsell, T., and Hujoel, P. (2010). Stability of treatment for anterior open-bite malocclusion: a meta-analysis. *American Journal of Orthodontics and Dentofacial Orthopedics*, **139**, 154–9. [DOI: 10.1016/j.ajodo.2010.10.019] [PubMed: 21300243].
Unfortunately, the authors were only able to find case series types of studies that satisfied the inclusion criteria, therefore their findings must be viewed with caution.

Kim, Y. H. (1987). Anterior open bite and its treatment with multi-loop edgewise archwire. *Angle Orthodontist*, **57**, 290–321. [DOI: 10.1043/0003-3219(1987)057<0290:AOAITW>2.0.CO;2] [PubMed: 3479033].

Lin, L. -H., Huang, G. -W., and Chen, C. -S. (2013). Etiology and treatment modalities of anterior open bite malocclusion. *Journal of Experimental and Clinical Medicine*, **5**, 1–4. [DOI: 10.1016/j.jecm.2013.01.004]
A good résumé of AOB malocclusions.

Linder-Aronson, S. (1970). Adenoids: their effect on mode of breathing and nasal airflow and their relationship to characteristics of the facial skeleton and dentition. *Acta Otolaryngologica (Supplement)*, **265**, 1–132. [PubMed: 5272140]

Lopez-Gavito, G., Wallen, T. R., Little, R. M., and Joondeph, D. R. (1985). Anterior open-bite malocclusion: a longitudinal 10-year postretention evaluation of orthodontically treated patients. *American Journal of Orthodontics*, **87**, 175–86. [DOI: 10.1016/0002-9416(85)90038-7] [PubMed: 3856391]

Mizrahi, E. (1978). A review of anterior open bite. *British Journal of Orthodontics*, **5**, 21–7.
A worthy review. [DOI: 10.1179/bjo.5.1.21] [PubMed: 284793].

Orton, H. S. (1990). *Functional Appliances in Orthodontic Treatment*. London: Quintessence Books.
A beautifully illustrated and informative book. The maxillary and buccal intrusion splints are described.

Tieu, L. D., Walker, S. L., Major, M. P., and Flores-Mir, C. (2013). Management of ankylosed primary molars with permanent successors – a systematic review. *Journal of the American Dental Association*, **114**, 602–11. [DOI: 10.14219/jada.archive.2013.0171]
A good review of the literature.

Vaden, J. L. (1998). Non-surgical treatment of the patient with vertical discrepancy. *American Journal of Orthodontics and Dentofacial Orthopedics*, **113**, 567–82. [DOI: 10.1016/S0889-5406(98)70268-9] [PubMed: 9598615]

 References for this chapter can also be found at: **www.oup.com/uk/orthodontics5e**. Where possible, these are presented as active links which direct you to the electronic version of the work, to help facilitate onward study. If you are a subscriber to that work (either individually or through an institution), and depending on your level of access, you may be able to peruse an abstract or the full article if available.

13
Crossbites
Benjamin R. K. Lewis

Chapter contents

13.1 Definitions

- **Crossbite:** a discrepancy in the buccolingual relationship of the upper and lower teeth. By convention, the transverse relationship of the arches is usually described in terms of the position of the lower teeth relative to the upper teeth. However, more recently, some clinicians describe the crossbite by using the individual upper teeth, as it is these teeth that often need to be moved to correct the crossbite.

- **Buccal crossbite:** the buccal cusps of the lower teeth occlude buccal to the buccal cusps of the upper teeth (Fig. 13.1).

- **Lingual crossbite:** the buccal cusps of the lower teeth occlude lingual to the lingual cusps of the upper teeth. This is also known as a scissors bite (Fig. 13.2).

- **Displacement:** on closing from the rest position, the mandible encounters a deflecting contact(s) and is displaced to the left or the right, and/or anteriorly, into maximum interdigitation (Fig. 13.3).

13.2 Aetiology

A variety of factors acting either singly or in combination can lead to the development of a crossbite.

13.2.1 Local causes

The most common local cause is crowding where one or two teeth are displaced from the arch. For example, a crossbite of an upper lateral incisor often arises due to lack of space between the upper central incisor and the deciduous canine, which forces the lateral incisor to erupt palatally and in linguo-occlusion with the opposing teeth. Posteriorly, early loss of a second deciduous molar may result in forward movement of the upper first permanent molar, with the resulting loss of space forcing the second premolar to erupt palatally. Also, the retention of

a primary tooth or the presence of a supernumerary tooth can deflect the eruption of the permanent successor leading to a crossbite.

13.2.2 Skeletal

Generally, the greater the number of teeth in crossbite, the greater the skeletal component of the aetiology. A crossbite of the buccal segments may be due to a true transverse discrepancy between the arches, or as a result of an anteroposterior discrepancy, which results in a relative mismatch of arch widths with a wider part of one arch occluding with a narrower part of the opposing jaw. For this reason, buccal crossbites of an entire buccal segment are most commonly associated with Class III malocclusions (Fig. 13.4), and lingual crossbites are associated

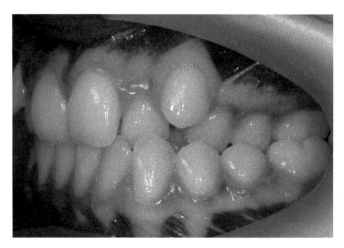

Fig. 13.1 A buccal crossbite.

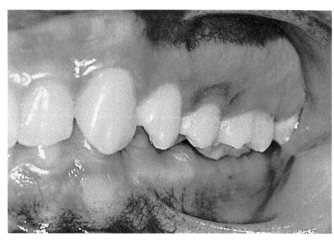

Fig. 13.2 A lingual (scissors) crossbite.

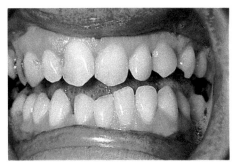
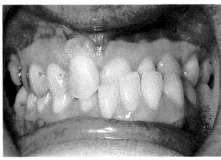

Fig. 13.3 Displacement on closure into crossbite.

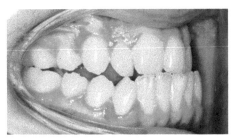
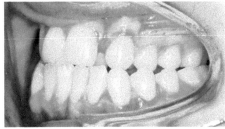

Fig. 13.4 A Class III malocclusion with buccal crossbite.

with Class II malocclusions. Anterior crossbites involving all the incisors are also predominantly associated with Class III skeletal patterns. Crossbites, usually unilateral, can also be associated with true skeletal asymmetry and/or asymmetric mandibular growth.

13.2.3 Soft tissues

Non-nutritive sucking habits are often associated with a posterior crossbite because the habit leads to a lowered position of the tongue with a negative pressure being generated intra-orally.

13.2.4 Rarer causes

These include cleft lip and palate, where growth in the width of the upper arch is restrained by the scar tissue of the cleft repair. Trauma to, or pathology of, the temporomandibular joints can lead to restriction of growth of the mandible on one side, leading to a skeletal asymmetry with an associated crossbite generation.

13.3 Types of crossbite

13.3.1 Anterior crossbite

An anterior crossbite is present when one or more of the upper incisors is in linguo-occlusion (i.e. in reverse overjet) relative to the lower arch (Fig. 13.5). Anterior crossbites involving only one or two incisors are considered in this chapter, whereas management of more than two incisors in crossbite is covered in Chapter 11 (Class III malocclusions). Anterior crossbites are frequently associated with displacement on closure which is important to identify to ensure correct diagnosis and treatment planning (see Fig. 13.3).

13.3.2 Posterior crossbites

Crossbites of the premolar and molar region, involving one or two teeth or an entire buccal segment, can be subdivided as follows (see Fig. 13.6).

Unilateral buccal crossbite with or without an associated mandibular displacement

This type of crossbite may affect only one or two teeth per quadrant, or the whole of the buccal segment. When a single tooth is affected, the problem usually arises because of the displacement of an individual tooth from the line of the arch, plus or minus the opposing tooth. This may lead to a deflecting contact on closure into the crossbite.

When the whole of the buccal segment is involved, the underlying aetiology is usually that the maxillary arch is of a similar width to the mandibular arch (i.e. it is too narrow) with the result that on closure from the rest position into maximum occlusion the buccal segment teeth initially meet cusp to cusp and, in order to achieve a more comfortable and efficient intercuspation, the patient displaces their mandible to the left or right. It is often difficult to detect this displacement on closure as the patient soon learns to close straight into the position of maximal interdigitation. This type of crossbite may be associated with a centreline shift in the lower arch in the direction of the mandibular displacement (Fig. 13.7).

Occasionally, a patient may present with the buccal segment teeth in unilateral crossbite with no associated mandibular displacement. This category of crossbite is less common and can arise as a result of a deflection of two (or more) opposing teeth during eruption, but the greater the number of teeth in a segment that are involved, the greater the likelihood that there is an underlying skeletal asymmetry.

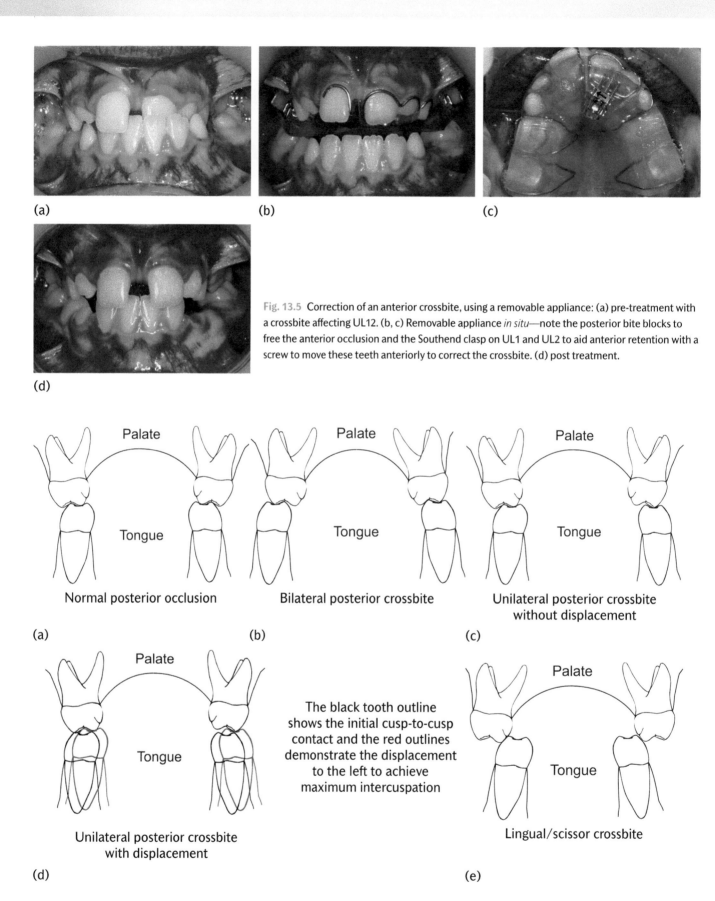

Fig. 13.5 Correction of an anterior crossbite, using a removable appliance: (a) pre-treatment with a crossbite affecting UL12. (b, c) Removable appliance *in situ*—note the posterior bite blocks to free the anterior occlusion and the Southend clasp on UL1 and UL2 to aid anterior retention with a screw to move these teeth anteriorly to correct the crossbite. (d) post treatment.

Palate

Tongue

Normal posterior occlusion

(a)

Palate

Tongue

Bilateral posterior crossbite

(b)

Palate

Tongue

Unilateral posterior crossbite without displacement

(c)

Palate

Tongue

Unilateral posterior crossbite with displacement

(d)

The black tooth outline shows the initial cusp-to-cusp contact and the red outlines demonstrate the displacement to the left to achieve maximum intercuspation

Palate

Tongue

Lingual/scissor crossbite

(e)

Fig. 13.6 (a–e) Diagrams representing the different types of posterior crossbite.

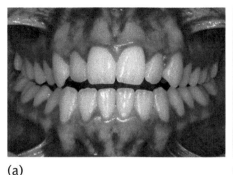
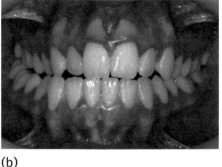

(a)
(b)

Fig. 13.7 Unilateral crossbite with displacement. (a) Initial contact of the teeth in a cusp-to-cusp relationship—note that the centrelines are coincident. (b) Mandibular displacement to the right to achieve maximum intercuspation—note lower centreline has also moved to the right.

Bilateral buccal crossbite

Bilateral crossbites (Fig. 13.8) are more likely to be associated with a skeletal discrepancy, either in the anteroposterior or transverse dimension, or in both.

Lingual crossbites

If this type of crossbite is associated with one or two teeth, then it is usually due to their individual displacement as a result of crowding or retention of the deciduous predecessor.

Where the whole buccal segment is involved, either unilaterally or bilaterally, then this is usually described as a scissor bite and there is typically an underlying skeletal component. This type is most often seen in Class II malocclusions where a wider part of the maxillary arch is further forward relative to the mandibular arch resulting in the lower buccal teeth occluding lingual to the maxillary palatal cusps.

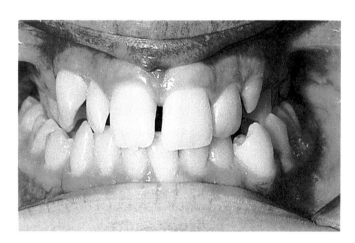

Fig. 13.8 A bilateral buccal crossbite.

13.4 Management

13.4.1 Rationale for treatment

There is some evidence that a mandibular displacement associated with a crossbite, sometimes known as a 'functional crossbite' *may* predispose towards temporomandibular joint dysfunction syndrome in a *susceptible* individual (see Chapter 1, Section 1.4.6). Recent work has also suggested that unilateral crossbites associated with mandibular displacement can result in asymmetric mandibular growth. Therefore, some argue that a crossbite which is associated with a mandibular displacement is a functional indication for orthodontic treatment. However, treatment for a bilateral crossbite without displacement should be approached with caution, as partial relapse may result in a unilateral crossbite with displacement. In addition, a bilateral crossbite is probably as efficient for chewing as the normal buccolingual relationship of the teeth. The same cannot be said of a lingual crossbite where the cusps of affected teeth do not meet together at all.

Anterior crossbites, as well as being frequently associated with displacement, can lead to movement of a lower incisor labially through the labial supporting tissues, resulting in gingival recession (Fig. 13.9). In this case, early treatment is advisable to reduce or eliminate these unwanted gingival effects.

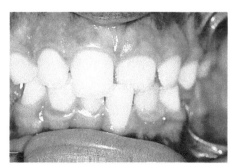
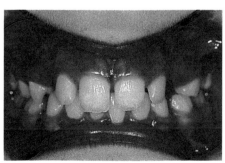

(a)
(b)

Fig. 13.9 An anterior crossbite which has resulted in forward movement of LL1 with associated gingival recession.

It is important to identify a mandibular displacement associated with any crossbite as it will potentially affect the treatment modality chosen to manage it.

13.4.2 Treatment of anterior crossbite

When deciding on the most appropriate treatment for an anterior crossbite, the following factors should be considered:

- What type of movement is required? If bodily or apical movement is required then fixed appliances are indicated; however, if in the mixed dentition, tipping movements will suffice, then a removable appliance can be considered.

- How much overbite is expected at the end of treatment? For treatment to be successful there must be some overbite present to retain the corrected incisor position. When planning treatment, it should be remembered that proclination of an upper incisor will result in a reduction of overbite compared with the pre-treatment position (see Fig. 11.11).

- Is there space available within the arch to accommodate the tooth/teeth to be moved? If not, are extractions required and if so, which teeth?

- Is reciprocal movement of the opposing tooth/teeth required?

In the mixed dentition, provided that there is sufficient overbite and tilting movements will suffice, treatment can often be accomplished with a removable appliance. The appliance should incorporate good anterior retention to counteract the displacing effect of the active element (where two or more teeth are to be proclined, a screw appliance may circumvent this problem – see Fig. 13.5) and buccal capping just thick enough to free the occlusion with the opposing arch and prevent any unwanted differential eruption of the posterior teeth which would inadvertently reduce the post-treatment overbite (see Chapter 17). A fixed appliance can also be used in the mixed dentition, and may be quicker, cheaper, and have less effect on speech.

An anterior crossbite can also be corrected in the permanent dentition, when comprehensive fixed appliance treatment can be carried out (Fig. 13.10). If there will be insufficient overbite to retain the corrected incisor(s), then consideration should be given to moving the lower incisors lingually within the confines of the soft tissue envelope in order to try and increase overbite (Fig. 11.12).

If the upper arch is crowded, the upper lateral incisor often erupts in a palatal position relative to the arch. If the lateral incisor is markedly bodily displaced, relief of crowding by extraction of the displaced tooth itself may sometimes be an option, but it is wise to seek a specialist opinion

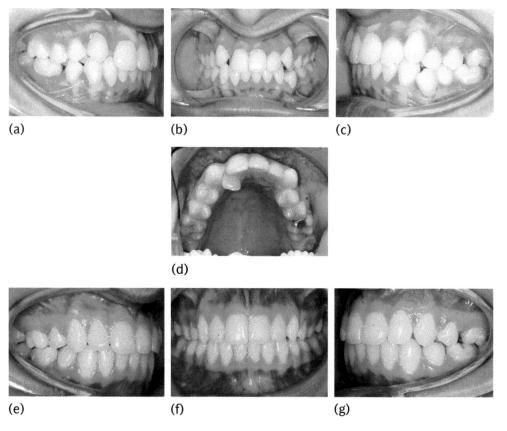

(a)　　　　(b)　　　　(c)

(d)

(e)　　　　(f)　　　　(g)

Fig. 13.10 A patient with a crossbite of the upper right lateral incisor who was treated by extraction of all four second premolars and fixed appliances: (a–d) prior to treatment; (e–g) post treatment.

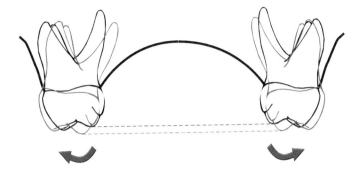

Fig. 13.11 Expansion of the upper arch results in the palatal cusps of the buccal segment teeth swinging down occlusally which can lead to an opening of the bite as highlighted by the difference between the black and red lines.

before taking this step due to the aesthetic and occlusal ramifications that this can have.

13.4.3 Treatment of posterior crossbite

It is important to consider the aetiology of this feature before embarking on treatment. For example, is the crossbite due to displacement of one tooth from the arch, in which case correction will involve aligning this tooth, or is reciprocal movement of two or more opposing teeth required? Also, if there is a skeletal component, will it be possible to compensate for this by tooth movement? The inclination of the affected teeth should also be evaluated. Upper arch expansion is more likely to be stable if the teeth to be moved were initially tilted palatally.

Expansion of the upper buccal segment teeth will result in some tipping down or 'dumping' of the palatal cusps (Fig. 13.11). This has the effect of hinging the mandible downwards leading to an increase in lower face height, which may be undesirable in patients who already have an increased lower facial height, and/or a reduced overbite. If expansion is indicated in these patients, fixed appliances are required to apply buccal root torque to the buccal segment teeth in order to try and resist this tendency, perhaps supported with high-pull headgear or temporary anchorage devices to enhance vertical control of the molar teeth.

Recent work has indicated that transverse problems which are amenable to orthodontic correction are best treated in the prepubertal growth spurt. But the actual timing of treatment will depend upon other features of the malocclusion.

As expansion will create additional space, it may be advisable to defer a decision regarding extractions until after the expansion phase has been completed (see Chapter 11, Fig. 11.13).

Where a crossbite is due to skeletal asymmetry, then a thorough assessment is required to determine the aetiology and contribution of both the maxilla and mandible to the presenting features. Full correction of the malocclusion may require a combined approach involving orthognathic surgery (see Chapter 22) once growth has slowed to adult levels.

Interestingly, a Cochrane review on this topic reported that due to a paucity of good quality evidence, the authors were only able to make limited conclusions. They found that there was some low- to moderate-quality evidence to suggest that the quadhelix appliance may be more successful than removable expansion plates at correcting posterior crossbites and expanding the inter-molar width for children in the early mixed dentition.

Unilateral buccal crossbite

Where this problem has arisen due to the displacement of one tooth from the arch, for example, an upper premolar tooth which has been crowded palatally, treatment will involve movement of the displaced tooth into the line of the arch, relieving crowding as required. If the tooth's displacement is marked, consideration can be given to extracting the displaced tooth itself.

If correction of a crossbite requires movement of the opposing teeth in opposite directions, this can be achieved by the use of cross elastics (Fig. 13.12) attached to bands or bonded brackets on the teeth involved. If this is the only feature of a malocclusion requiring treatment, it is wise to leave the attachments *in situ* following correction, stopping the elastics for a month to review whether the corrected position is stable. If the crossbite relapses, the cross elastics can be reinstituted and an alternative means of retention or more comprehensive treatment considered.

A unilateral crossbite involving all the teeth in the buccal segment is usually associated with a mandibular displacement, and treatment is directed towards expanding the upper arch so that it fits around the lower arch at the end of treatment, correcting the transverse discrepancy and eliminating the associated mandibular displacement. If the upper buccal teeth are tilted palatally, this can be accomplished with an upper removable appliance incorporating a midline screw and buccal capping. More commonly, a quadhelix appliance (see Fig. 13.13 and Section 13.4.4) can be used, particularly if comprehensive fixed appliance treatment is indicated. As a degree of relapse can be anticipated, some slight overexpansion of the upper arch is advisable. It is wise to

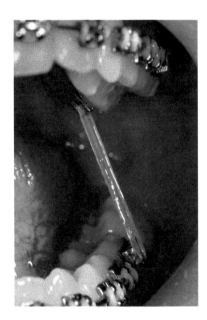

Fig. 13.12 Correction of an isolated crossbite of the first molars on the left-hand side using cross elastics from an attachment on the palatal surface of the maxillary first molar to the hook on the tube on the mandibular first molar.

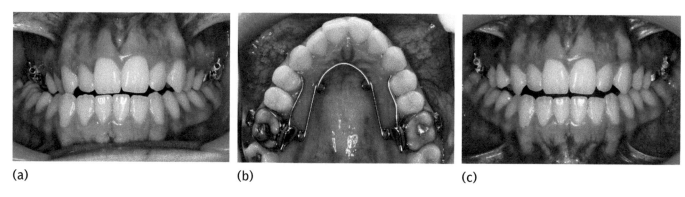

(a)　　　　　　　　　　　　(b)　　　　　　　　　　　　(c)

Fig. 13.13 A removable quadhelix appliance used to correct a unilateral crossbite with displacement. (a) Initial presentation—note the lower centre-line shift to the right; (b) removable quadhelix appliance secured with blue separating elastics; (c) corrected posterior crossbite—note the centrelines are now coincident.

remember that stability is aided by good cuspal interdigitation and that it is important to avoid too much overexpansion as a lingual crossbite or fenestration of the buccal periodontal support may result.

Bilateral buccal crossbite

Unless the upper buccal segment teeth are tilted palatally to a significant degree, bilateral buccal crossbites are often better accepted. Rapid maxillary expansion (RME) (see Section 13.4.6) can be used to try and expand the maxillary basal bone, but even with this technique, a degree of relapse in the buccopalatal tooth position occurs following intervention, with the risk of developing a unilateral crossbite with associated mandibular displacement. Surgically assisted RME can also be considered (see Fig. 13.20).

Bilateral buccal crossbites are common in patients with a repaired cleft of the palate. Expansion of the upper arch by stretching of the scar tissue is often indicated in these cases (see Chapter 24) and is readily achieved using a quadhelix appliance (Fig. 13.14).

Lingual crossbite

If a single tooth is affected, this is often the result of displacement due to crowding. If extraction of the displaced tooth itself is not indicated

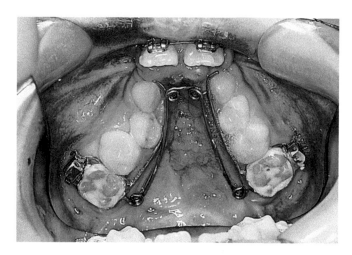

Fig. 13.14 Expansion of a repaired cleft maxilla with a quadhelix appliance.

to relieve crowding, then fixed appliances can be used to move the affected tooth into the line of the arch. More severe cases with a greater skeletal element usually need a combination of buccal movement of the affected lower teeth and palatal movement of the upper teeth with fixed appliances. Treatment is not straightforward and should only be tackled by the experienced orthodontist, particularly as a scissors bite will often dislodge fixed attachments on the buccal aspect of the lower teeth until the crossbite is eliminated. Fig. 13.15 demonstrates the correction of a unilateral scissor bite with an upper removable appliance to provide inter-occlusal space and cross elastics to correct the crossbite.

13.4.4 The quadhelix appliance

The quadhelix is a very efficient, fixed, slow expansion appliance. The quadhelix appliance can be adjusted to give more expansion anteriorly or posteriorly as required, and can also be used to de-rotate rotated molar teeth. When active expansion is complete, it can be made passive to aid retention of the expansion.

A quadhelix is fabricated in 1 mm stainless steel wire and comprises four loops which increase the overall length of wire, giving the appliance more flexibility. It is attached to the teeth by bands cemented to a molar tooth on each side. Preformed types are available, made of 0.9 mm stainless steel, which slot into rectangular palatal attachments welded onto bands on the molars and can be readily removed by the operator for adjustment. An additional advantage of removable quadhelix appliances is that, because it inserts into rectangular slots, it can be manipulated so that additional torque can be more easily placed onto the first molars to limit unwanted tipping of the palatal cusps or to help achieve asymmetry expansion (Fig. 13.16). The appliance can also be custom-made in a laboratory.

The usual activation is about half a tooth width each side. Overexpansion can occur readily if the appliance is overactivated, and therefore its use should be limited to those who are experienced with fixed appliances.

A tri-helix has only one anterior coil and is therefore less efficient. Its use is limited to cases with narrow and/or high palatal vaults, for example, in cleft lip and palate patients.

Fig. 13.15 Cross elastics to correct a lingual crossbite. (a) Initial presentation; (b, c) cross elastics with an upper removable appliance to create occlusal space; (d) corrected scissor bite—note the tipping of the posterior teeth towards each other and their extrusion has generated an anterior open bite and left posterior open bite; (e) fixed appliances *in situ* 4 weeks after initial placement which has corrected the open bites; (f) following the completion of active treatment.

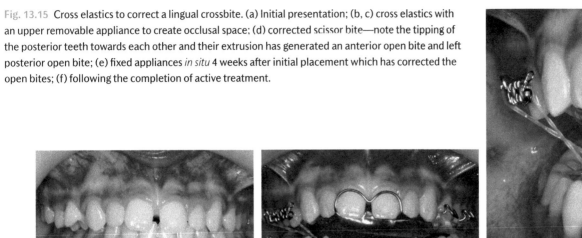

(a)　　　　　　　　(b)　　　　　　　　(c)

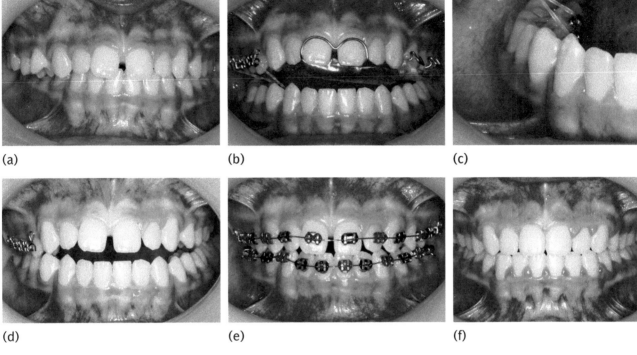

(d)　　　　　　　　(e)　　　　　　　　(f)

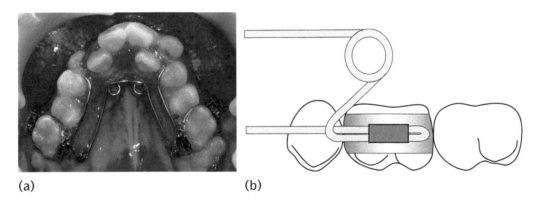

(a)　　　　　　　　(b)

Fig. 13.16 A removable quadhelix appliance. (a) Appliance *in situ*—note it is secured with metal ties to prevent it inadvertently becoming detached. (b) Diagram showing the connection into the rectangular sleeves on the palatal aspect of the first molar teeth which allows the application of torque.

13.4.5 The expansion arch

The expansion or E arch (Fig. 13.17) is a 0.9–1.135 mm diameter wire that is placed into the headgear tubes buccal to the fixed appliances and can be kept away from the brackets by a small inset bend placed mesial to the first molars. It is secured via a metal ligature between the central incisors. Additional circles can be bent into the wire mesial to the maxillary first molars to allow for metal ligatures to be secured from the hooks on the first molar brackets. This appliance is made at the chairside and can be a used as an alternative to the quadhelix appliance. However, it can result in more buccal tipping of the crowns.

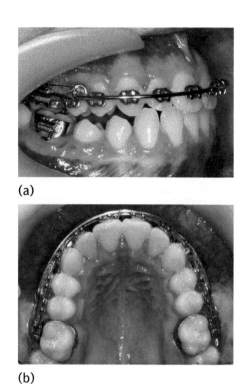

(a)

(b)

Fig. 13.17 (a, b) Expansion arch *in situ*.

13.4.6 Rapid maxillary expansion

This upper appliance incorporates a Hyrax screw (similar to the type used for expansion in removable appliances) soldered to bands, usually to both a premolar and molar tooth on both sides. The screw is turned twice daily, resulting in expansion of the order of 0.2–0.5 mm/day, usually over an active treatment period of 2 weeks (Figs 13.18 and 13.19). The large force generated is designed to open the midline palatal suture and expand the upper arch, particularly more anteriorly, by skeletal expansion rather than by movement of the teeth. For this reason, some advocate limiting this approach to patients in their early teens before

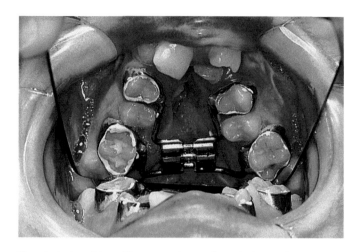

Fig. 13.18 A rapid maxillary expansion appliance being used to expand a repaired cleft maxilla.

the suture fuses, or in cleft palate patients where it can be utilized to expand the cleft segments by stretching the scar tissue. If considering this approach, it is advisable to check that there is adequate supporting buccal bone and soft tissues. The patient should also be warned of the temporary appearance of a midline diastema.

Once expansion is complete, the appliance is left *in situ* as a retainer, usually for several months. Bony infill of the expanded suture has been demonstrated but in the long term it has been shown that approximately 50% of the skeletal expansion which has been gained is subsequently lost, and for this reason some overexpansion is indicated. This appliance should only be used by the experienced clinician.

Surgically assisted RME (Fig. 13.20) or surgically assisted rapid palatal expansion (SARPE) is gaining acceptance as it is believed that this technique delivers a greater amount of skeletal expansion; however, claims of reduced periodontal support loss (compared with conventional expansion) and improved nasal airflow are unsubstantiated. This approach involves surgically cutting the mid-palatal suture and buccal corticotomies prior to expansion (see Chapter 22).

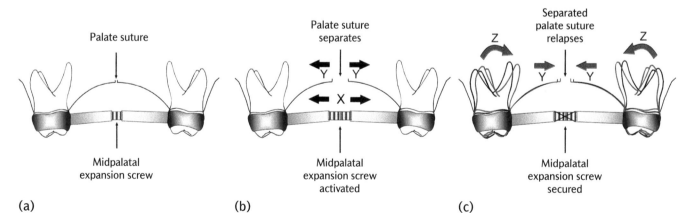

(a)   (b)   (c)

Fig. 13.19 Diagram demonstrating the effects of RME. (a) RME device *in situ*. (b) Expansion of the screw (X) results in lateral movement of the buccal teeth and the palatal shelves, separating the mid-palatal suture (Y). (c) During the healing period, some loss of the skeletal expansion occurs (Y) due to the stretched gingival and palatal mucosa exerting a medial force, which also results in some tipping of the buccal teeth (Z) as the intermolar width is fixed—these changed are shown in red.

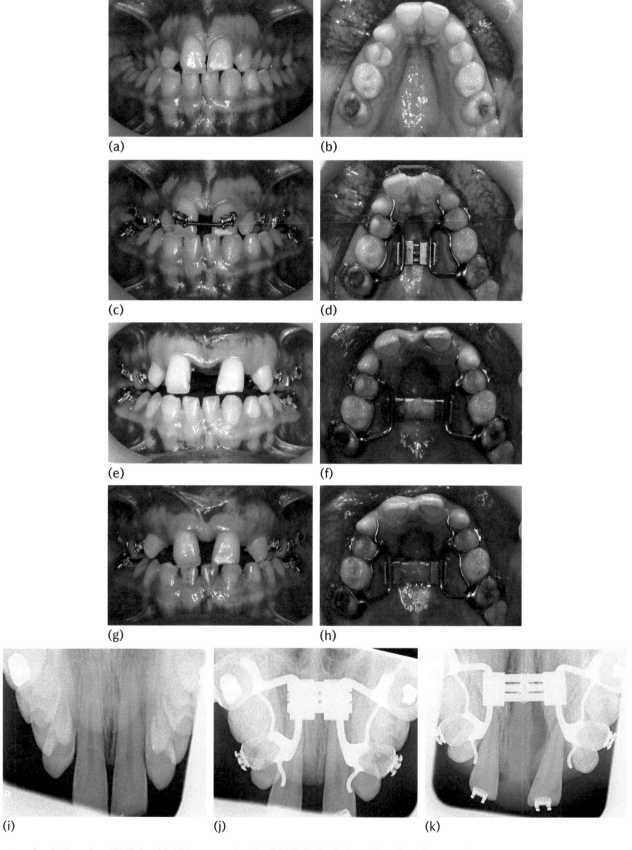

Fig. 13.20 Surgically assisted RME. (a, b) Initial presentation. (c, d) RME device *in situ* and sectional fixed appliances have created a midline diastema to allow the surgical access to cut the mid-palatal suture. (e, f) Post expansion with device secured. (g, h) After 3 months of healing—note the spontaneous reduction in the size of the midline diastema. (i) Initial occlusal radiograph. (j) Occlusal radiograph prior to expansion. (k) Occlusal radiograph post expansion—note bony void between palatal shelves.

Relevant Cochrane review

Agostino, P., Ugolini, A., Signori, A., Silvestrini-Biavati, A., Harrison, J. E., and Riley, P. (2014). Orthodontic treatment for posterior crossbites. *Cochrane Database of Systematic Reviews*, Issue 8, Art. No.: CD000979. DOI: 10.1002/14651858.CD000979.pub2 https://www.cochranelibrary.com/cdsr/doi/10.1002/14651858.CD000979.pub2/full

The authors concluded that there is some evidence which suggests the quadhelix appliance may be more successful than removable expansion plates at correcting posterior crossbites and expanding the intermolar width for children in the early missed dentition (aged 8–10 years).

Principal sources and further reading

Birnie, D. J. and McNamara, T. G. (1980). The quadhelix appliance. *British Journal of Orthodontics*, **7**, 115–20. [DOI: 10.1179/bjo.7.3.115] [PubMed: 7002208].
The fabrication, management, and modifications of the quadhelix appliance are described in this paper.

Bucci, R., D'Antò, V., Rongo, R., Valletta, R., Martina, R., and Michelotti, A. (2016). Dental and skeletal effects of palatal expansion techniques: a systematic review of the current evidence from systematic reviews and meta-analyses. *Journal of Oral Rehabilitation*, **43**, 543–64. [DOI: **10.1111/joor.12393**] [PubMed: 27004835]
An interesting systematic review which looked at all the previous systematic reviews on this topic. They concluded that palatal expansion is effective in the correction of posterior crossbites in the short term. There is more evidence to support the use of RME rather than slow maxillary expansion. The amount of skeletal expansion is less than dentoalveolar expansion. More evidence is required on the long-term effects.

Hermanson, H., Kurol, J., and Ronnerman, A. (1985). Treatment of unilateral posterior crossbites with quadhelix and removable plates. A retrospective study. *European Journal of Orthodontics*, **7**, 97–102. [DOI: 10.1093/ejo/7.2.97] [PubMed: 3926519].
In this study it was found that the clinical results achieved were similar with the two types of appliance. However, the number of visits and chairside time were greater for the removable appliance. The authors calculated that the mean cost of treatment was 40% greater for the removable appliance compared with the quadhelix.

Herold, J. S. (1989). Maxillary expansion: a retrospective study of three methods of expansion and their long-term sequelae. *British Journal of Orthodontics*, **16**, 195–200. [DOI: 10.1179/bjo.16.3.195] [PubMed: 2669948].

Kilic, N., Kiki, A., and Oktay, H. (2008). Condylar asymmetry in unilateral posterior crossbite patients. *American Journal of Orthodontics and Dentofacial Orthopedics*, **133**, 382–7. [DOI: 10.1016/j.ajodo.2006.04.041] [PubMed: 18331937].

Lagravère, M. O., Carey, J., Heo, G., Toogood, R. W., and Major, P. W. (2010). Transverse, vertical and anteroposteior changes from bone-anchored maxillary expansion vs traditional rapid maxillary expansion; a randomised clinical trial. *American Journal of Orthodontic and Dentofacial Orthopedics*, **137**, 304.e1–12. [DOI: 10.1016/j.ajodo.2009.09.016] [PubMed: 20197161]

Lee, R. (1999). Arch width and form: a review. *American Journal of Orthodontics and Dentofacial Orthopedics*, **115**, 305–13. [DOI: 10.1016/S0889-5406(99)70334-3] [PubMed: 10066980].

Linder-Aronson, S. and Lindgren, J. (1979). The skeletal and dental effects of rapid maxillary expansion. *British Journal of Orthodontics*, **6**, 25–9. [DOI: 10.1179/bjo.6.1.25] [PubMed: 396941].

Marshall, S. D., English JD Jr, Huang GJ, Messersmith ML, Nah HD, Riolo ML, et al. (2008). Ask us – long term stability of maxillary expansion. *American Journal of Orthodontics and Dentofacial Orthopedics*, **133**, 780–1. [DOI: 10.1016/j.ajodo.2008.02.001] [PubMed: 18538225]

McNally, M. R., Spary, D. J., and Rock, W. P. (2005). A randomized controlled trial comparing the quadhelix and the expansion arch for the correction of crossbite. *Journal of Orthodontics*, **32**, 29–35. [DOI: 10.1179/146531205225020769] [PubMed: 15784941]
This study found that both appliances were equally effective, but that the expansion arch could be made at the chair side, did not require additional attachments, and was cheap to fabricate. However, 70% of patients disliked the appearance of the expansion arch.

References for this chapter can also be found at: **www.oup.com/uk/orthodontics5e**. Where possible, these are presented as active links which direct you to the electronic version of the work, to help facilitate onward study. If you are a subscriber to that work (either individually or through an institution), and depending on your level of access, you may be able to peruse an abstract or the full article if available.

14
Canines

L. Mitchell

Chapter contents

14.1 Facts and figures

Development of the upper and lower canines commences between 4 and 5 months of age. The upper canines erupt, on average, at 11–12 years of age. The lower canines erupt, on average, at 10–11 years of age.

In a Caucasian population (Gorlin et al. 1990): congenital absence of upper canines, 0.3%; congenital absence of lower canines, 0.1%; impaction of upper canines, 1–2%, of which 8% are bilateral; impaction of lower canines, 0.35%; resorption of upper incisors due to impacted canine, 0.7% of 10–13-year-olds. A recent meta-analysis found a prevalence of transposition of 0.33%.

14.2 Normal development

The development of the maxillary canine commences around 4–5 months of age, high in the maxilla. Crown calcification is complete around 6–7 years of age. The permanent canine then migrates forwards and downwards to lie buccal and mesial to the apex of the deciduous canine before erupting down the distal aspect of the root of the upper lateral incisor. Pressure from the unerupted canine on the root of the lateral incisor, leads to flaring of the incisor crowns, which resolves as the canine erupts. In normal development, the maxillary canines should be palpable in the labial sulcus by age 11 years.

14.3 Aetiology of maxillary canine displacement

Canine displacement is generally classified into buccal or palatal displacement. More rarely, canines can be found lying horizontally above the apices of the teeth of the upper arch (Fig. 14.1) or displaced high adjacent to the nose (Fig. 14.2).

The aetiology of canine displacement is still not fully understood (see also Box 14.1). The following have been suggested as possible causative factors:

- **Displacement of the crypt.** This is the probable aetiology behind the more marked displacements such as those shown in Figs 14.1 and 14.2.

- **Long path of eruption.**
- **Short-rooted or absent upper lateral incisor.** A 2.4-fold increase in the incidence of palatally displaced canines in patients with absent or short-rooted lateral incisors has been reported (Becker et al. 1981) (Fig. 14.1). It has been suggested that a lack of guidance during eruption is the reason behind this association. Because of the association

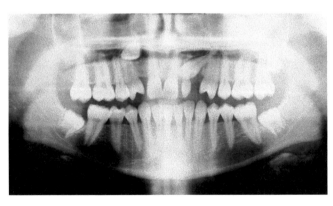

Fig. 14.1 Ectopic upper maxillary canines—with the upper right being significantly displaced. NB: absent upper right lateral incisor, a peg-shaped upper left lateral incisor.

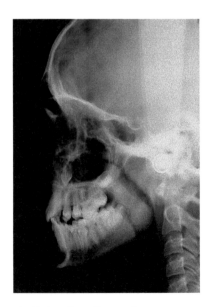

Fig. 14.2 Severely displaced maxillary canine.

Box 14.1 Aetiology of canine displacements

- *Palatal*:
  - Polygenic
  - Multifactorial
- *Buccal*: crowding.

of palatal displacement of an upper canine with missing or peg-shaped lateral incisors, it is important to be particularly observant in patients with this anomaly.

- Crowding. Jacoby (1983) found that 85% of buccally displaced canines were associated with crowding, whereas 83% of palatal displacements had sufficient space for eruption. If the upper arch is crowded, this often manifests as insufficient space for the canine, which is the last tooth anterior to the molar to erupt. In normal development, the canine comes to lie buccal to the arch and in the presence of crowding will be deflected buccally.

- Retention of the primary deciduous canine. This usually results in mild displacement of the permanent tooth buccally. However, if the permanent canine itself is displaced, normal resorption of the deciduous canine will not occur. In this situation, the retained deciduous tooth is an indicator, rather than the cause, of displacement.

- Genetic factors. It has been suggested that palatal displacement of the maxillary canine is an inherited trait with a pattern that suggests polygenic inheritance. The evidence cited for this includes:

(a) the prevalence varies in different populations with a greater prevalence in Europeans than other racial groups

(b) affects females more commonly than males

(c) familial occurrence

Box 14.2 Dental anomalies associated with palatally displaced canines

- Hypodontia
- Tooth size reduction including peg-shaped lateral incisors
- Transposition
- Impacted upper first permanent molars
- Ectopic position of other teeth
- Infra-occluded deciduous molars
- Late developing dentition.

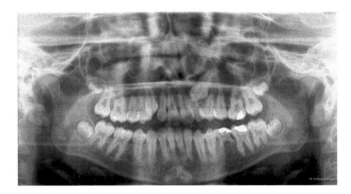

Fig. 14.3 OPT radiograph of patient with a displaced upper left canine and absent lower second premolars.

(d) occurs bilaterally with a greater than expected frequency

(e) occurs in association with other dental anomalies (Figs 14.1 and 14.3; Box 14.2).

14.4 Interception of displaced canines

Because management of ectopic canines is difficult and early detection of an abnormal eruption path gives the opportunity, if appropriate, for interceptive measures, it is essential to routinely palpate for unerupted canines when examining any child aged 10 years and older. It is also important to locate the position of the canines before undertaking the extraction of other permanent teeth.

Canines, which are palpable in the normal developmental position (buccal and slightly distal to the upper lateral incisor root), have a good prognosis for eruption. Clinically, if a definite hollow, or asymmetry, or both are found on palpation, further investigation is warranted. On occasion, routine panoramic radiographic examination may demonstrate asymmetry in the position and development of the canines.

A number of studies have investigated the widely held belief that extraction of the deciduous canine facilitates an improvement in the position of a palatally displaced canine (Fig. 14.4) where the unerupted tooth is not markedly ectopic. However, a recent Cochrane review concluded that there were deficiencies in the design and reporting of these studies and that there is currently no robust evidence to support this

practice. It must be borne in mind that this is not to say that extracting the deciduous canine does not favour improvement, rather that there is currently no data from controlled trials upon which to base this approach. Clinical experience suggests that interceptive measures are more successful between the developmental ages of 10–13 years and when there is space available for the unerupted canine, therefore space maintenance or even space creation should be considered in crowded dentitions if this approach is being contemplated.

If a palatally displaced canine is detected in the mixed dentition, then the orthodontist should discuss with the patient and their parent/guardian:

- the evidence base (including clinical experience)
- the potential benefits (i.e. successful eruption of the permanent canine or improvement in its position)
- the negative aspects (i.e. an extraction and the commitment to proceed to exposure and orthodontic alignment if the hoped for improvement in position does not occur).

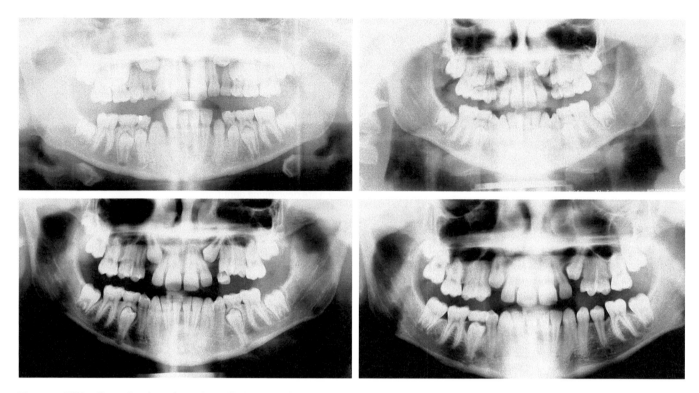

Fig. 14.4 OPT radiographs of a patient whose displaced maxillary permanent canines improved following the extraction of the upper deciduous canines.

14.5 Assessing maxillary canine position

The position of an unerupted canine should initially be assessed clinically, followed by radiographic examination if displacement is suspected.

14.5.1 Clinically

It is usually possible to obtain a good estimate of the likely location of an unerupted maxillary canine by palpation (in the buccal sulcus and palatally) and by the inclination of the lateral incisor (Fig. 14.5).

14.5.2 Radiographically

The views commonly used for assessing ectopic canines (Box 14.3) include the following.

> **Box 14.3 The radiographic assessment of a displaced canine should include the following**
>
> • Location of the position of both the canine crown and the root apex relative to adjacent teeth and the arch.
> • Prognosis of adjacent teeth and the deciduous canine, if present.
> • Presence of resorption, particularly of the adjacent central and/or lateral incisors.

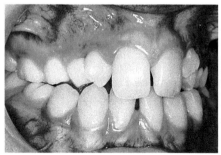

(a)

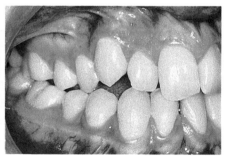

(b)

Fig. 14.5 (a) Patient aged 9 years showing distal inclination of the upper lateral incisor caused by the position of the unerupted canine; (b) the same patient aged 13 years showing the improvement that has occurred in the inclination of the lateral incisor following eruption of the permanent canine.

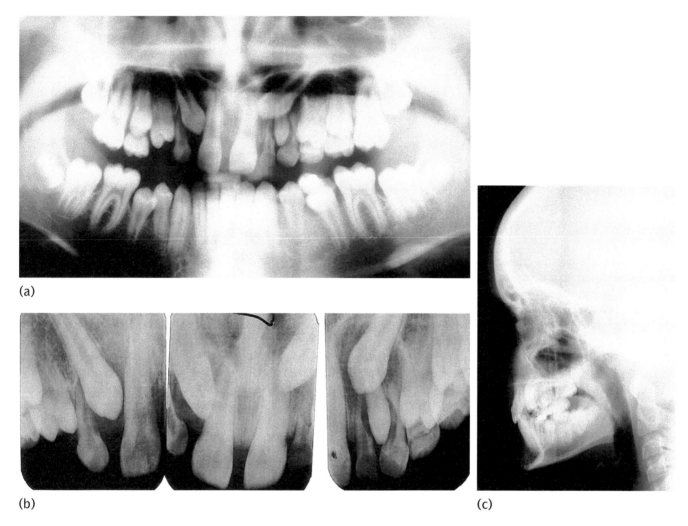

(a)

(b)   (c)

Fig. 14.6 The radiographs of a patient with displaced maxillary canines (note that the upper right lateral incisor is absent and the upper left lateral incisor is peg shaped): (a) OPT radiograph; (b) periapical radiographs (note that both maxillary canines are palatally positioned as their position changes in the same direction as the tube shift); (c) lateral cephalometric radiograph.

- Dental panoramic tomogram (OPT, OPG, or DPT). This film gives a good overall assessment of the development of the dentition and canine position. However, this view suggests that the canine is further away from the midline and at a slightly less acute angle to the occlusal plane (i.e. more favourably positioned for alignment) than is actually the case (Fig. 14.6a). This view should be supplemented with an intra-oral view.

- Periapical. This view is useful for assessing the prognosis of a retained deciduous canine and for detecting resorption (Fig. 14.6b).

- Upper anterior occlusal. To facilitate the use of vertical parallax in conjunction with an OPT radiograph, the angle of the tube should be increased to 70–75° (rather than the customary 60–65°).

- Lateral cephalometric. For accurate localization, this view should be combined with an anteroposterior view (e.g. an OPT) (Fig. 14.6c).

- Cone beam computed tomography (CBCT). Although there is an increased radiographic dose with this view, the three-dimensional (3D) images produced provide useful information on the exact position of the impacted tooth, especially in relation to other teeth and whether there is any associated root resorption. However, clinicians need to be able to justify the increased dosage and follow CBCT guidelines when using this type of investigation (see Chapter 5, Fig. 5.17).

The principle of parallax can be used to determine the position of an unerupted tooth relative to its neighbours. To use parallax, two radiographs are required with a change in the position of the X-ray tube between them. The object furthest away from the X-ray beam will appear to move in the same direction as the tube shift. Therefore, if the canine is more palatally positioned than the incisor roots it will move with the tube shift (Fig. 14.6b). Conversely, if it is buccal it will move in the opposite direction to the tube shift. Examples of combinations of radiographs which can be used for parallax include two periapical radiographs (horizontal parallax) and an OPT and an upper anterior occlusal (vertical parallax).

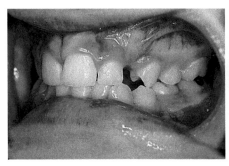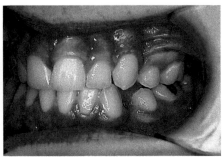

Fig. 14.7 Mildly buccally displaced maxillary canine which erupted spontaneously into a satisfactory position following relief of crowding.

14.6 Management of buccal displacement

NB: the width of the maxillary canine is greater than that of the first premolar which in turn is greater than that of the deciduous canine.

Buccal displacement is usually associated with crowding, and therefore relief of crowding prior to eruption of the canine will usually effect some spontaneous improvement (Fig. 14.7). Buccal displacements are more likely to erupt than palatal displacements because of the thinner buccal mucosa and bone. Erupted, buccally displaced canines are managed by relief of crowding, if indicated, and alignment—usually with a fixed appliance.

In severely crowded cases where the upper lateral incisor and first premolar are in contact and no additional space exists to accommodate the wider canine tooth, extraction of the canine itself may be indicated. In some patients, the canine is so severely displaced that a good result is unlikely, necessitating removal of the canine tooth and the use of fixed appliances to close any residual spacing.

More rarely, a buccally displaced canine tooth does not erupt or its eruption is so delayed that treatment for other aspects of the malocclusion is compromised. In these situations, exposure of the impacted tooth may be indicated. If the crown is located below the mucogingival junction, an open procedure to expose the crown is sufficient. However, if the crown is above the mucogingival junction, then a different approach is required. To ensure an adequate width of attached gingiva either an apically repositioned or, preferably, a replaced flap should be used. In the latter case, in order to be able to apply traction to align the canine, an attachment can be bonded to the tooth at the time of surgery. A gold chain or a stainless steel ligature can be attached to the bond and used to apply traction.

14.7 Management of palatal displacement

The treatment options available are as follows (see also Box 14.4).

14.7.1 Surgical removal of canine

This option can be considered under the following conditions:

- The retained deciduous canine has an acceptable appearance and the patient is happy with the aesthetics and/or reluctant to embark on more complicated treatment (Fig. 14.8). The clinician must

ensure that the patient understands that the primary canine will be lost eventually and a prosthetic replacement required. However, if the occlusion is unfavourable, for example, a deep and increased

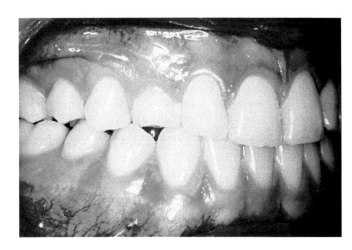

Fig. 14.8 This patient decided that the appearance of her retained deciduous canine was satisfactory and elected to have her unerupted displaced maxillary canine removed.

Box 14.4 Factors affecting treatment decision

- Patient's opinion of appearance and motivation towards orthodontic treatment.
- Malocclusion.
- Position of displaced canine: is it within range of orthodontic alignment?
- Presence of spacing/crowding.
- Condition of retained deciduous canine, if present.
- Condition of adjacent teeth.

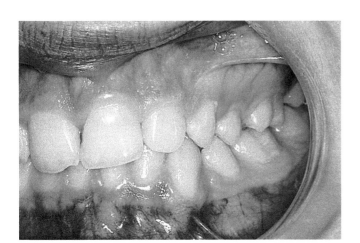

Fig. 14.9 Aesthetic result following removal of the displaced upper left permanent canine.

overbite is present, this may affect the feasibility of bridgework later, necessitating the exploration of alternative options.

- The upper arch is very crowded and the upper first premolar is adjacent to the upper lateral incisor. Provided that the first premolar is not mesio-palatally rotated, the aesthetic result can be acceptable (Fig. 14.9).
- The canine is severely displaced. Depending upon the presence of crowding and the patient's wishes, either any residual spacing can be closed by forward movement of the upper buccal segments with fixed appliances, or a prosthetic replacement can be considered.

If space closure is not planned, it may be preferable to keep the unerupted canine under biannual radiographic observation until the fate of the third molars is decided. However, if any pathology, for example, resorption of adjacent teeth or cyst formation, intervenes, removal should be arranged as soon as possible.

14.7.2 Surgical exposure and orthodontic alignment

Indications are as follows:

- Well-motivated patient
- Well-cared-for dentition
- Favourable canine position
- Space available (or can be created).

Whether orthodontic alignment is feasible or not depends upon the 3D position of the unerupted canine:

- **Height:** the higher a canine is positioned relative to the occlusal plane, the poorer the prognosis. In addition, the access for surgical exposure will be more restricted. If the crown tip is at or above the apical third of the incisor roots, orthodontic alignment will be very difficult.
- **Anteroposterior position:** the nearer the canine crown is to the midline, the more difficult alignment will be. Most operators regard canines which are more than halfway across the upper central incisor to be outside the limits of orthodontics.

- **Position of the apex:** the further away the canine apex is from normal, the poorer the prognosis for successful alignment. If it is distal to the second premolar, other options should be considered.
- **Inclination:** the smaller the angle with the occlusal plane, the greater the need for traction.

If these factors are favourable, the usual sequence of treatment is as follows:

1. Make space available (although some operators are reluctant to embark on permanent extractions until after the tooth has been exposed and traction successfully started).
2. Arrange exposure.
3. Allow the tooth to erupt for 2–3 months.
4. Commence traction.

With deeply buried canines there is a danger that the gingivae may cover the tooth again. If this is likely to be a problem, either an attachment plus the means of traction (e.g. a wire ligature or gold chain) can be bonded to the tooth at the time of exposure or about 2 days after pack removal.

Traction can be applied using either a removable appliance (Fig. 14.10) or a fixed appliance (Fig. 14.11). To complete alignment, a fixed appliance is necessary, as movement of the root apex buccally is required to complete positioning of the canine into a functional relationship with the lower arch. The chances of success are reduced and the duration of traction increased in adult patients.

14.7.3 Transplantation

In the past, the long-term results of transplantation have been disappointing. Recent work has highlighted the importance of timing, in view of the stage of root development of the canine and careful surgical technique. Transplantation should be carried out when the canine root is two-thirds to three-quarters of its final length; unfortunately, by the time most ectopic canines are diagnosed, root development is further advanced.

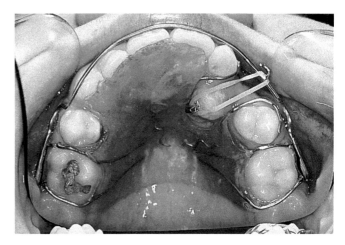

Fig. 14.10 Traction applied to an exposed canine using a removable appliance.

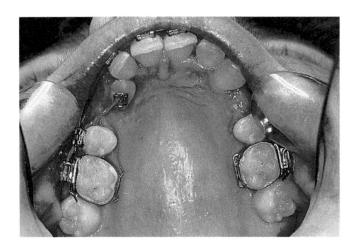

Fig. 14.11 A fixed appliance being used to move an exposed canine towards the line of the arch.

If transplantation is to be attempted, it must be possible to remove the canine intact and there must be space available to accommodate the canine within the arch and occlusion. In some cases, this will mean that some orthodontic treatment will be required prior to transplantation.

The main causes of failure of transplanted canines are replacement resorption and inflammatory resorption. Replacement resorption, or ankylosis, occurs when the root surface is damaged during the surgical procedure and is promoted by rigid splinting of the transplanted tooth, which encourages healing by bony rather than fibrous union. A more recent study has indicated that a careful surgical technique is essential to prevent damage to the root surface and the transplanted canine should be positioned out of occlusion and splinted with a sectional archwire for 6 weeks.

Inflammatory resorption follows death of the pulpal tissues, and therefore the vitality of the transplanted tooth must be carefully monitored.

Generally speaking, this approach is usually one of last resort.

14.8 Resorption

Unerupted and impacted canines can cause resorption of adjacent lateral incisor roots and may sometimes progress to cause resorption of the central incisor. The increasing use of CBCT has shown that the prevalence of root resorption is greater than previously thought. A recent study indicated that two-thirds of upper lateral incisors associated with ectopic canines showed signs of resorption. This sequela is more common in females than males.

Swift intervention is essential, as resorption often proceeds at a rapid rate. If it is discovered on radiographic examination, specialist advice should be sought quickly. Extraction of the canine may be necessary to halt the resorption. However, if the resorption is severe, it may be wiser to extract the affected incisor(s), and if appropriate, exposure and traction to bring the canine into the arch (Fig. 14.12).

14.9 Transposition

Transposition is the term used to describe interchange in the position of two teeth. This anomaly is comparatively rare, but almost always affects the canine tooth. It affects males and females equally and is more common in the maxilla. In the upper arch, the canine and the first premolar are most commonly involved; however, transposition of the canine and lateral incisor is also seen (Fig. 14.13). In the mandible,

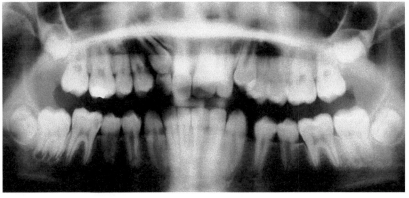

(a)

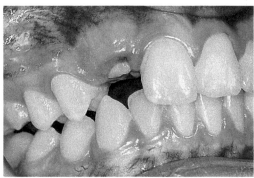

(b)

Fig. 14.12 (a) Resorption of the upper right lateral incisor by an unerupted maxillary canine; (b) following extraction of the lateral incisor the canine erupted adjacent to the central incisor.

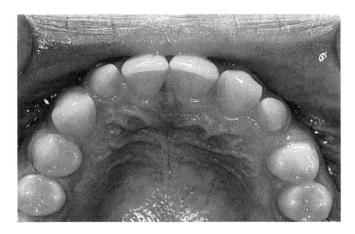

Fig. 14.13 Transposition of the upper left maxillary canine and lateral incisor.

the canine and lateral incisor appear to be almost exclusively affected (Fig. 14.14). The aetiology of this condition is not understood.

Management depends upon whether the transposition is complete (i.e. the apices of the affected teeth are transposed), or partial; the malocclusion; and the presence or absence of crowding. Possible treatment options include acceptance (particularly if transposition is complete), extraction of the most displaced tooth if the arch is crowded, or orthodontic alignment. In the last case, the relative positions of the root apices will be a major factor in deciding whether the affected teeth are corrected or aligned in their transposed arrangement.

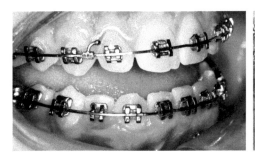 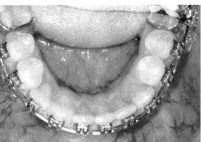

Fig. 14.14 Patient with transposition of lower left canine and lateral incisor.

Key points

- It is important that the position of the maxillary canine is assessed from age 10 years onwards and if displacement is suspected, further investigation instigated.
- Palatal displacement is associated with a number of common dental anomalies therefore it is especially important to check the position of the canine in patients with these anomalies.

Relevant Cochrane reviews

Parkin, N., Benson, P. E., Thind, B., Shah, A., Khalil, I., and Ghafoor, S. (2017). Open versus closed surgical exposure of canine teeth that are displaced in the roof of the mouth. *Cochrane Database of Systematic Reviews*, Issue 8, Art. No.: CD006966. DOI: 10.1002/14651858.CD006966.pub3 https://www.cochranelibrary.com/cdsr/doi/10.1002/14651858.CD006966.pub3/full
This review concluded that currently, there is no evidence to support one surgical technique over the other in terms of dental health, aesthetics, economics, and patient factors.

Principal sources and further reading

Armstrong, C., Johnstone, C., Burden, D., and Stevenson, M. (2003). Localising ectopic maxillary canines – horizontal or vertical parallax. *European Journal of Orthodontics*, **25**, 585–9. [DOI: 10.1093/ejo/25.6.585] [PubMed: 14700264].

Brough, E., Donaldson, A. N., and Naini, F. B. (2010). Canine substitution for missing maxillary lateral incisors: the influence of canine morphology, size, and shade on perceptions of smile attractiveness. *American Journal of Orthodontics and Dentofacial Orthopedics*, **138**, 705–7. [DOI: 10.1016/j.ajodo.2010.08.004] [PubMed: 21130320].
An interesting question and answer exchange between the editor of the journal and the authors.

Fleming, P. S., Sharma, P. K., and DiBiase, A. T. (2010). How to . . . mechanically erupt a palatal canine. *Journal of Orthodontics*, **37**, 262–71. [DOI: 10.1179/14653121043200] [PubMed: 21186306]
A well-illustrated paper that describes the practical steps in aligning a palatal canine following exposure.

Gorlin, R. J., Cohen, M. M., and Levin, L. S. (1990). *Syndromes of the Head and Neck* (3rd edn). Oxford: Oxford University Press.
This excellent reference book includes, among a wealth of other information, data on the development and incidence of canine anomalies.

Hussain, J., Burden, D., and McSherry, P. (2016). *Management of the Palatally Ectopic Maxillary Canine*. London: Faculty of Dental Surgery of the Royal College of Surgeons of England (https://www.rcseng.ac.uk/dental-faculties/fds/publications-guidelines/clinical-guidelines/).
This recently updated review evaluates the evidence relating to the management of palatally displaced canines.

Jacobs, S. G. (1999). Localisation of the unerupted maxillary canine: how to and when to. *American Journal of Orthodontics and Dentofacial Orthopedics*, **115**, 314–22. [DOI: 10.1016/S0889-5406(99)70335-5] [PubMed: 10066981].
An interesting discussion of different radiographic approaches to localizing unerupted maxillary canines.

Kokich, G. and Mathews, D. P. (2014). *Orthodontic and Surgical Management of Impacted Teeth*. Chicago, IL: Quintessence.
A beautifully illustrated book which covers the whole gamut of possible impactions

McSherry, P. F. (1998). The ectopic maxillary canine: a review. *British Journal of Orthodontics*, **25**, 209–16. [DOI: 10.1093/ortho/25.3.209] [PubMed: 9800020]

McSherry, P. F. and Richardson, A. (1999). Ectopic eruption of the maxillary canine quantified in three dimensions on cephalometric radiographs between the ages of 5 and 15 years. *European Journal of Orthodontics*, **21**, 41–8. [DOI: 10.1093/ejo/21.1.41] [PubMed: 10191576]
This interesting study found that differences in the eruption pattern of palatally ectopic canines were evident from as early as 5 years of age.

Naoumova, J., Kurol, R., and Kjellberg, H. (2015). Extraction of the deciduous canine as an interceptive treatment in children with palatally displaced canines – part I: shall we extract the canine or not? *European Journal of Orthodontics*, **37**, 209–18. [DOI: 10.1093/ejo/cju040] [PubMed: 25246604]

Naoumova, J., Kurol, R., and Kjellberg, H. (2015). Extraction of the deciduous canine as an interceptive treatment in children with palatally displaced canines – part II possible predictors of success and cut-off points for a spontaneous eruption. *European Journal of Orthodontics*, **37**, 219–29. [DOI: 10.1093/ejo/cju102] [PubMed: 25700993]
The results of this well-designed randomized controlled trial appear to support the extraction of the deciduous canine to improve the position of palatally impacted permanent canines.

Parkin, N. and Benson, P. (2011). Current ideas on the management of palatally displaced canines. *Faculty Dental Journal*, **2**, 24–9. [DOI: 10.1308/204268510X12888692969905]
An excellent article by the authors of the two Cochrane reviews putting their findings into context.

References for this chapter can also be found at: **www.oup.com/uk/orthodontics5e**. Where possible, these are presented as active links which direct you to the electronic version of the work, to help facilitate onward study. If you are a subscriber to that work (either individually or through an institution), and depending on your level of access, you may be able to peruse an abstract or the full article if available.

15

Anchorage planning

Benjamin R. K. Lewis

Chapter contents

15.1 Introduction

Orthodontic anchorage is defined as the resistance to unwanted tooth movement.

Orthodontic tooth movement is achieved through the forces generated by an orthodontic appliance. However, the desired force which is generated has an equal and opposite reactionary force, as described by Newton's third law, which will be spread over the other teeth that are contacted by the appliance and which can result in unwanted tooth movement. The aim of controlling orthodontic anchorage is to resist these reactionary forces to minimize the unwanted tooth movement and maximize the desired tooth movements.

An analogy which may help to simplify this difficult concept is that of ice skating. Imagine that you are standing on the ice and push against the barrier of the rink. You will move backwards and the barrier will remain stationary. The barrier, in this instance, is analogous to absolute anchorage (see Section 15.3), for example, an ankylosed tooth or osseointegrated implant.

If two skaters push against each other equally, and they themselves are of similar size, both will move backwards by an equal amount. This is an equal and opposite reaction. If one skater is larger than the other, the smaller skater will be pushed away, whereas the larger skater will only move slightly, or not at all. However, if the larger skater now pushes against two smaller skaters then the larger skater will move more. This can be considered similar to pitting one larger tooth against a smaller

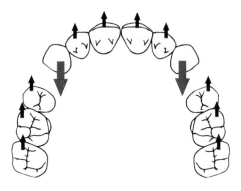

Fig. 15.1 Diagram showing the effect upon the anchor teeth of retracting upper canines with a fixed appliance.

tooth, or against two smaller teeth. The more teeth you try to move, the more likely your anchorage unit will move as well.

A clinical scenario is the retraction of upper canines using a fixed appliance, with all the available teeth involved in the appliance. An equal and opposite force to that being generated by retracting canines will also be acting on the remaining upper arch teeth to move them anteriorly, which can compromise the anchorage unit causing unwanted forward tooth movement of the rest of the dentition (Fig. 15.1).

15.2 Assessing anchorage requirements

Anchorage requirements should be considered in all three dimensions: anteroposteriorly, vertically, and transversely. Planning anchorage is a fundamental part of treatment planning and needs to be undertaken as part of managing the space requirements of orthodontic treatment. When considering anchorage management, it is important to assess the following factors.

15.2.1 Space requirements

The amount of crowding or spacing should be assessed as part of treatment planning. This can be done using either a visual assessment or more formally using a structured space analysis (see Chapter 7, Section 7.7). The results of this assessment will guide the clinician when deciding the most appropriate method of space creation, the potential treatment mechanics, and also the need for any anchorage reinforcement. For example, the extraction of maxillary first premolar teeth will result in 7 mm of space being generated on each side which can be used for

tooth alignment or retraction of the upper labial segment. This may be too much space, the exact amount required, or too little. If it results in too much space, then the clinician needs to plan the controlled loss of anchorage to allow the posterior teeth to move mesially while the anterior teeth are being retracted into the optimum position. If the space created by the extractions is just sufficient, then the clinician needs to maintain all the space for tooth alignment or retraction of the incisors, ensuring good anchorage control of the posterior teeth. If the extraction space is insufficient, then additional space needs to be generated with further extractions, expansion, interproximal enamel reduction, or distalization of posterior teeth.

15.2.2 The type of tooth movement to be achieved

There are six different types of tooth movement: tipping, bodily movement, rotation, torqueing, intrusion, and extrusion. Tipping occurs

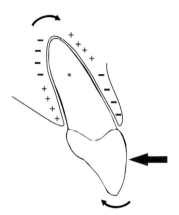

Fig. 15.2 Diagram showing the effect of a tipping force applied to the crown of a tooth (+ = pressure; – = tension). The red circle represents the tooth's centre of resistance.

when the crown of a tooth moves in one direction and the root apex moves, by a lesser amount, in the opposite direction rotating around the tooth's centre of resistance (Fig. 15.2). Bodily movement occurs when both the crown and the root move in the same direction equally (Fig. 15.3). In practice, this is often achieved by a series of small tipping and uprighting movements due to the 'play' between the archwire and the bracket slot (see Chapter 18). Rotational movement occurs when a force is applied mesially or distally to the labial aspect of a tooth.

Teeth have a centre of resistance around which movement occurs. If force is applied directly through the centre of resistance then the tooth will move bodily, however, because the centre of resistance lies within the root this cannot occur. A simple force applied to the crown of a tooth with a round wire will cause the tooth to tip (see Chapter 18, Fig. 18.1); however, with a fixed appliance in place, the built-in programme of the bracket interacting with a rectangular orthodontic wire causes the force to act as a 'couple', which can be used to change the inclination of teeth or to produce bodily tooth movement.

Bodily movement requires more force to be placed onto a tooth than tipping movements and is therefore more anchorage demanding on the remaining teeth.

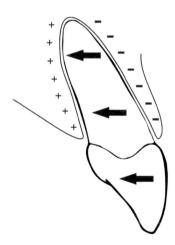

Fig. 15.3 Diagram showing the distribution of the applied force with bodily movement (+ = pressure; – = tension).

15.2.3 The number of teeth to be moved

As the number of teeth to be moved increases, so does the anchorage demand. If the anchorage requirements of treatment are high, then consideration should be given to moving a single tooth in stages or only a few teeth at a time to conserve anchorage. However, although the theoretical principles are sound and this is a commonly applied method of preventing unwanted tooth movement, there is some debate within the literature about the level of anchorage conservation that this technique actually achieves by the end of treatment when all the active tooth movements have been completed.

15.2.4 The distance of the movement required

The greater the distance the teeth are to be moved, the greater the strain on the anchorage, and the greater the risk of unwanted tooth movement.

15.2.5 Aims of treatment

The aims of treatment can fundamentally alter the complexity of treatment and also the prognosis for success. The aims of treatment need to be specific and achievable, with the treatment mechanics that will be required to achieve the aims being acceptable to the individual patient. The fewer teeth that need to be moved to achieve the aims of treatment then the less the anchorage demand; however, if treatment is complex and multiple teeth are to be moved, there will be a greater anchorage demand and often a greater demand on the level of cooperation from the patient. In cases with a Class II molar relationship on initial presentation, the anchorage needs will be far greater if a Class I molar (and canine) relationship is to be achieved rather than a Class II molar (and Class I canine) relationship at the end of treatment (Fig. 15.4). The need to achieve a Class I canine relationship is usually

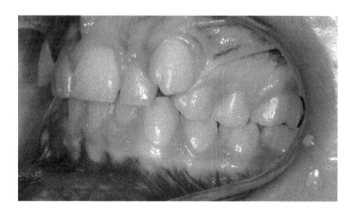

Fig. 15.4 Anchorage requirements will alter dramatically in this patient depending on whether you aim to treat Class I or Class II molars, as to achieve a Class I molar relationship will require active distal movement of the maxillary molars. For both potential outcomes, this is a high anchorage case as the initial molar relationship is a full unit Class II and so no mesial movement can be allowed without resulting in a compromised occlusal finish.

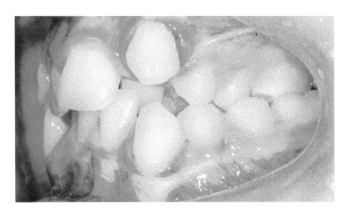

Fig. 15.5 This case demonstrates significant upper and lower arch crowding. Extractions will therefore be required in both arches with the lower canines moving distally during treatment to allow the alignment of the lower incisors. In order to achieve a Class I canine relationship at the end of treatment, the upper canines will require significant distal movement and anchorage reinforcement, for example, with headgear or temporary anchorage devices, is indicated.

very important for treatment success, therefore it is critical that anchorage planning should focus not only on the intended molar movements but also on the required movements of the canines to achieve this goal (Fig. 15.5).

15.2.6 Root surface area of the teeth to be moved

The size of the root surface area of the tooth or teeth to be moved influences the anchorage requirements—the larger the root surface area, the greater the demand (Fig. 15.6). Teeth are maintained in a position of balance between the opposing forces of the lips and tongue, with the periodontal ligament, and the surrounding bone, resisting any tooth movement; therefore, for tooth movement to occur, a threshold of force must be achieved. This applies equally to the teeth in the anchorage unit, and if the threshold is exceeded, unwanted movement of the anchor teeth will occur and anchorage will be lost. As such, the forces applied to achieve the desired tooth movements must be carefully selected to try and ensure they remain below the threshold of the teeth acting as the anchorage unit. Increasing the number of teeth acting in an anchorage unit (e.g.

including the second molars in a fixed appliance) is one method of increasing this threshold.

15.2.7 Growth rotation and skeletal pattern

An increased rate of tooth movement has been associated with patients who have an increased vertical dimension or backward growth rotation. It has been suggested that space closure or anchorage loss may occur more rapidly in these high-angled cases and so the requirement for anchorage reinforcement needs to be considered in these individuals. Conversely, in a patient with reduced vertical dimensions or a forward growth rotation, space closure or anchorage loss may be slower; therefore, the planned extraction pattern or the treatment mechanics may need to be altered to accommodate this. One hypothesis which has been proposed for this observation is the relative strength of the facial muscles, with individuals with reduced vertical dimensions having a stronger musculature.

15.2.8 Occlusal interdigitation and occlusal interferences

Occlusal interdigitation or occlusal interferences can prevent or slow down tooth movement. This can lead to an increased anchorage demand which may prevent the desired tooth movement and increase the likelihood of unwanted tooth movement. This phenomenon can be utilized to an orthodontist's advantage, as it has been suggested that if teeth in the anchorage unit have a good interdigitation with the opposing dentition, this may increase their anchorage value by reducing mesial movement of the anchorage unit.

15.2.9 Bone quality

Maxillary bone is less dense than mandibular bone so the threshold for tooth movement in the maxillary teeth is lower than that in the mandibular teeth. Teeth move more readily through cancellous bone than cortical bone and the anchorage value of teeth can be increased by moving their roots closer to the cortical plate; however, this can put them at increased risk of root resorption, and as such, should be done with care. Certain groups of patients, such as individuals with hypodontia or previous experience of periodontal disease, can have reduced quantity and/ or quality of alveolar bone. This will affect the anchorage balance when undertaking orthodontic treatment and must also be taken into consideration when planning the retention phase of treatment.

15.3 Classification of anchorage

- **Simple anchorage:** one tooth pitted against another.
- **Reciprocal anchorage:** two teeth or groups of teeth of equal size or equivalent anchorage value are pitted against each other, resulting in movement of both units by a similar amount. For example, a quad-helix used to expand the maxillary arch (Fig. 15.7) or applying power chain on an upper fixed appliance to two central incisors to close a median diastema (Fig. 15.8).

- **Anchorage reinforcement:** a variety of methods can be utilized:
  - **Intramaxillary compound anchorage:** multiple teeth are used in an anchorage unit within the same arch, for example, using a molar and a second premolar as an anchorage unit for the retraction of a canine.
  - **Intermaxillary compound anchorage:** multiple teeth in opposing arches, for example, the use of intermaxillary elastics (Fig. 15.9).

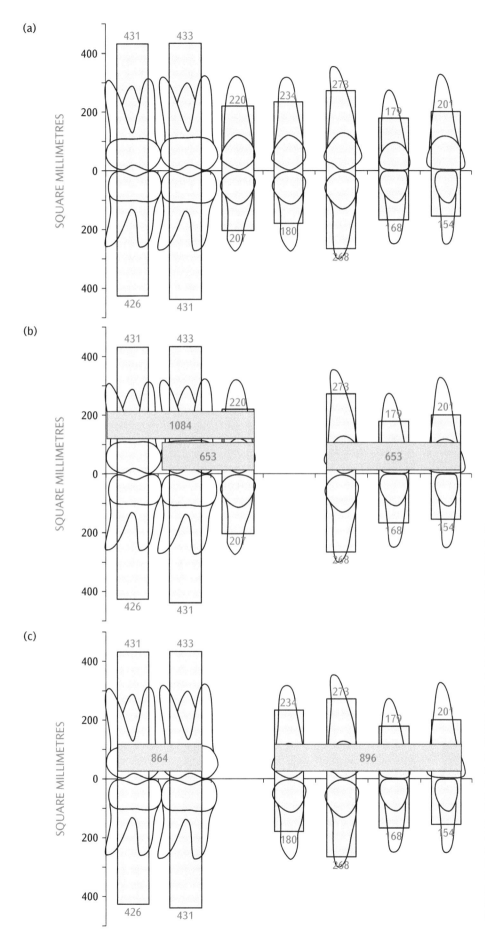

Fig. 15.6 Diagrammatic representation of the relative root surface areas of the permanent dentition and the effect on anchorage requirements. (a) Root surface areas for the permanent dentition (excluding third molars). (b) Anchorage balance following the extraction of all four first premolars. If the second molars are not included then space closure will occur equally from the posterior teeth moving mesially and the anterior teeth moving distally, due to the similar root surface areas of the anterior teeth, and the second premolar and first permanent molar. However, if the second permanent molar is included in the appliance then the anchorage balance will be shifted to favour distal movement of the anterior teeth. (c) Anchorage balance following removal of second premolars. If the second permanent molars are not included in the appliance, most of the space closure will occur by the first permanent molars moving mesially. Adapted from *Acta Odontologica Scandinavica*, 21, Jepsen, A., Root surface measurement and a method for X-ray determination of root surface areas, pp. 35–46. Copyright © Acta Odontologica Scandinavica Society, reprinted by permission of Taylor & Francis Ltd, www.tandfonline.com on behalf of Acta Odontologica Scandinavica Society.

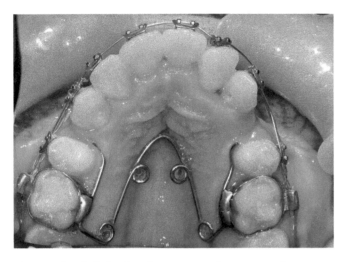

Fig. 15.7 Quadhelix fixed appliance to expand the upper arch.

- **Differential tooth movements:** tipping movements are less anchorage demanding than bodily movement. This concept can be utilized when planning tooth movements to increase the relative anchorage value of specific teeth.
- **Use of intra-oral adjuncts:** this incorporates non-tooth structures such as the palatal vault when using a Nance button in conjunction with a transpalatal arch (Fig. 15.10), or bone when using temporary anchorage devices (TADs).
- **Use of extra-oral adjuncts:** this incorporates devices utilizing extra-oral structures to place a force upon the teeth. For example, headgear systems.
- **Stationary/absolute anchorage:** this can only be achieved when using an osseointegrated implant or ankylosed tooth as an anchorage unit.

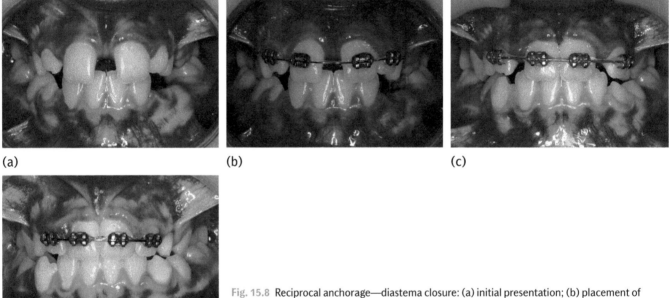

(a) (b) (c)

(d)

Fig. 15.8 Reciprocal anchorage—diastema closure: (a) initial presentation; (b) placement of sectional fixed appliances; (c) approximation of the central incisors; (d) approximation of the lateral incisors.

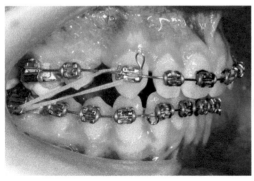

(a)

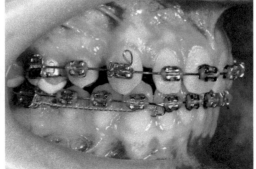

(b)

Fig. 15.9 (a, b) Use of intermaxillary elastics to retract a canine.

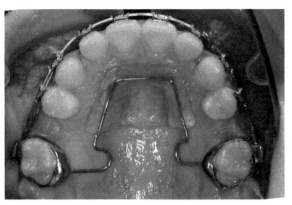 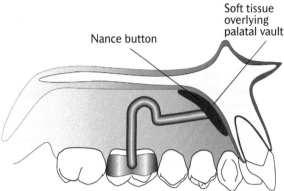

Soft tissue
overlying
palatal vault

Nance button

Fig. 15.10 (a, b) Transpalatal arch with Nance button. The anterior palatal vault is used as additional anchorage with the addition of an acrylic button.

15.4 Intra-oral anchorage

Anchorage reinforcement can be achieved by utilizing the teeth, soft tissues, and skeletal structures intra-orally.

15.4.1 Increasing the number of teeth in the anchorage unit

Incorporating as many teeth as possible into an anchorage unit will aid in reducing anchorage loss. If the anchorage demand is high, then consideration should be given to moving one tooth at a time to prevent strain of the anchorage unit (conserving anchorage). This will also allow better monitoring of any anchorage loss, allowing additional anchorage re-enforcing mechanics to be utilized if required.

15.4.2 Differential extraction pattern

The extraction pattern planned for the patient can influence the anchorage balance of a case. Extracting teeth closer to the area of crowding reduces the amount of tooth movement required and thus the risk of anchorage loss. Also, by careful selection of the appropriate teeth to be extracted, the anchorage balance can be changed in such a way that it is possible to make some teeth more resistant to unwanted movement (Fig. 15.6).

A differential extraction pattern, between arches, can aid in anchorage management. One such example is the treatment of Class II division 1 cases where the upper first premolars are extracted to aid reduction of an overjet and correction of the canine relationship to Class I. This becomes possible as the anchorage unit is greater posteriorly in the maxilla with the upper first molars and second premolars incorporated within the appliance. In the lower arch, the extraction of the lower second premolars will not only reduce the retraction of the lower labial segment but also work favourably for molar correction with the lower molars more likely to move mesially. These desired tooth movements can be enhanced with inter-arch (Class II) elastic use. This extraction pattern can be reversed in the treatment of Class III cases with the extraction of lower first premolars and upper second premolars. This differential extraction pattern will aid the camouflage of the reverse overjet with retroclination of the lower labial segment.

15.4.3 Care with initial intra-arch orthodontic mechanics

A number of factors may increase the demands on the anchorage units, such as the engagement of severely displaced teeth in the early stages of alignment. Anchorage loss will also occur if there is friction in the system as a greater force needs to be exerted to overcome friction and achieve the planned tooth movement. As a result of this higher applied force, the reactionary force is greater, which may result in unwanted tooth movement of the anchorage unit.

15.4.4 Bodily movement of teeth

Bodily movement requires more force than tipping movements and is therefore more anchorage demanding. Use of large, rectangular stainless steel archwires will ensure bodily movement occurs rather than tipping, as the archwire will fill more of the bracket slot (see Chapter 18, Fig. 18.4). Differential tooth movements can be undertaken in an effort to limit unwanted tooth movements. This involves restricting the anchorage teeth to bodily movement while allowing the teeth you do wish to move to tip into place. As tipping movements occur more readily, differential tooth movement should occur. This is a concept which is fundamental to certain appliance systems such as Begg and Tip-Edge (see Chapter 18, Section 18.6.2).

15.4.5 Transpalatal and lingual arches

Both a transpalatal arch (usually connecting the upper first molars) and a lower lingual arch (usually connecting the lower first molars) can be used to reinforce anchorage by linking contralateral molar teeth (Figs 15.11 and 15.12). The teeth are joined with an arch bar, usually 1 mm diameter stainless steel, which connects across the vault of the palate or around the lingual aspect of the lower arch. This linking of teeth helps to prevent or reduce unwanted mesial molar movement. By fixing the intermolar width, which aids transverse anchorage, any mesial movement of the molars means that the buccal roots are more likely to come into contact with the cortical plate of the bone which,

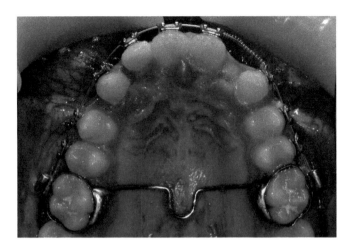

Fig. 15.11 Transpalatal arch.

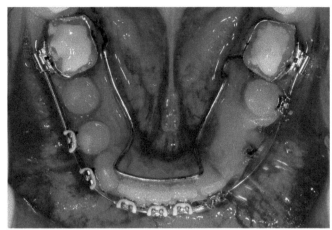

Fig. 15.12 Lingual arch.

as mentioned previously, resists subsequent mesial tooth movement, but can also increase the risk of root resorption. Anchorage can potentially be further increased by adding an acrylic button, or Nance button, which lightly contacts the anterior palatal mucosa (Fig. 15.10). Caution should be taken with all these appliances, because if anchorage is lost and the molars move mesially then the lingual arch can cause proclination of the lower labial segment, or the U-loop of the transpalatal arch or acrylic of the Nance button may become engaged in the palatal mucosa. It is with this in mind that the palatal loop of the transpalatal arch would normally face distally.

The amount of anchorage reinforcement these devices provide has been questioned in the literature and it is advisable for the clinician to carefully monitor for any anchorage loss during treatment.

15.4.6 Intermaxillary anchorage

Anchorage from one arch can be used to reinforce anchorage in the other. In addition to occlusal interlocking mentioned earlier, the two main adjuncts which can be utilized to achieve this is with the use of intermaxillary elastic traction (see Chapter 18, Section 18.3.4) or Class

II correctors, which are metal pistons connected between the arches. Intra-oral elastics are available in a variety of sizes and strengths. Class II elastics will be run from an anterior attachment in the upper arch to a posterior attachment in the lower arch. Class III elastics are the reverse, located anteriorly in the lower to posteriorly in the upper (Figs 15.13 and 15.14).

As with any force applied there can be unwanted effects, and intermaxillary traction is not without this problem. Class II or Class III elastics can lead to extrusion of the molars, which will in turn reduce the overbite and can also cause an increase in the face height, this might be beneficial in a few patients but for the majority these movements would be unwanted. The other significant consequence is that in an unspaced lower arch, the use of Class II elastics and Class II correctors will result in proclination of the lower labial segment.

15.4.7 Removable and functional appliances

Removable appliances can be used alone or in conjunction with a fixed appliance to reinforce anchorage (Fig. 15.15). By virtue of their palatal coverage, they have an increased anchorage value to resist unwanted

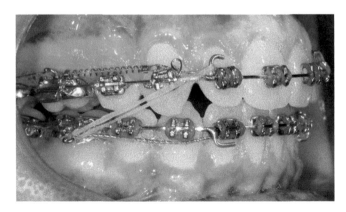

Fig. 15.13 Class II intermaxillary traction (elastics).

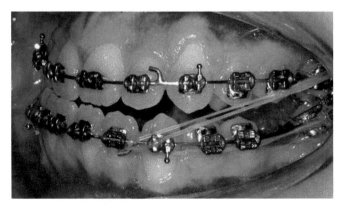

Fig. 15.14 Class III intermaxillary traction (elastics).

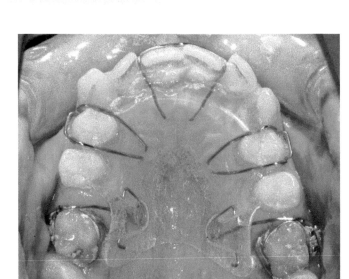

Fig. 15.15 Nudger removable appliance used as an adjunct to fixed appliance treatment. The nudger is worn full time, holding the distal movement achieved during the part-time (12–14 hours) headgear wear.

tooth movement. Other design features which reinforce anchorage include the following:

- **Anteroposteriorly:** by colleting around the posterior teeth with acrylic, inclined bite-blocks, or the use of incisor capping.
- **Transversely:** the pitting of one side of the arch against the other can reinforce transverse anchorage, typically seen where an expansion screw is used for increasing the palatal transverse dimension (Fig. 15.16), usually resulting in reciprocal anchorage.
- **Vertically:** by either reducing the vertical dimensions during treatment of a high-angle patient by intruding the posterior teeth, often aided with high-pull headgear (see Chapter 12, Section 12.3.1); or

Box 15.1 Classification of TADs

- Osseointegration
- Mechanical retention:
  - Plate design
  - Screw design.

increasing the vertical dimension by allowing differential tooth eruption with the use of an anterior bite-plane.

All of these three-dimensional features can be incorporated into functional appliances, which additionally can be used to gain anchorage in the anteroposterior direction to aid in the treatment of a Class II malocclusion, often reducing the complexity during the fixed appliance phase of treatment.

15.4.8 Temporary anchorage devices

The use of temporary anchorage devices (TADs), also known as orthodontic bone anchorage devices, is becoming increasingly common in contemporary orthodontics. They first became popular in the 1990s and were developed from the dental implants used in restorative dentistry and maxillofacial bone plates. There are three distinct types (Box 15.1):

- **Osseointegrated implants**

  These were modified from dental implants, making them shorter, with a wider diameter than those used in restorative dentistry. Osseointegrated implants can be used to provide maximum anchorage and are useful if large or difficult tooth movements are required. This type of implant, placed in the mid-palatal region and attached to a palatal arch (Fig. 15.17), was compared with conventional headgear in a randomized controlled trial. The authors concluded that mid-palatal implants are an acceptable technique for reinforcement of anchorage.

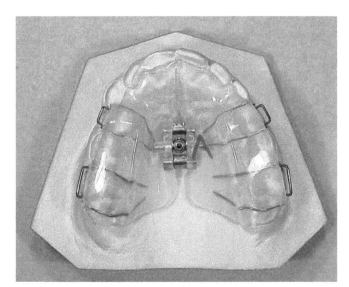

Fig. 15.16 Upper removable appliance with midline expansion screw—demonstrates reciprocal anchorage.

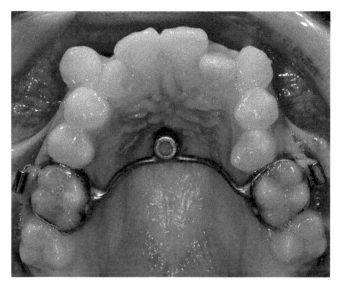

Fig. 15.17 Osseointegrated mid-palatal implant used in conjunction with a transpalatal arch to achieve absolute anchorage.

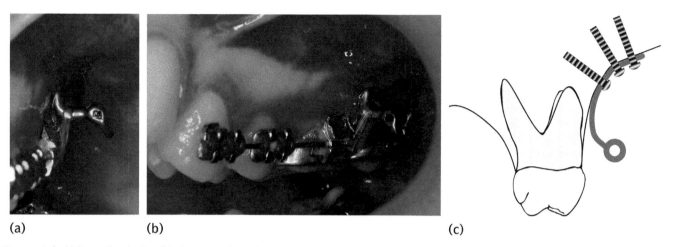

(a)   (b)   (c)

Fig. 15.18 (a, b) Bone plate *in situ* with the exposed attachment bucco-gingival to the maxillary first molars. (c) Diagram showing a miniplate *in situ*.

They have three principal disadvantages:

(1) They need to be left for 3 months after placement to allow osseointegration.

(2) Due to their size, they are restricted to being used in edentulous areas.

(3) Since the implant osseointegrates, it requires a complex surgical procedure together with bone removal at the completion of treatment and some patients may find this unacceptable.

● Miniplate systems

These are based on maxillofacial bone plates, with a transmucosal portion projecting into the mouth to allow connection to the fixed appliance. They can provide reliable anchorage, but require a surgical procedure to both place and remove them (Fig. 15.18).

● Mini-screws

These were developed from the screws of maxillofacial plating systems, but are smaller in size (typically 6–12 mm in length and 1.2–2 mm in diameter), hence the term mini-screw. No osseointegration is required (or desired) which means that they do not provide absolute anchorage as there is the possibility that they can move during treatment. Their head and neck configuration has been adapted to facilitate placement of auxiliaries to the fixed appliance (Fig. 15.19).

Due to their ease of use—for both the patient and the orthodontist—the mini-screw approach is now the most popular. There is a range of different systems available with various claimed strengths and weaknesses. Their designs and the associated treatment mechanics are under constant review. They are usually placed under local anaesthesia and can often be removed at the end of treatment without requiring any anaesthetic.

Bone anchorage devices have the ability to provide anchorage in three dimensions: anteroposteriorly, vertically, and transversely. They can provide anchorage either directly or indirectly:

● *Direct anchorage* is achieved when forces are applied directly to the TAD (Fig. 15.20).

● *Indirect anchorage* is achieved when the TAD is linked to the anchorage teeth, and then the orthodontic forces are applied to this anchorage unit (Fig. 15.21).

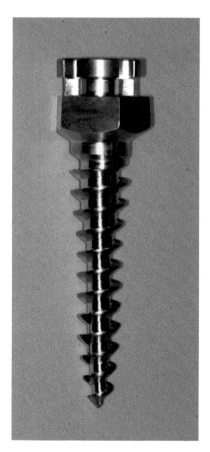

Fig. 15.19 Mini-screw temporary anchorage device with modified head to allow the attachments of orthodontic auxiliaries.

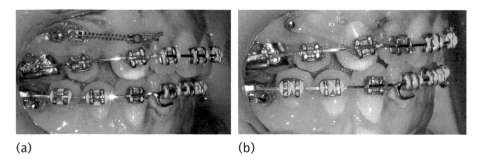

Fig. 15.20 Direct anchorage using a temporary anchorage device to conserve anchorage in maximum anchorage case: (a) at commencement of space closure; (b) 3 months later.

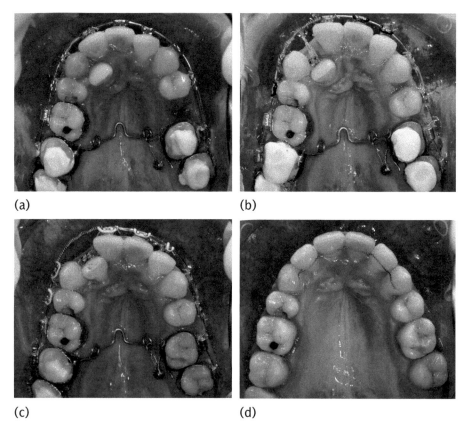

Fig. 15.21 (a–d) Indirect anchorage using a temporary anchorage device attached to a TPA to reinforce the posterior anchorage following the enforced extraction of a compromised maxillary left second premolar, allowing arch alignment and centreline correction.

The benefit of using TADs for indirect anchorage is that conventional treatment mechanics can be utilized, however, the disadvantage is that if the TAD moves or becomes loose between visits, then some anchorage loss could have occurred before it is noticed and rectified.

The use of TADs is allowing different approaches to anchorage, as well as possibly altering the scope of what was previously thought possible with fixed appliances. However, as with all these adjuncts, there are risks associated with their use which the patients must be made aware of. These include the risk of damage to adjacent structures such as blood vessels, nerves, and tooth roots; the risk of fracture; the risk of gingival inflammation; and the risk of them becoming loose with subsequent anchorage loss or need for replacement/use of other means of anchorage reinforcement.

15.5 Extra-oral anchorage

15.5.1 General principles

Headgear can be used for:

- extra-oral anchorage
- extra-oral traction.

Extra-oral anchorage holds the posterior teeth in position, preventing unwanted mesial movement of the anchorage unit.

Extra-oral traction applies a force to the posterior teeth to achieve tooth movement, usually in a distal direction. Traction can also be used to attempt to achieve an orthopaedic effect by using conventional headgear to restrict the growth of the maxilla in a forwards and downwards direction, or using reverse headgear (see Section 15.5.4) to protract the maxilla. In simple terms, traction requires greater forces, for longer periods of time, than that required to maintain the position of the posterior teeth.

There are three directions of pull that can be achieved with headgear and these should be considered at the time of treatment planning (Box 15.2):

- High- or occipital-pull headgear which helps to control the vertical as well as anteroposterior anchorage and is typically used in cases with increased vertical proportions (Fig. 15.22).

Box 15.2 Factors that need to be considered for effective headgear planning

1. Forces:
    (a) Direction
    (b) Magnitude
    (c) Duration
2. Centre of resistance.

- Straight- or combination-pull headgear which controls the anteroposterior and is typically used in cases with average vertical proportions (Fig. 15.23).
- Low- or cervical-pull headgear which aids in the control of anteroposterior anchorage but is also used to increase the vertical dimension by having an extrusive effect on the molars in cases of reduced vertical proportions (Fig. 15.24). Care should be taken with low-pull headgear in a Class II skeletal pattern as extrusion of the maxillary molars may lead to a clockwise rotation of the mandible making the class II skeletal pattern worse as the mandible rotates downwards and backwards.

The amount of force applied to the headgear is controlled by adjusting the attachment straps and should be carefully monitored at each

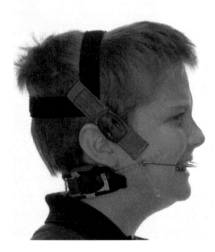

Fig. 15.23 Combination headgear using high pull and cervical pull together.

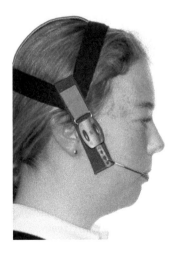

Fig. 15.22 High-pull headgear attached to face-bow with snap-away design.

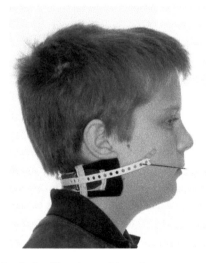

Fig. 15.24 Cervical-pull headgear with neck strap.

visit. For orthodontic change, it is normal to apply 250–350 g to achieve anchorage reinforcement, increasing to 400–450 g to obtain extra-oral traction. For orthopaedic change, often termed maxillary restraint, the forces are increased to 500 g.

The duration of force also varies according to the purpose. Extra-oral anchorage requires a minimum of 10 hours per day, which is usually best achieved at bedtime. Extra-oral traction requires an increased duration and a minimum of 12 hours of wear per day is required though most operators ask for 14 hours. For orthopaedic changes, the duration of wear requested is also normally 14 hours, but the length of treatment with the headgear appliance is longer when compared to extra-oral traction (which may be achieved, in a cooperative patient, within 6–9 months).

The effect of a force depends on where it is applied in relation to the centre of resistance. If the force passes directly through the centre of resistance then pure translation will occur. If not, then tipping will arise.

The centre of resistance for forces applied to the upper first molars is felt to be at the trifurcation of their roots. The centre of resistance for the maxilla as a whole is further forward, and is suggested to be between the premolar roots. Adjustment of the direction of force applied by the headgear relative to the centre of resistance of the first molar will influence how the molar will move.

In theory, intrusion of the upper incisors can be attempted by applying headgear to the anterior labial segment of a working archwire, though the forces used must be light to avoid possible root resorption of the upper incisors. Due to concerns over safety, this technique has now been largely abandoned.

Headgear can be added to a removable appliance or a functional appliance, such as a twin-block appliance, usually with the aim of achieving orthopaedic changes. In these cases, the forces are kept above the occlusal plane, not only to control the vertical dimension, but also to prevent dislodging the appliance.

15.5.2 Components of headgear

The components of headgear have been modified dramatically in the last 20 years to improve safety (see Section 15.5.3). Where headgear is to be used in conjunction with a fixed appliance, patients first need to be fitted with upper molar orthodontic bands with buccal headgear tubes. Where headgear is being used with a removable or functional appliance then headgear tubes need to be added to either the molar clasps or incorporated into the acrylic (see Chapter 17, Fig. 17.7).

- **Face-bow:** the face-bow slots into the headgear tubes. The original face-bow was called a Kloehn bow, however, due to safety concerns about the unprotected intra-oral ends, its use is now largely historic. Currently the face-bow of choice is a Nitom™ locking face-bow produced with a specialized safety catch (Fig. 15.25). A less complex safety version is the Hamill face-bow with a reverse loop attachment (Fig. 15.26); however, although the Hamill type can reduce the degree of soft tissue injury, there is a much higher risk of accidental disengagement from the headgear tube when compared to the Nitom™ face-bow.

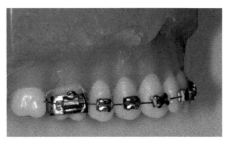

(a)

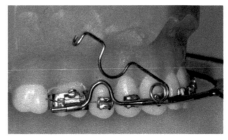

(b)

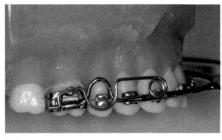

(c)

Fig. 15.25 A Nitom™ locking face-bow: (a) band on the first molars with a headgear tube; (b) the intra-oral arm of the face-bow inserted into the headgear tube; (c) the Nitom™ locking attachment secures behind the headgear tube, preventing the face-bow's accidental disengagement.

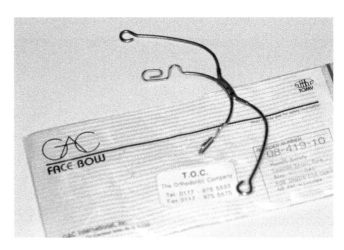

Fig. 15.26 Hamill safety face-bow with reverse loop attachment.

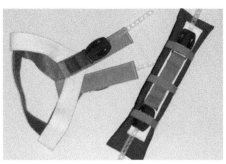
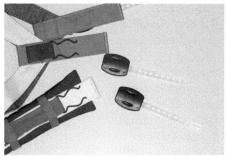

Fig. 15.27 Safety release headgear with a snap-away spring mechanism which breaks apart when excessive force is applied.

- **Headcap or neck strap:** a headcap or neck strap can be used independently or together to achieve the direction of pull required.
  - *High/occipital pull*: use of the headcap only (Fig. 15.22). This produces intrusive forces and either leads to intrusion of the molars or prevents them from extruding during treatment. This approach is useful where no increase in the vertical proportions can be tolerated during treatment.
  - *Combination pull*: uses the headcap and neck strap together (Fig. 15.23). In this situation, it is anticipated that the movements of the molars will be more translational with no intrusive or extrusive effects. Greater forces are applied with the headcap (250–300 g) than the neck strap (100–150 g) as teeth are more easily extruded with orthodontic treatment.
  - *Low/cervical pull*: use of neck strap alone (Fig. 15.24). The force produced will be downwards and backwards with an extrusive element. Useful in patients with deep bites and low mandibular plane angles as this direction will tend to extrude the molars resulting in an increase in the lower face height and reduction of the overbite.
- **Spring mechanism or strap:** this element connects the face-bow to the headcap or neck strap. Adjustment to this allows for an increase in the magnitude of the force applied. Elastics are rarely used due to their tendency to break.

15.5.3 Headgear safety

Injuries associated with headgear have been reported in the past. Most notably these include serious ocular injuries, reportedly resulting in blindness, which was as a result of the ends of the face-bow coming out of the mouth and causing direct trauma to the eyes. This can occur if the face-bow is pulled out of the mouth and recoils back into the face, but has also been reported after spontaneous disengagement at night.

It is therefore essential that safety features are incorporated when fitting headgear to prevent injuries. The British Orthodontic Society recommends that at least two safety features are incorporated into the headgear. These can take several forms including a snap-away, safety release spring strap mechanism, rigid neck strap, locking face-bow, or safety face-bow (Figs 15.27 and 15.28).

The simplest safety element is the Masel strap (Fig. 15.28), which resists dislodgement of the face-bow. However, evidence suggests that this is not a foolproof method as head posture will affect the fit of the strap and still allow detachment of the face-bow (Fig. 15.29).

Success with extra-oral anchorage is dependent on good patient cooperation. Even with the use of charts for the patients to complete, a number of studies have indicated that patients will often not wear the headgear for the prescribed duration. This has led to a reduction of the use of headgear within clinical practice especially following the introduction of TADs which

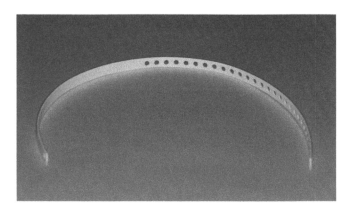

Fig. 15.28 Rigid Masel safety strap.

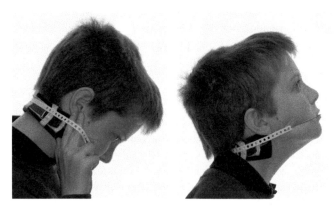

Fig. 15.29 Masel safety strap in use demonstrating how head extension can alter its effectiveness.

have been found to have a good level of acceptance by patients and clinicians, and also reduce the cooperation demands placed upon a patient.

15.5.4 Reverse headgear

A face-mask or reverse/protraction headgear has two uses.

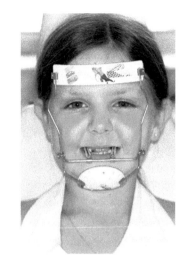

- *Tooth movement*: moving the posterior maxillary teeth mesially, thereby closing up excess space typically found in hypodontia cases, however this use has diminished due to the increasing use of TADs.
- *Skeletal changes*: advancement of the maxilla can be achieved in patients, where a face-mask is fitted and worn a minimum of 14 hours per day (Fig. 15.30). This approach is discussed further in Chapter 11.

Fig. 15.30 Reverse headgear/ face-mask.

15.6 Monitoring anchorage during treatment

15.6.1 Single-arch treatments

If an appliance is used in one arch only (e.g. an upper removable appliance to retract a buccally placed canine, or a quadhelix to expand the upper arch prior to comprehensive appliance treatment) then the lower arch, which is not actively being altered orthodontically, can be used as a reference guide to monitor anchorage during treatment. In these cases, a record at each visit of the molar and canine relationships bilaterally should be made, together with overjet, overbite, or any centreline changes. In this way, any adverse tooth movements can be identified and dealt with.

15.6.2 Definitive orthodontic treatment with upper and lower fixed appliances

In this situation, tooth movements are occurring in both arches simultaneously making assessment of any anchorage loss more complex.

Careful recording of molar and canine relationships, together with overjet, overbite, centrelines, and residual spacing, are essential for these cases. Once alignment has been achieved, and prior to commencing space closure, anchorage requirements should be reassessed with regard to the original aims of treatment. In many cases anchorage can be reinforced using either Class II or Class III elastic traction between the arches. Failure to assess the case correctly at this stage may lead to a compromised result. Some clinicians advocate taking a lateral cephalogram at this stage to enable comparison with the pre-treatment cephalogram; however, this is certainly not required for all patients and, in view of the radiation dose, should be prescribed with care and only undertaken if the outcome is likely to alter the planned treatment mechanics.

15.7 Common problems with anchorage

Anchorage problems arise when the following occurs:

- Failure to correctly plan anchorage requirements at the start of treatment.
- Poor patient compliance, repeated breakages, or failure to wear intermaxillary elastics as instructed will have deleterious effects on the treatment. Lack of headgear wear will necessitate finding alternative methods of anchorage reinforcement, perhaps with the use of TADs or resorting to extractions in a previously non-extraction case.

There is no harm in being overcautious with anchorage requirements at the start of treatment. A transpalatal arch can be easily removed when the canines are Class I, headgear wear can be reduced. However, to tell a patient that headgear is needed some 6 months into treatment or extractions are now required, when not previously discussed, makes a compromise more likely.

15.8 Summary

Orthodontic anchorage planning is fundamentally the balance between maximizing the tooth movements required to achieve the correction of a malocclusion and limiting the undesirable movement of any other teeth. The type of tooth movement undertaken will determine the strain placed upon the anchorage unit. Anchorage can be increased by maximizing the number of teeth (and surface area of their roots) resisting the active tooth movement, either within the same arch (intramaxillary anchorage) or in the opposing arch (intermaxillary anchorage). Extra-oral forces with headgear can also be used, although there is an increasing use of TADs which are reducing the need for patient compliance.

Key points

- Orthodontic anchorage is the resistance to unwanted tooth movement.
- The forces needed to orthodontically move a tooth will vary depending on the type of tooth, its periodontal condition, the distance of movement planned, as well as the type of orthodontic tooth movement desired.
- Goals of anchorage management are to maximize desired tooth movement and minimize unwanted tooth movement.
- Anchorage is not just an anteroposterior phenomenon; unwanted tooth movements can also occur in the vertical and transverse dimensions.
- Anchorage control needs to be continually monitored during treatment to obtain the optimum aesthetic and occlusal result. The earlier any problems with anchorage control are identified, the less undesirable tooth movement will have occurred and the more scope there will be for correction.

Relevant Cochrane reviews

Jambi, S., Walsh, T., Sandler, J., Benson, P. E., Skeggs, R. M., and O'Brien, K. D. (2014). Reinforcement of anchorage during orthodontic brace treatment with implants or other surgical methods. *Cochrane Database of Systematic Reviews*, Issue 8, Art. No.: CD005098. DOI: 10.1002/14651858.CD005098. pub3 https://www.cochranelibrary.com/cdsr/doi/10.1002/14651858. CD005098.pub3/full
This review included 15 studies and concluded there was strong evidence that surgical anchorage, especially with the use of mini-screw implants, was a more effective method of controlling anchorage than traditional approaches.

Jambi, S., Thiruvenkatachari, B., O'Brien, K. D., and Walsh, T. (2013). Orthodontic treatment for distalising upper first molars in children and adolescents. *Cochrane Database of Systematic Reviews*, Issue 10, Art. No.: CD008375. DOI: 10.1002/14651858.CD008375.pub2 https://www. cochranelibrary.com/cdsr/doi/10.1002/14651858.CD008375.pub2/full
This review included ten studies and concluded that the use of intra-oral appliances to distalize maxillary molars was more effective than extra-oral appliances (headgear). However, the use of intraoral appliances was counteracted by a loss of anterior anchorage which did not occur when headgear was used.

Principal sources and further reading

Antoszewska-Smith, J. I., Sarul, M., Łyczek, J., Konopka, T., and Kawala, B. (2017). Effectiveness of orthodontic miniscrew implants in anchorage reinforcement during en-masse retraction: a systematic review and meta-analysis. *American Journal of Orthodontics and Dentofacial Orthopedics*, **151**, 440–55. [DOI: 10.1016/j.ajodo.2016.08.029] [PubMed: 28257728]

Bowden, D. E. J. (1978). Theoretical considerations of headgear therapy; a literature review. 1. Mechanical principles. *British Journal of Orthodontics*, **5**, 145–52. [DOI: 10.1179/bjo.5.3.145] [PubMed: 385036].

Bowden, D. E. J. (1978). Theoretical considerations of headgear therapy: a literature review. 2. Clinical response and usage. *British Journal of Orthodontics*, **5**, 173–81. [DOI: 10.1179/bjo.5.4.173] [PubMed: 385038]
These two papers provide an authoritative review of the principles of headgear.

Cousley, R. (2005). Critical aspects in the use of orthodontics palatal implants. *American Journal of Orthodontics and Dentofacial Orthopaedics*, **127**, 723–9. [DOI: 10.1016/j.ajodo.2004.01.027] [PubMed: 15953898]

Crismani, A. G., Berti, M. H., Celar, A. G., Bantleton, H. P., and Burstone, C. J. (2010). Mini-screws in orthodontic treatment: review and analysis of published clinical trials. *American Journal of Orthodontics and Dentofacial Orthopedics*, **137**, 108–13. [DOI: 10.1016/j.ajodo.2008.01.027] [PubMed: 20122438]
This review indicated that mini-screws (TADs) can be used to reinforce anchorage with a failure rate of less than one in five.

Firouz, M., Zernik, J., and Nanda, R. (1992). Dental and orthopaedic effects of high-pull headgear in treatment of Class II, division 1 malocclusion. *American Journal of Orthodontics and Dentofacial Orthopedics*, **102**, 197–205.

Kerschen, R. H., O'Higgins, E. A., and Lee, R. T. (2000). The Royal London Space Planning: an integration of space analysis and treatment planning: Part I: Assessing the space required to meet treatment objectives. *American Journal of Orthodontics and Dentofacial Orthopedics*, **118**, 448–55.

Kerschen, R. H., O'Higgins, E. A., and Lee, R. T. (2000). The Royal London Space Planning: an integration of space analysis and treatment planning: Part II: The effect of other treatment procedures on space. *American Journal of Orthodontics and Dentofacial Orthopedics*, **118**, 456–61.

Papadopoulos, M. A., Papageorgiou, S. N., and Zogakis, I. P. (2011). Clinical effectiveness of orthodontics miniscrew implants: a meta-analysis. *Journal of Dental Research*, **90**, 969–76.

Postlethwaite, K. (1989). The range and effectiveness of safety products. *European Journal of Orthodontics*, **11**, 228–34.

Prahbu, J. and Cousley, R. R. J. (2006). Current products and practice: bone anchorage devices in orthodontics. *Journal of Orthodontics*, **33**, 288–307.
This paper is an overview of available bone anchorage devices.

Proffit, W. R., Fields, H. R., and Sarver, D. M. (2012). *Contemporary Orthodontics* (5th edn). St Louis, MO: Mosby.

Reynders, R., Ronchi, L., and Bipat, S. (2009). Mini-implants in orthodontics: a systematic review of the literature. *American Journal of Orthodontics and Dentofacial Orthopaedics*, **135**, 564.e1–19.

Sandler, J., Benson, P. E., Doyle, P., Majumder, A., O'Dwyer, J., Speight, P., et al. (2008). Palatal implants are a good alternative to headgear: a randomised trial. *American Journal of Orthodontics and Dentofacial Orthopedics*, **133**, 51–7.
Randomised clinical trial to compare headgear wear with mid-palatal implants. Using clinical and radiographic interpretation, the mid-palatal implant was found to be very effective.

Stivaros, N., Lowe, C., Dandy, N., Doherty, B., and Mandall, N. A. (2010). A randomized clinical trial to compare the Goshgarian and Nance palatal arch. *European Journal of Orthodontic*, **32**, 171–6.

Samuels, R. H. (1996). A review of orthodontic face-bow injuries and safety equipment. *American Journal of Orthodontics and Dentofacial Orthopedics*, **110**, 269–72.

Samuels, R. H. (1997). A new locking face-bow. *Journal of Clinical Orthodontics*, **31**, 24–7.

Upadhyay, M., Yadav, S., Nagaraj, K., and Patil, S. (2008). Treatment effects of mini-implants for en-masse retraction of anterior teeth in bialveolar dental protrusion patients: a randomized controlled trial. *American Journal of Orthodontics Dentofacial Orthopaedics*, **134**, 18–29.

Upadhyay, M., Yadav, S., Nagaraj, K., Uribe, F., and Nanda, R. (2012). Mini-implants vs fixed functional appliances for treatment of young adult Class II female patients. *The Angle Orthodontist*, **82**, 294–303.

Zablocki, H. L., McNamara, J. A. Jr., Franchi, L., and Baccetti, T. (2008). Effect of the transpalatal arch during extraction treatment. *American Journal of Orthodontics and Dentofacial Orthopedics*, **133**, 852–60.

 References for this chapter can also be found at: **www.oup.com/uk/orthodontics5e**. Where possible, these are presented as active links which direct you to the electronic version of the work, to help facilitate onward study. If you are a subscriber to that work (either individually or through an institution), and depending on your level of access, you may be able to peruse an abstract or the full article if available.

16
Retention

S. J. Littlewood

Chapter contents

16.1 Introduction

It is often suggested that the commonest risk of orthodontic treatment is relapse. Retainers are used to minimize this relapse. Orthodontic retention is an essential part of treatment and needs to be planned and discussed with the patient as part of the initial treatment plan.

16.2 Definition of relapse and post-treatment changes

Relapse is officially defined by the British Standards Institute as the return, following correction, of the features of the original malocclusion. However, what is more relevant to patients are any post-treatment changes in tooth position, which can be defined as any changes from the final tooth position at the end of treatment. Post-treatment changes may be a return towards the original malocclusion, but may also be movement caused by age changes, unrelated to the orthodontic treatment.

16.3 Aetiology of post-treatment changes

The exact causes of post-treatment changes are difficult to identify, but four broad areas have been suggested as possible reasons (Fig. 16.1):

- Gingival and periodontal factors
- Occlusal factors
- Soft tissues factors
- Growth factors.

These factors are discussed below, including some suggestions as to how these problems may be overcome.

16.3.1 Gingival and periodontal factors

When teeth are moved, the periodontal ligament and associated alveolar bone remodels. Until the periodontium adapts to the new position, there is a tendency for the stretched periodontal fibres to pull the tooth back to its original position. Different parts of the periodontal ligament complex remodel at different rates (Fig. 16.2). The alveolar bone remodels within a month, the principal fibres rearrange in 3–4 months, and the collagen fibres in the gingivae reorganize after 4–6 months. However, elastic fibres in the dento-gingival and interdental fibres, around the neck of the tooth, can take more than 8 months to remodel. Until the fibres have remodelled there is a tendency for the tooth to be pulled back to its original position.

In practice, this means that teeth need to be held long enough to allow the periodontal fibres to remodel to their new position. This is particularly important for rotated teeth. By correcting any rotated teeth early, this ensures that they are held in the correct position for longer by the fixed appliance. An alternative approach is to actively cut the interdental and dento-gingival fibres above the alveolar bone. This process is known as pericision (see Section 16.7.1).

16.3.2 Occlusal factors

The way the teeth occlude at the end of treatment may affect stability. It has been suggested that if the teeth interdigitate well at the end of

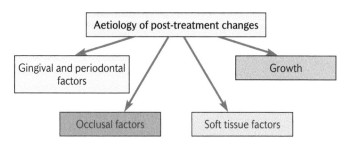

Fig. 16.1 Aetiology of post-treatment changes.

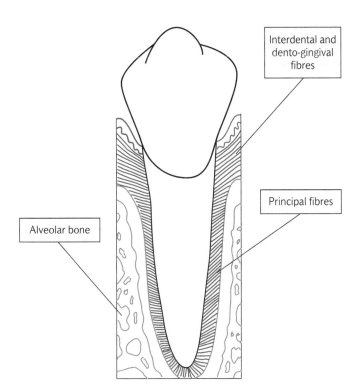

Fig. 16.2 Gingival and periodontal fibres.

Interdental and dento-gingival fibres

Principal fibres

Alveolar bone

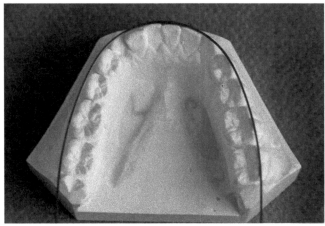

Fig. 16.3 Maintaining the original lower archform to reduce relapse.

treatment then the result is likely to be more stable. While theoretically this sounds sensible, this has not yet been proved clinically, though gross occlusal interferences will predispose to unwanted post-treatment changes.

One of the few occasions when no retainers are required at all uses the occlusion. This is when a labial crossbite is corrected and the result is maintained by the overbite.

16.3.3 Soft tissues

The teeth lie in an area of balance between the tongue on the lingual aspect and the cheeks and lips on the buccal and labial aspects. This area of balance is sometimes referred to as the neutral zone. Although the forces from the tongue are stronger, the activity of a healthy periodontium will resist proclination of the teeth. However, the further teeth are moved out of this zone of stability, the more unstable they are likely to be. This is particularly true for the lower labial segment. If this is either proclined or retroclined excessively, relapse is more likely. In the same way, if the archform (overall shape of the arch) is markedly changed, it is more likely to relapse due to soft tissue pressures. Changes in a patient's intercanine width are more unstable than changes in the intermolar width, which in turn are more unstable than changes in the interpremolar width. Where possible, the original lower archform is therefore maintained throughout treatment, and the upper archform is then planned around the lower (Fig. 16.3).

Although the theory about placing the teeth in the neutral zone is useful, practically there are two major problems for the clinician. Firstly, we do not know exactly where the neutral zone is and how big it is.

Secondly, it is likely that due to changes in muscle tone with age, the neutral zone will change as the patient gets older.

16.3.4 Growth

Although the majority of a patient's growth is complete by the end of puberty, it is now known that small age changes may be occurring throughout life. Subtle changes in the relative positions of the maxilla and the mandible mean that the oral environment and therefore the pressures on the dentition are constantly changing. If the pressures on the teeth are always changing, then it is perhaps not surprising that there is a risk of relapse of the teeth as the patient gets older. These late, small growth changes may at least partly explain the late lower incisor crowding that is seen in patients who have had, but also in those who have not had, orthodontic treatment.

16.3.5 Can the orthodontist prevent post-treatment changes in the long term?

If a patient has a healthy periodontium, the orthodontist can influence periodontal risk factors for relapse by maintaining the teeth in position for long enough to allow fibres to remodel, or by cutting the supracrestal fibres in a process known as pericision (see Section 16.7.1). Occlusal risk factors can also be minimized by the orthodontist, who has the ability to position teeth in the correct occlusal relationships.

The orthodontist, however, cannot prevent long-term growth and soft tissue changes, which perhaps should be regarded as normal age changes. At the present time we are unable to predict the nature of these late changes, which remain an unpredictable cause of post-treatment changes throughout life. These late changes may have little or nothing to do with the orthodontic treatment, but patients may attribute the unwanted post-treatment changes to their orthodontic treatment. During the consent process for orthodontic treatment, it is important that patients are informed about the effects of these unpredictable late age changes, and how they can be minimized.

16.4 How common are post-treatment changes?

Long-term studies of post-treatment changes following fixed appliances have shown that 10 years after retainers are stopped, up to 70% of patients may need retreatment due to these post-treatment changes. These changes continue to get worse over the following decades.

It is difficult to predict, on an individual basis, what post-treatment changes in tooth position will occur. At the present time we are not able to identify which patients will have teeth that will remain in a reasonably stable position, and which patients will not, so we have to presume every patient has the potential to show post-treatment changes. As a result, a contemporary approach is to recommend long-term retention (in the form of fixed retainers, or long-term wear of removable retainers) for as long as the patient wants to keep their teeth stable. This information must be passed onto the patient as part of the informed consent process.

16.5 Consent and the responsibilities of retention

The process of obtaining valid consent requires patients to understand all their options for treatment, including their commitments, and the risks and benefits involved (see Chapter 7, Section 7.8). Post-treatment changes and the need for retention is a vital part of this consent discussion before treatment begins. Arguably the aspect of orthodontics that requires the most commitment from patients is the need to wear and maintain retainers in the long term. A patient who is unwilling, or unable, to commit to retention may not be suitable for treatment.

The clinician is responsible for:

- informing the patient of the need for retainers
- choosing a retention regimen appropriate for each individual patient
- providing advice about how to minimize risks caused by the retainers
- making arrangements for their long–term maintenance, informing the patient of any costs involved.

The patient is responsible for:

- wearing the retainers as advised, including how often to wear the retainers and ensuring they look after them as advised in order to minimize risks
- arranging regular checks of their retainers for as long as they are wearing them, to make sure they are maintained in a condition that ensures they are safe and can successfully reduce relapse. There may be cost implications for the patient for this long-term maintenance.

16.6 Retainers

Retainers are used to reduce relapse. The clinician is faced with a multitude of different options when choosing which retainer to use. When choosing the retention regimen, the following factors should be considered:

- Likely stability of the result
- Initial malocclusion
- Oral hygiene
- Quality of the result (is any settling of the occlusion required?)
- Compliance of patient
- Patient expectations
- Patient preference
- Ease of maintenance.

Retainers can either be removable or fixed. The potential advantages and disadvantages of these will be considered, followed by a detailed look at the most popular retainers in current use.

16.6.1 Removable or fixed retainers?

There are potential advantages to both fixed and removable retainers. The benefits of removable retainers are that they are:

- easier for oral hygiene (they can be removed by the patient for cleaning)
- capable of being worn part-time if required
- predominantly the responsibility of the patient, not the orthodontist (if a patient chooses not to wear their removable retainer, it is the patient's responsibility, whereas if a patient's fixed retainer fails, the orthodontist carries some responsibility).

The potential advantages of fixed retainers include the fact that:

- patients do not need to remember to wear them
- they are useful when the result is very unstable.

There are certain cases where the final result will be extremely unstable. In these cases, it is essential that a retainer is *in situ* full-time, otherwise relapse could occur. In these cases, a fixed retainer is recommended (see Box 16.1).

Box 16.1 High-risk relapse cases where a full-time (bonded) retainer is advisable

- Closure of spaced dentition (including median diastema).
- Following correction of severely rotated teeth.
- Where there has been substantial movement of the lower labial segment, either excessive proclination or retroclination, or a significant change in the intercanine width.
- Where an overjet has been reduced, but the lips are still incompetent.
- Combined periodontal and orthodontic cases, where reduced periodontal support makes relapse more likely (see Chapter 20).

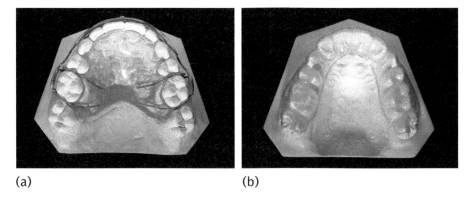

(a)   (b)

Fig. 16.4 Removable retainers. (a) Upper Hawley retainer; (b) upper clear plastic retainer.

16.6.2 Introduction to removable retainers

There are many different types of removable retainers, including Hawley (Fig. 16.4a), clear plastic (Fig. 16.4b), Begg, and Barrer. A removable detailing appliance called a positioner is sometimes also included as a type of removable retainer, but it is really an active appliance made of an elastomeric material. Positioners are used in cases where detailing is required, and the teeth are not well intercuspated at the end of treatment. The teeth are cut off the cast and repositioned and the positioner is then made over this corrected cast. As the patient clenches on the positioner the teeth can be guided into a better occlusion. The positioner can then be worn long term as a retainer. Positioners have the disadvantages of being expensive to construct and long-term patient compliance may be a problem.

16.6.3 How often should removable retainers be worn?

We have already mentioned that due to the unpredictable nature of post-treatment changes, long-term wear is advisable. However, how many hours per day should patients wear removable retainers? The best quality research evidence suggests that both Hawley and clear plastic retainers only need to be worn at night. This of course excludes cases with a high risk of relapse, when full-time wear using a fixed retainer is indicated (see Box 16.1).

16.6.4 Hawley retainer

The Hawley retainer is the original removable retainer. It is a simple and robust appliance made from an acrylic baseplate with a metal labial bow (Fig. 16.5). It was originally designed as an active removable appliance, but it became clear that it could be used as a retainer to maintain the teeth in the correct position after treatment. It has the advantages of being simple to construct, reasonably robust, rigid enough to maintain transverse corrections, and it is easy to add a prosthetic tooth. When replacing missing teeth, it is advisable to put rigid metal stops on the retainer mesial and distal to any prosthetic tooth, to prevent relapse (Fig. 16.6). Hawley retainers also allow more rapid vertical settling of teeth than clear plastic retainers, due to the lack of complete occlusal coverage.

Various adaptations are possible, depending on the case:

- Acrylic facing can be added to the labial bow to help control rotations.
- A reverse U-loop can be used to control the canine position.

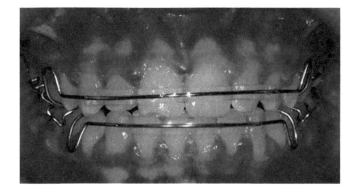

Fig. 16.5 Hawley retainers. These upper and lower Hawley retainers have an acrylic facing added to the labial bow. This acrylic provides increased contact with the teeth and is designed to reduce relapse, particularly with rotated teeth.

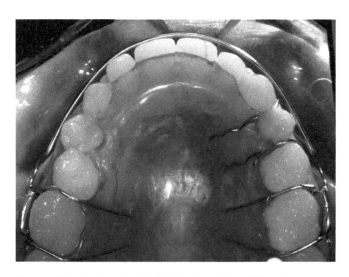

Fig. 16.6 Prosthetic tooth added to Hawley retainer. This patient presented with missing upper left first premolar and both upper second premolars. It was decided to maintain the second deciduous molars, which had good roots. A space was localized in the area of the upper left first premolar, and this Hawley was fitted with a prosthetic tooth in that region. Note the presence of the mesial and distal stops either side of the prosthetic tooth to reduce the relapse potential.

- A passive bite-plane can be added to maintain corrections of deep overbites.

- The labial bow can be soldered to the cribs, so there are fewer wires to cross the occlusal surfaces and interfere with the occlusion.

- Clear polyethylene bow to provide improved aesthetics (see Fig. 16.7).

16.6.5 Clear plastic retainers

Clear plastic retainers (Fig. 16.8) offer a number of potential advantages over traditional Hawley retainers:

- Superior aesthetics

- Less interference with speech

- More economical and quicker to make

- Less likely to break

- Ease of fabrication

- Superior retention of the lower incisors.

Both Hawley and clear plastic retainers are equally successful in the upper arch, but the clear plastic retainers are better at preventing relapse in the lower arch.

Clear plastic retainers only need to be worn at night, every night. It is important that the patient is instructed never to drink with the clear plastic retainer *in situ*, particularly cariogenic drinks (Fig. 16.9). The retainer can act like a reservoir, holding the cariogenic drink in contact with the incisal edges and cuspal tips and leading to decalcification.

Clear plastic retainers may be contraindicated in patients with poor oral hygiene. This is because these types of retainers are retained by the plastic engaging the undercut gingival to the contact point. If the oral hygiene is poor, then hyperplastic gingivae can obliterate these areas of undercut, which means the retainer may be loose.

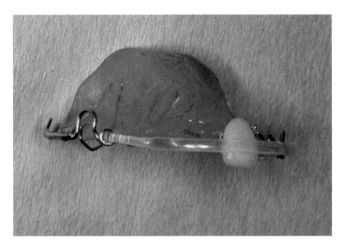

Fig. 16.7 Hawley retainer with aesthetic polyethylene bow. This is a Hawley retainer with an aesthetic polyethylene bow with stainless steel joint (Clearbow®, PWG Orthodontic Specialists, Dorval, Canada). This allows the patient to wear a removable retainer with a prosthetic tooth, with an aesthetic labial bow.

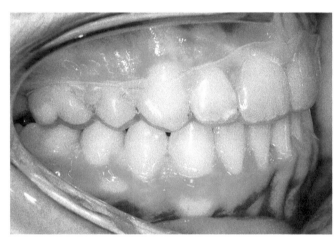

Fig. 16.8 Upper clear plastic retainer. The upper vacuum-formed retainer has been trimmed to finish 1–2 mm above the gingival margin. The exception is the area cut away over the canine to make it simpler for the patient to remove the retainer.

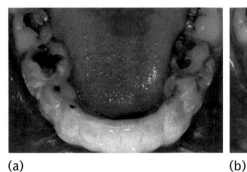

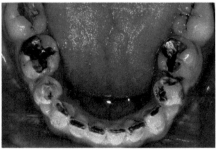

(a)   (b)

Fig. 16.9 Cariogenic drinks and clear plastic retainers. It is vital that patients are instructed not to wear clear plastic retainers when eating or drinking. This patient wore a clear plastic retainer full-time (a), while regularly drinking fizzy drinks, leading to substantial tooth surface loss and caries (b). Reproduced from Chapter 37 Stability and retention, in *Orthodontics: Principles and Practice*, D.S. Gill and F.B. Naini (Eds). Copyright (2011) with permission from John Wiley & Sons, Ltd.

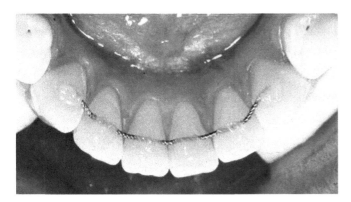

Fig. 16.10 Multistrand bonded retainer. This multistrand stainless steel retainer is bonded to each tooth from lower canine to lower canine, using composite resin. The diameter of the round wire is 0.0195 inches which allows some flexibility between the teeth. This flexibility allows the teeth to move very slightly in function.

16.6.6 Fixed retainers

Fixed or bonded retainers are usually attached to the palatal aspect of the upper or lower labial segment, using normal acid-etch composite bonding. There are different types of bonded retainers:

- Multistrand retainers bonded to each tooth (Fig. 16.10)
- Flexible chain retainers bonded to each tooth
- Nickel titanium computer-assisted design/manufacture (CAD/CAM) retainer (Fig. 16.11)
- Rigid canine-and-canine retainers, which are only bonded to the canine teeth
- Reinforced fibres.

The multistrand 'twistflex' wire type, bonded to each tooth in the labial segment, is the commonest type of retainer. In rare situations, activity may develop in these wires, causing unwanted tooth movement, which has led to the development of flexible chain retainers and nickel-titanium CAD/CAM retainers (Fig. 16.11) to ensure a passive fit.

Fixed retainers bonded only to the canine teeth allow easier cleaning. These canine-and-canine retainers are more rigid, and are sometimes referred to as 'fail-safe'. This because if one attachment fails, the patient will immediately know about it and get it repaired. The disadvantage with the canine-and-canine retainers is that they may result in relapse of the incisors, which are not bonded to the wire. The reinforced fibre retainers are not recommended as they tend to fracture more frequently due to lack of flexibility.

Bonding retainers is a very technique-sensitive process. The tooth surface should be thoroughly cleaned before bonding, in particular removing any calculus lingual to the lower labial segment (etching alone is often not sufficient). A dry field needs to be maintained and the wire held passively in position while being bonded to the teeth with a composite resin using the acid-etch technique. If the bonded retainer is not passive when bonded, or is distorted *in situ*, it can cause unwanted tooth movement, which can compromise aesthetics and dental health (see section on 'Principal sources and further reading').

The most common problem with bonded retainers is localized relapse if there is partial debond of the retainer. To overcome this, some

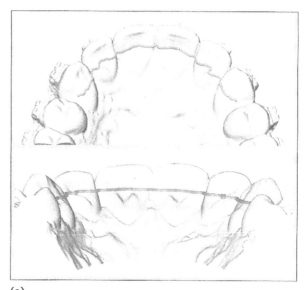

(a)

(b)

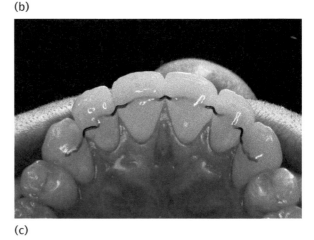

(c)

Fig. 16.11 Nickel-titanium CAD/CAM Memotain® retainer. (a) Digital scan of proposed retainer sent for approval to clinician. After sending off an impression or a digital scan to the manufacturers, this digital design is sent to the clinician to approve the retainer design. Note the accuracy of the wire as it conforms to the exact shape of the palatal surfaces. (b) Nickel-titanium fixed retainer, with positioning jig, sealed onto the cast. The use of nickel-titanium aims to allow flexibility and shape memory when in physiological use. (c) Nickel-titanium CAD/CAM fixed bonded in place.

clinicians use dual retention—using a bonded retainer, backed up with a removable retainer at night. This 'belt and braces' approach ensures that if a bonded retainer partially debonds, the teeth can be maintained in position until it can be repaired (Fig. 16.12).

16.6.7 Care of retainers

In the past, patients were asked to wear retainers for only 1–2 years. However, now that we have a better understanding of the risk of relapse, we need to ask our patients to wear them for longer. It is therefore essential that the patients have a clear understanding of how to look after the retainers.

Removable retainers are easier to care for, as they can be removed to allow oral hygiene intra-orally, in addition to easier cleaning of the retainers themselves. Although toothpaste can be used to clean acrylic-based retainers, like the Hawley retainer, many clear plastic retainers need to be cleaned with special cleaning materials that do not degrade the plastic. Some clinicians provide a spare retainer for each arch, in case the original is lost. This is particularly the case with clear plastic retainers, which are cheaper to fabricate. Box 16.2 shows an example of a patient information sheet for clear plastic retainers.

Fixed retainers have the potential to cause both periodontal disease and caries unless they are well maintained. Fixed retainers can be used safely in the long term, provided patients are properly instructed how to look after them. They should be shown how to clean interdentally—either by using floss that can be threaded under the wire, or by the gentle use of small interdental brushes or other similar interdental cleaning aids. Fixed retainers need to be reviewed on a regular basis by the orthodontist or dental practitioner to check for any bond failure, or unwanted tooth movement caused by fixed retainers that have become active.

It is the orthodontist's responsibility to ensure that the patient is fully informed on how to look after their retainers in the long term to avoid any adverse effects.

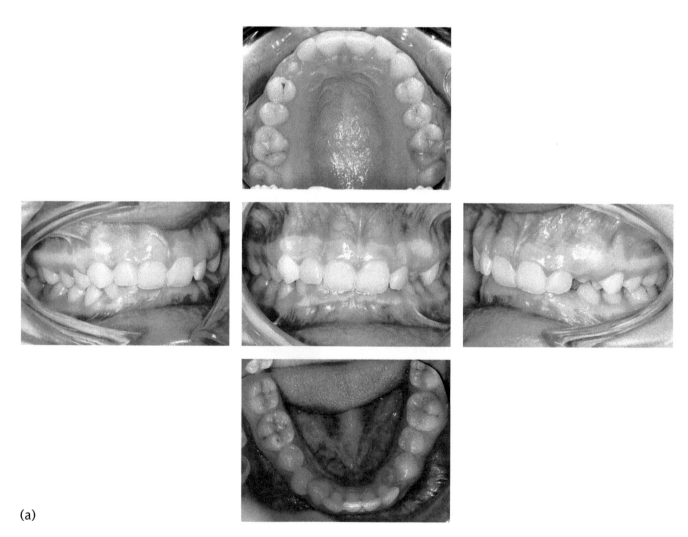

(a)

Fig. 16.12 (a) Initial presentation. This patient presented with a Class II division 2 incisor relationship. It was decided to treat the case as non-extraction, using some enamel stripping in the lower arch and accepting some proclination of the lower labial segment. This would help to reduce the overbite, but would increase the risk of instability. The patient was therefore informed that she would require permanent retention of the lower labial segment at the end of treatment.

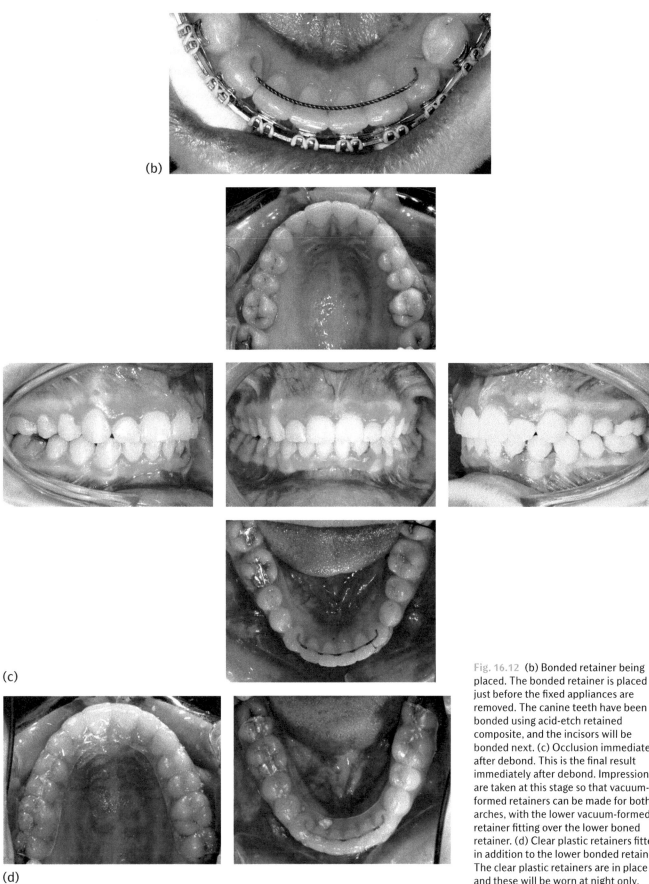

(b)

(c)

(d)

Fig. 16.12 (b) Bonded retainer being placed. The bonded retainer is placed just before the fixed appliances are removed. The canine teeth have been bonded using acid-etch retained composite, and the incisors will be bonded next. (c) Occlusion immediately after debond. This is the final result immediately after debond. Impressions are taken at this stage so that vacuum-formed retainers can be made for both arches, with the lower vacuum-formed retainer fitting over the lower boned retainer. (d) Clear plastic retainers fitted in addition to the lower bonded retainer. The clear plastic retainers are in place and these will be worn at night only.

Box 16.2 Patient information sheet about clear plastic retainers

1. **Your retainers are as important as your braces.**
   If you do not wear your retainers as instructed, your teeth will move back towards how they were before treatment. If you cannot wear your retainers, please contact …

2. **How often do I wear them?**
   You should wear the retainers at night, *every* night.

3. **How long do I have to wear them?**
   The best way to reduce the risk of teeth going crooked is to continue wearing the retainers at night. This is because we now know that teeth move all through our life.

4. **How do I keep them clean?**
   Clean your retainers with a toothbrush and water but *do not use toothpaste* on the retainer. Toothpaste will discolour and degrade the retainer. Your orthodontist may recommend using a special retainer cleaner.

5. **Do not eat or drink with the retainer in.**
   You should never eat or drink when you are wearing the retainer.

6. **Keep the retainer safe**
   When you are not wearing the retainer, keep it safely in a protective box.

7. **What do I do if I miss wearing it for a night?**
   You must try and wear the retainers every night. If you do forget, then wear the retainer full-time except meals for 2 days. This is often enough to squeeze the teeth back into place.

8. **What do I do if I lose a retainer?**
   If you lose a retainer, wear the spare we have provided. Then contact the department and if you bring the models back in we will be able to make another spare for you. There will be a small charge to make the replacement.

9. **What do I do if the retainer rubs?**
   If the retainer rubs, you can smooth it with an emery board used to file nails. If this doesn't work, then contact us.

10. **Bring your retainers to every appointment**
    It is important that you bring your retainers to every appointment, so that we can check and adjust them if needed.

This information can be given to patients who are prescribed clear plastic retainers. This sheet can be downloaded from: www.oup.com/uk/orthodontics5e.

16.7 Adjunctive techniques used to reduce post-treatment changes

Adjunctive techniques are additional soft and hard tissue procedures, usually used in addition to retainers, to help enhance stability:

- Pericision
- Interproximal reduction.

16.7.1 Pericision

This is also known as circumferential supracrestal fibreotomy. The principle is to cut the interdental and dento-gingival fibres above the level of the alveolar bone (Fig. 16.2). The elastic fibres within the interdental and dento-gingival fibres have a tendency to pull the teeth back towards their original position. This is particularly true with teeth that have been de-rotated.

Pericision is a simple procedure undertaken under local anaesthetic and requires no periodontal dressing afterwards. The cuts are made vertically into the periodontal pocket, severing the supra-alveolar fibres around the neck of the teeth, but taking care not to touch the alveolar bone. The technique has been shown to reduce rotational relapse by up to 30% and is most effective in the maxilla. There are no adverse effects on the periodontal health, provided there is no evidence of inflammation or periodontal disease before the pericision.

16.7.2 Interproximal reduction

This is also known as reproximation or enamel stripping (see Chapter 7, Section 7.7.5). The removal of small amounts of enamel mesiodistally has been used to reshape teeth and to create small amounts of space (see Chapter 7, Fig. 7.7). It has been suggested that by flattening the interdental contacts, this will increase the stability between adjacent teeth. It may also be the case that by removing small amounts of tooth tissue any minor crowding is relieved, avoiding possible proclination of the lower labial segment and increase in the intercanine width, both of which are potentially unstable movements.

16.8 Conclusions about retention

Retention is an important part of almost every case of orthodontic treatment. This is because post-treatment changes in tooth position are an unpredictable risk for every patient. Post-treatment changes can be due to orthodontic factors, but it can also be due to factors out of the control of the orthodontist, such as further growth and changes in soft tissues. The patient needs to be made aware of the long-term risk of these unwanted changes and informed of ways of reducing the risk of this happening. This should be discussed before treatment.

Reducing post-treatment changes usually means the patient wearing a retainer. The choice of retainer is affected by the likely stability of the result, the original presenting malocclusion, patient compliance, patient expectations, and the quality of the result.

The patient must be given information about possible post-treatment changes and how to look after and maintain the retainers, so that the patient can take responsibility for the retention phase of treatment.

The orthodontist is responsible for:

- ensuring the patient recognizes the need for and importance of retainers

- choosing an appropriate retention regimen suitable for each individual patient

- informing each patient how to wear and look after their retainers safely, making sure the patient appreciates the need for the long-term maintenance of retainers.

Key points about retention

- Relapse is an unpredictable risk for every orthodontic patient.
- Relapse can be due to orthodontic factors, but can also be due to age changes out of the orthodontist's control.
- As part of the informed consent process, the patient needs to be aware of the long-term risk of relapse and informed of ways of reducing this risk.

- Removable and fixed retainers can be used to reduce relapse, in addition to adjunctive techniques such as pericision.
- Removable retainers only need to be worn at night.
- The patient must recognize their responsibilities in the retention phase of treatment.

Relevant Cochrane review

Littlewood, S. J., Millett, D. T., Doubleday, B., Bearn, D. R., and Worthington, H. V. (2016). Retention procedures for stabilising tooth position after treatment with orthodontic braces. *Cochrane Database of Systematic Reviews*, Issue 1, Art. No.: CD002283. DOI: 10.1002/14651858.CD002283. pub4 https://www.cochranelibrary.com/cdsr/doi/10.1002/14651858.CD002283.pub4/full
This systematic review discusses the best evidence for different approaches to reducing relapse.

Principal sources and further reading

Hichens, L., Rowland, H., Williams, A., Hollinghurst, S., Ewings, P., Clark, S., et al. (2007). Cost-effectiveness and patient satisfaction: Hawley and vacuum-formed retainers. *European Journal of Orthodontics*, **29**, 372–8. [DOI: 10.1093/ejo/cjm039] [PubMed: 17702797]

Rowland, H., Hichens, L., Williams, A., Hills, D., Killingback, N., Ewings, P., et al. (2007). The effectiveness of Hawley and vacuum-formed retainers: a single-center randomized controlled trial. *American Journal of Orthodontics and Dentofacial Orthopedics*, **132**, 730–7. [DOI: 10.1016/j.ajodo.2006.06.019] [PubMed: 18068589]
These two papers describe a well-designed randomized controlled trial comparing Hawley retainers and vacuum-formed retainers.

Kucera, J. and Marek, I. (2016). Unexpected complications associated with mandibular fixed retainers: a retrospective study. *American Journal of Orthodontics and Dentofacial Orthopedics*, **149**, 202–11. [DOI: 10.1016/j.ajodo.2015.07.035] [PubMed: 26827976]
This paper describes the side effects of bonded retainers, including unwanted tooth movement with the retainer still in situ.

Little, R. M., Wallen, T. R., and Riedel, R. A. (1981). Stability and relapse of mandibular alignment – first four premolar extraction cases treated by traditional edgewise orthodontics. *American Journal of Orthodontics and Dentofacial Orthopedics*, **80**, 349–65. [DOI: 10.1016/0002-9416(81)90171-8]
A classic paper that demonstrates the high risk of relapse after orthodontic treatment.

Littlewood, S. J. (2017). Responsibilities and retention. *APOS Trends in Orthodontics*, **7**, 211–14. [DOI: 10.4103/apos.apos_82_17]
This paper provides an overview of the important roles and responsibilities of the patient, orthodontist, and general dental practitioner in retention.

References for this chapter can also be found at: **www.oup.com/uk/orthodontics5e**. Where possible, these are presented as active links which direct you to the electronic version of the work, to help facilitate onward study. If you are a subscriber to that work (either individually or through an institution), and depending on your level of access, you may be able to peruse an abstract or the full article if available.

17

Removable appliances

L. Mitchell

Chapter contents

Learning objectives for this chapter

- Gain an understanding of the limitations of removable appliances.
- Gain an appreciation of contemporary use of removable appliances.
- Gain an understanding of the design, insertion, and adjustment of removable appliances.

This chapter concerns those appliances that are fabricated mainly in acrylic and wire, and can be removed from the mouth by the patient. Functional appliances are made of the same materials, but work primarily by exerting intermaxillary traction and so are considered separately in Chapter 19. Removable retainers, such as Hawley retainers, are discussed in Chapter 16 and removable, clear orthodontic aligners are considered in Chapter 21.

17.1 Mode of action of removable appliances

Removable appliances are capable of the following types of tooth movement:

- Tipping movements—because a removable appliance applies a single-point contact force to the crown of a tooth, the tooth tilts around a fulcrum, which in a single-rooted tooth is approximately 40% of the root length from the apex.
- Movements of blocks of teeth—because removable appliances are connected by a baseplate (see Section 17.5) they are more efficient at moving blocks of teeth than fixed appliances.
- Influencing the eruption of opposing teeth—this can be achieved by use of either:
  (a) a flat anterior bite-plane, which frees the occlusion of the lower molars allowing their eruption. This is useful in overbite reduction (see Section 17.5.2), or
  (b) buccal capping, which frees contact between the incisors, thereby eliminating incisor interferences (see Section 17.5.3). This may also be of value when intrusion of the buccal segments is required (see Chapter 12, Section 12.3.1).

17.1.1 Indications for the use of removable appliances

Although widely utilized in the past as the sole appliance to treat a malocclusion, with the increasing availability and acceptance of fixed appliances, the limitations of the removable appliance have become more apparent. The removable appliance is only capable of producing tilting movements of individual teeth (see Chapter 15, Fig. 15.2), which can be used to advantage where simple tipping movements are required,

but can lead to a compromise result if employed where more complex tooth movements are indicated. As a result, the role of the removable appliance has changed and it is now widely used as an adjunct to fixed appliance treatment.

Removable appliances provide a useful means of applying extra-oral traction to segments of teeth, or an entire arch, to help achieve intrusion and/or distal movement. Removable appliances are also employed for arch expansion, which is another example of their usefulness in moving blocks of teeth. Removable appliances are particularly helpful where a flat anterior bite-plane or buccal capping is required to influence development of the buccal segment teeth and/or to free the occlusion with the lower arch.

Removable appliances are also utilized in a passive role as space maintainers following permanent tooth extractions and also as retaining appliances following fixed appliance treatment. They are particularly helpful when space has been created for missing teeth as pontic teeth can be included.

The advantages and disadvantages of removable appliances are summarized in Table 17.1.

Lower removable appliances are generally less well tolerated by patients. This is due in part to their encroachment upon tongue space, but also the lingual tilt of the lower molars makes retentive clasping difficult.

Although less likely to cause iatrogenic damage, for example, root resorption or decalcification, removable appliances can be detrimental to the patient if used inappropriately. Skill is required to judge the situations where their use is applicable and to carry out tooth movement effectively.

Table 17.1 Advantages and disadvantages of removable appliances

Advantages	Disadvantages
Can be removed for tooth-brushing	Appliance can be left out
Palatal coverage increases anchorage	Only tilting movements possible
Easy to adjust	Good technician required
Less risk of iatrogenic damage (e.g. root resorption) than with fixed appliances	Affects speech
Acrylic can be thickened to form flat anterior bite-plane or buccal capping	Intermaxillary traction more difficult
Useful as passive retainer or space maintainer	Lower removable appliances are difficult to tolerate
Can be used to transmit forces to blocks of teeth	Inefficient for multiple individual tooth movements

17.2 Designing removable appliances

17.2.1 General principles

The design of an appliance should never be delegated to a laboratory as they are only able to utilize the information provided by the plaster casts. Success depends upon designing an appliance that is easy for the patient to insert and wear, and is relevant to the occlusal aims of treatment.

17.2.2 Steps in designing a removable appliance

Four components need to be considered for every removable appliance:

- Active component(s)
- Retaining the appliance
- Anchorage
- Baseplate.

A detailed consideration of each of these components is given in the following sections.

Generally, extractions should be deferred until after an appliance is fitted. The rationale for this is twofold:

1. If the extractions are carried out first, there is a real risk that the teeth posterior to the extraction site will drift forward, resulting in an appliance that does not fit well or even does not fit at all. This is most noticeable when upper first permanent molars have been extracted or there is a conspicuous delay before the appliance is fitted.

2. Occasionally a patient decides after an appliance is fitted that they do not wish to continue wearing it and therefore decide against continuing with treatment. It is obviously preferable if this change of mind occurs before any extractions have been undertaken.

Rarely, it is necessary to carry out extractions first, for example, when a displaced tooth will interfere with the design of the appliance. However, even in these cases it is preferable to take impressions for the fabrication of the appliance before the extractions and to instruct the technician to remove the tooth concerned from the model. The appliance should then be fitted as soon as practicable after the tooth, or teeth, are extracted.

17.3 Active components

17.3.1 Springs

Springs are the most commonly used active component. Their design can readily be adapted to the needs of a particular clinical situation and they are inexpensive. However, a skilled technician is required to fabricate a spring that works efficiently with the minimum of adjustment on fitting.

The expression for the force F exerted by an orthodontic spring is one of only a few formulae remembered by the author of this chapter and on this basis is recommended to the reader as being worthwhile:

$$F \propto \frac{dr^4}{l^3}$$

where d is the deflection of the spring on activation, r is the radius of the wire, and l is the length of the spring.

Thus even small changes in the diameter or length of wire used in the construction of a spring will have a profound impact upon the force delivered, for example, doubling the radius of the wire increases the force by a factor of 16. It is obviously desirable to deliver a light (physiological) force (see Chapter 4, Section 4.10) over a long activation range, but there are practical restrictions upon the length and diameter of wire used to construct a spring. The span of a spring is usually constrained by the size of the arch or the depth of the sulcus. However, incorporating a coil into the design of a spring increases the length of wire and therefore results in the application of a smaller force for a given deflection. A spring with a coil will work more efficiently if it is activated in the direction that the wire has been wound, so that the coil unwinds as the tooth moves.

In practice, the smallest diameter of wire that can be used for spring construction is 0.5 mm. However, wire of this diameter is liable to

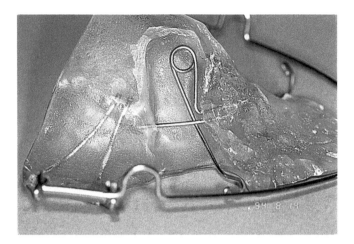

Fig. 17.1 Palatal finger spring. Note that the spring is boxed in with acrylic and a guard wire is present to help prevent distortion.

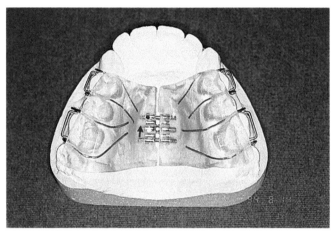

Fig. 17.3 Screw appliance to expand the upper arch.

distortion or breakage and therefore some designs are protected by acrylic, for example, the palatal finger spring (Fig. 17.1), or strengthened by being sleeved in tubing (Fig. 17.2).

It is essential that a spring is adjusted to ensure that the point of application will give the desired direction of movement. The further the spring is from the centre of resistance of the tooth, the greater the degree of tilting. Therefore, a spring should be adjusted so that it is as near the gingival margin as possible without causing gingival trauma. If the spring is overactivated, this increases the force on the tooth and has the effect of moving the centre of resistance more apically (therefore more tipping occurs).

17.3.2 Screws

Screws are less versatile than springs, as the direction of tooth movement is determined by the position of the screw in the appliance. They are also bulky, more expensive, and require patients to remember to turn it. However, a screw appliance may be useful when it is desirable to utilize the teeth to be moved for additional clasping to retain the appliance. This is helpful when a number of teeth are to be moved together,

for example, in an appliance to expand the upper arch (Fig. 17.3), or in the mixed dentition where retaining an appliance is always difficult.

The most commonly used type of screw consists of two halves on a threaded central cylinder (Fig. 17.4) turned by means of a key which separates the two halves by a predetermined distance, usually about 0.25 mm for each quarter turn.

Activation of a screw is limited by the width of the periodontal ligament, as to exceed this would result in crushing the ligament cells and cessation of tooth movement (see Chapter 4, Section 4.10). One quarter-turn opens the two sections of the appliance by 0.25 mm.

17.3.3 Elastics

Special intra-oral elastics are manufactured for orthodontic use (see Chapter 18, Fig. 18.20). These elastics are usually classified by their size, ranging from ⅛ inch to ¾ inch, and the force that they are designed to deliver, usually 2, 3.5, or 4.5 ounces. Selection of the appropriate size and force is based upon the root surface area of the teeth to be moved and the distance over which the elastic is to be stretched. The elastics should be changed every day. Latex-free alternatives are now widely available.

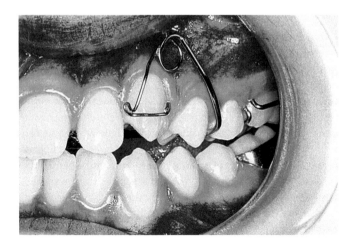

Fig. 17.2 Buccal canine retractor (distal section sleeved in tubing).

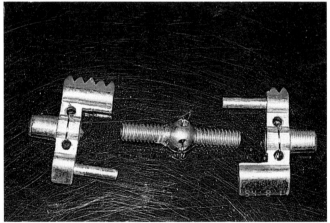

Fig. 17.4 Components of a screw.

17.4 Retaining the appliance

17.4.1 Adams clasp

This crib was designed to engage the undercuts present on a fully erupted first permanent molar at the junctions of the mesial and distal surfaces with the buccal aspect of the tooth (Fig. 17.5). The crib is usually fabricated in hard 0.7 mm stainless steel wire and should engage about 1 mm of undercut. In practice, this means that in children the arrowheads will lie at or just below the gingival margin. However, in adults with some gingival recession, the arrowheads should lie part way down the crown of the tooth (Fig. 17.6).

This crib can also be used for retention on premolars, canines, central incisors, and deciduous molars. However, it is advisable to use 0.6 mm wire for these teeth. When second permanent molars have to be utilized for retention soon after their eruption, it is wise to omit the distobuccal arrowhead, as little undercut exists and if included it may irritate the cheek.

The reason for the popularity of the Adams crib is its versatility as it can be easily adapted:

- Extra-oral traction tubes, labial bows, or buccal springs can be soldered onto the bridge of the clasp (Fig. 17.7).
- Hooks or coils can be fabricated in the bridge of the clasp during construction.
- Double cribs can be constructed which straddle two teeth.

Adjustment: the crib can be adjusted in two places. Bends in the middle of the flyover will move the arrowhead down and in towards the tooth. Adjustments near the arrowhead will result in more movement towards the tooth and will have less effect in the vertical plane (Fig. 17.8).

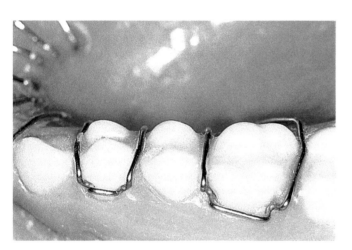

Fig. 17.5 Adams clasp.

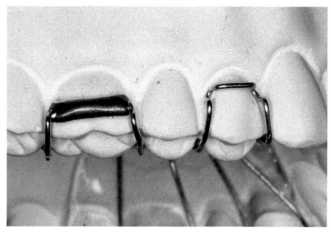

Fig. 17.7 A tube for an extra-oral face-bow has been soldered onto the bridge of this Adams crib.

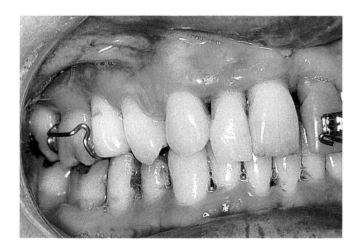

Fig. 17.6 Ideally the Adams clasp should engage about 1 mm of undercut. Therefore, in adults with some gingival recession, the arrowheads will probably lie part way down the crown of the tooth.

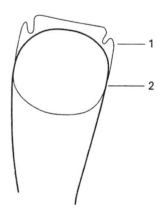

1 Arrowhead moves horizontally in towards tooth

2 Arrowhead moves in towards tooth and also vertically towards gingival crevice

Fig. 17.8 Adjustment of an Adams clasp.

17.4.2 Other methods of retention

Southend clasp

This clasp (Fig. 17.9) is designed to utilize the undercut beneath the contact point between two incisors. It is usually fabricated in 0.7 mm hard stainless steel wire.

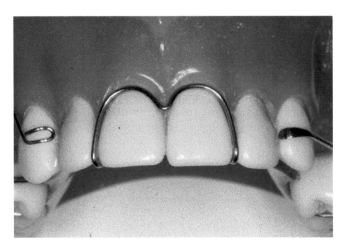

Fig. 17.9 Southend clasp.

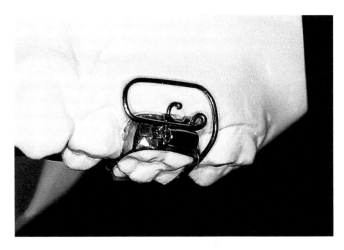

Fig. 17.10 Plint clasp.

Adjustment: retention is increased by bending the arrowhead in towards the teeth.

Ball-ended clasps

These clasps are designed to engage the undercut interproximally. This design affords minimal retention and can have the effect of prising the teeth apart.

Adjustment: the ball is bent in towards the contact point between the teeth.

Plint clasp

This clasp (Fig. 17.10) is used to engage under the tube assembly on a molar band or bracket.

Adjustment: by moving the clasp under the molar tube.

Labial bows

A labial bow (Fig. 17.11) is useful for anterior retention.

Adjustment: this will depend upon the exact design of an individual bow. However, the most commonly used type with U-loops is adjusted by squeezing together the legs of the U-loop and then adjusting the height of the labial bow by a bend at the anterior leg to compensate (Fig. 17.12).

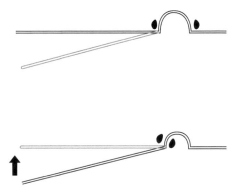

Fig. 17.12 Diagram illustrating how to tighten a labial bow. The first adjustment is to squeeze together the two legs of the U-loop. This causes the anterior section of the bow to move occlusally and therefore a second adjustment is required to lift it back to the desired horizontal position.

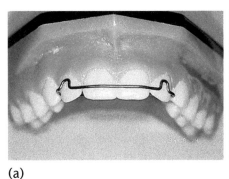
(a)

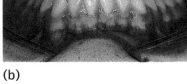
(b)

Fig. 17.11 Two types of labial bow.

17.5 Baseplate

The individual components of a removable appliance are connected by means of an acrylic baseplate, which can be a passive or active component of the appliance.

17.5.1 Self-cure or heat-cure acrylic

Heat-curing of polymethylmethacrylate increases the degree of polymerization of the material and optimizes its properties, but is technically more demanding to produce. It is common practice to make the majority of appliances in self-cure acrylic, retaining heat-cure acrylic for those situations where additional strength is desirable, for example, some functional appliances.

17.5.2 Anterior bite-plane

Increasing the thickness of acrylic behind the upper incisors forms a bite-plane onto which the lower incisors occlude. A bite-plane is prescribed when either the overbite needs to be reduced by eruption of the lower buccal segment teeth or elimination of possible occlusal interferences is necessary to allow tooth movement to occur.

Anterior bite-planes are usually flat. Inclined bite-planes may lead to proclination or retroclination of the lower incisors, depending upon their angulation.

When prescribing a flat anterior bite-plane, the following information needs to be given to the technician:

- How far posteriorly the bite-plane should extend. This is most easily conveyed by noting the overjet.
- The depth of the bite-plane. To increase the likelihood that the patient will wear the appliance, the bite-plane should result in a separation of only 1–2 mm between the upper and lower molars. The depth is prescribed in terms of the height of the bite-plane against the upper incisors, for example: '½ height of the upper incisor'.

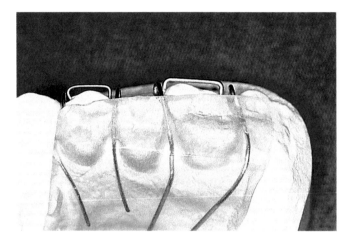

Fig. 17.13 Buccal capping.

17.5.3 Buccal capping

Buccal capping is prescribed when occlusal interferences need to be eliminated to allow tooth movement to be accomplished and reduction of the overbite is undesirable. Buccal capping is produced by carrying the acrylic over the occlusal surface of the buccal segment teeth (Fig. 17.13) and has the effect of propping the incisors apart. The acrylic should be as thin as practicably possible to aid patient tolerance. During treatment it is not uncommon for the capping to fracture and it is wise to warn patients of this, advising them to return if a sharp edge results. However, if as a result a tooth is left free of the acrylic and is liable to over-erupt, a new appliance will be necessary (as additions to buccal capping are rarely successful).

17.6 Commonly used removable appliances

17.6.1 To correct anterior crossbite in mixed dentition

Movement labially of upper incisors in the mixed dentition can be accomplished either using a spring or screw design depending upon the number of incisors to be moved. To move a single incisor buccally, a Z-spring is commonly used (Fig. 17.14). This design is also known as a double-cantilever spring when it is used for moving more than one tooth. A Z-spring for a single tooth should be fabricated in 0.5 mm wire, but for longer spans 0.6 or 0.7 mm is advisable. Good anterior retention is required to resist the displacing effect of this spring.

Activation is by pulling the spring about 1–2 mm away from the baseplate at an angle of approximately 45° in the direction of desired movement (so that the spring is not caught on the incisal edge(s) as the appliance is inserted).

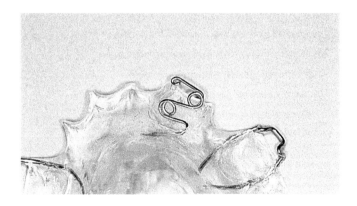

Fig. 17.14 Z-spring.

Buccal capping is usually incorporated into this appliance to free the occlusion with the lower arch.

17.6.2 Screw appliance to expand upper arch

As mentioned above, a design incorporating a screw is useful for moving blocks of teeth and has the additional advantage that the teeth being moved can also be clasped for retention. Again, buccal capping is also used to free occlusion with the lower arch (Fig. 17.3).

Activation: this is by means of turning the screw by one quarter-turn. One quarter-turn opens the two sections of the appliance by 0.25 mm. For active movement the patient should turn the screw twice a week (e.g. on a Wednesday and a Saturday). If opened too far, the screw will come apart; therefore patients should be warned that if the screw portion becomes loose they should turn it back one turn and not advance the screw again.

17.6.3 Nudger appliance

This appliance is used in conjunction with headgear to bands on the first molar teeth (Fig. 17.15). It is usually used to achieve distal movement of the molar teeth when it is intended to go onto fixed appliances to complete alignment. The appliance incorporates palatal finger springs (in 0.5 mm wire) to retract the first permanent molars. The appliance is worn full-time and the patient is asked to wear the headgear for 12–16 hours per day. The palatal finger springs are only lightly activated with the aim of minimizing forward movement of the molar when the headgear is not worn. This appliance is also very useful if unilateral distal movement is required. In this case, the contralateral molar can be clasped to aid retention. If overbite reduction is required

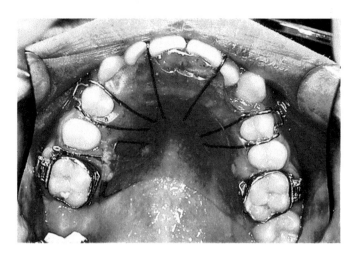

Fig. 17.15 Nudger appliance for unilateral movement of the upper right first permanent molar.

then a bite-plane can be included in the appliance. It is advisable to fit the bands on the molar teeth and then take an impression to fabricate the appliance.

17.6.4 Expansion and Labial Segment Alignment Appliance (ELSAA)

This appliance is used in Class II division 2 malocclusions prior to functional appliance therapy to correct an anteroposterior discrepancy (see Chapter 10, Section 10.4.5 and Fig. 10.22).

17.7 Fitting a removable appliance

It is always useful to explain again to the patient (and their parent/guardian) the overall treatment plan and the role of the appliance that is to be fitted. It is also prudent to delay any permanent extractions until after an appliance has been fitted and the patient's ability to achieve full-time wear has been demonstrated.

Fitting an appliance can be approached in the following way (see also Box 17.1):

1. Check that you have the correct appliance for the patient in the chair and that your prescription has been followed.
2. Show the appliance to the patient and explain how it works.
3. Check the fitting surface for any roughness.
4. Try in the appliance. If it does not fit, check the following:
   - Have any teeth erupted since the impression was taken? If necessary, adjust the acrylic.
   - Have any teeth moved since the impression was recorded? This usually occurs if any extractions have been recently carried out.
   - Has there been a significant delay between taking the impression and fitting the appliance?
5. Adjust the retention until the appliance just clicks into place.
6. If the appliance has a bite-plane or buccal capping, this will need to be trimmed so that it is active but not too bulky.

> **Box 17.1 Instruments which are useful for fitting and adjusting removable appliances**
>
> - Adams pliers (no. 64)
> - Spring-forming pliers (no. 65)
> - Maun's wire cutters
> - Pair of autoclavable dividers
> - Steel rule
> - A straight handpiece and an acrylic bur (preferably tungsten carbide)
> - A pair of robust hollow-chop pliers is a useful addition, but not essential.

7. The active element(s) should be gently activated, provided that extractions are not required to make space available into which the teeth are to be moved.

8. Give the patient a mirror and demonstrate how to insert and remove the appliance. Then let the patient practise.

9. Go through the instructions with the patient (and parent or guardian), stressing the importance of full-time wear. A sheet outlining the important points and containing details of what to do in the event of problems is advisable. Medico-legally, it is prudent to note in the patient's records if instructions have been given.

10. Arrange the next appointment.

If a working model is available, it is wise to store this with the patient's study models as it may prove helpful if the appliance has to be repaired.

17.8 Monitoring progress

Ideally, patients wearing active removable appliances should be seen around every 4 weeks. Passive appliances can be seen less frequently, but it is advisable to check, and if necessary adjust, the retention of the clasps every 3 months.

During active treatment it is important to establish that the patient is wearing the appliance as instructed. Indications of a lack of compliance include the following:

- The appliance shows little evidence of wear and tear.
- The patient lisps (ask the patient to count from 65 to 70 with, and without, their appliance).
- No marks in the patient's mouth around the gingival margins palatally or across the palate.
- Frequent breakages.

If wear is satisfactory, the following should be considered:

- Check the treatment plan (and progress onto the next step if indicated).
- The patient's oral hygiene.
- Record the molar relationship, overjet, and overbite.
- Reassess anchorage.
- Tooth movement since the last visit.
- Retention of the appliance (see Section 17.4).
- Whether the active elements of the appliance need adjustment.
- Whether the bite-plane or buccal capping need to be increased and/or adjusted.
- Record what action needs to be undertaken at the next visit.

17.8.1 Common problems during treatment

Slow rate of tooth movement

Normally, tooth movement should proceed at approximately 1 mm per month in children, and slightly less in adults. If progress is slow, check the following:

- Is the patient wearing the appliance full-time? If the appliance is not being worn as much as required, the implications of this need to be discussed with the patient (and if applicable, the parent). If poor cooperation continues, resulting in a lack of progress, consideration will have to be given to abandoning treatment.
- If the active element is a spring—is this correctly positioned and optimally activated?
- If the active element is a screw—is the patient adjusting this correctly, at the frequency requested?
- Is tooth movement obstructed by the acrylic or wires of the appliance? If this is the case, these should be removed or adjusted.
- Is tooth movement prevented by occlusion with the opposing arch? It may be necessary to increase the bite-plane or buccal capping to free the occlusion.

Frequent breakage of the appliance

The main reasons for this are as follows:

- The appliance is not being worn full-time.
- The patient has a habit of clicking the appliance in and out (this habit also results in an appliance that rapidly becomes loose).
- The patient is eating inappropriate foods while wearing the appliance. Success lies in dissuading the patient from eating hard and/or sticky foods altogether. Partial success is a patient who removes their appliance to eat hard or sticky foods!

Anchorage loss

This can be increased by the following:

- Part-time appliance wear, thus allowing the anchor teeth to drift forwards.
- The forces being applied by the active elements exceed the anchorage resistance of the appliance. Care is required to ensure that any springs are not being overactivated or that too much active tooth movement is being attempted at a time.

If anchorage loss is a problem see Chapter 15.

Palatal inflammation

This can occur for two reasons:

1. Poor oral hygiene. In the majority of cases, the extent of the inflammation exactly matches the coverage of the appliance and is caused by a mixed fungal and bacterial infection (Fig. 17.16). This may occur in conjunction with angular cheilitis. Management of this condition must address the underlying problem, which is usually poor oral hygiene. However, in marked cases it may be wise to supplement this with an antifungal agent (e.g. nystatin, amphotericin, or miconazole gel) which is applied to the fitting surface of the appliance four times daily. If associated with angular cheilitis, miconazole cream may be helpful.

2. Entrapment of the gingivae between the acrylic and the tooth/teeth being moved.

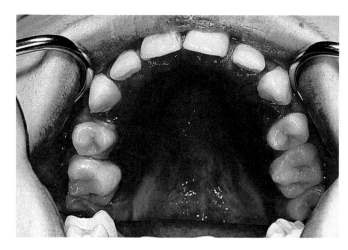

Fig. 17.16 Inflammation of the palate corresponding to the coverage of a removable appliance.

17.9 Appliance repairs

Before arranging for a removable appliance to be repaired, the following should be considered:

- How was the appliance broken? If a breakage has been caused by the patient failing to follow instructions, it is important to be sure any cooperation problems have been overcome before proceeding with the repair.
- Would it be more cost-effective to make a new appliance?
- Occasionally it is possible to adapt what remains of the spring or another component of the appliance to continue the desired movement.

- Is the working model available, or is an up-to-date impression required to facilitate the repair?
- How will the tooth movements which have been achieved be retained while the repair is being carried out? Often there is no alternative but to try and carry out the repair in the shortest possible time.

See also Chapter 25.

Key points

Removable appliances are:

- only capable of tipping movements of individual teeth
- useful for moving blocks of teeth
- useful for freeing the occlusion with the opposing arch
- useful as passive appliances (e.g. for retention)
- more commonly used nowadays as an adjunct to fixed appliances.

Further reading

Littlewood, S. J., Tait, A. G., Mandall, N. A., and Lewis, D. H. (2001). The role of removable appliances in contemporary orthodontics. *British Dental Journal*, **191**, 304–10. [DOI: 10.1038/sj.bdj.4801170] [PubMed: 11587502]
A readable and well-illustrated article.

Ward, S. and Read, M. J. F. (2004). The contemporary use of removable appliances. *Dental Update*, **May**, 215–7. [DOI: 10.12968/denu.2004.31.4.215] [PubMed: 15188527].
Another useful article.

 References for this chapter can also be found at: **www.oup.com/uk/orthodontics5e**. Where possible, these are presented as active links which direct you to the electronic version of the work, to help facilitate onward study. If you are a subscriber to that work (either individually or through an institution), and depending on your level of access, you may be able to peruse an abstract or the full article if available.

18

Fixed appliances

Benjamin R. K. Lewis

Chapter contents

18.1 Principles of fixed appliances

Fixed orthodontic appliances are adhered to teeth via a chemical or micromechanical attachment. This allows the clinician to obtain a far greater range of tooth movements than can be achieved with removable appliances. The combination of the tooth attachment, usually a bracket or a tube, along with an orthodontic archwire can result in tooth movements in all three planes of space. The use of a round archwire results in tipping and vertical tooth movements (Fig. 18.1), and the interaction between the archwire and the walls of the bracket allow the creation of a 'force couple' which can provide apical and rotational movements (Fig 18.2). The use of a rectangular archwire provides additional control of the root apex in the buccolingual direction, known as torque (Fig. 18.3). The closer the fit between the archwire and the bracket slot, the greater the degree of control (Fig. 18.4).

The 'edgewise' appliance was invented by Edward Angle, an American orthodontist, who is often described as the 'father of

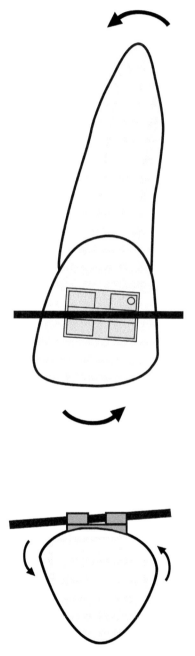

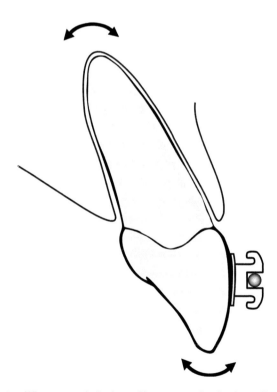

Fig. 18.1 When a round wire is used in a rectangular slot, buccolingual forces tip the tooth around a fulcrum within the root.

Fig. 18.2 Generation of a force couple by the interaction between the bracket slot and the archwire.

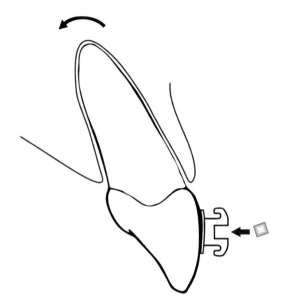

Fig. 18.3 When a rectangular wire is used with a rectangular slot, more control of buccolingual root movement is achieved, allowing bodily and torquing movements to be accomplished.

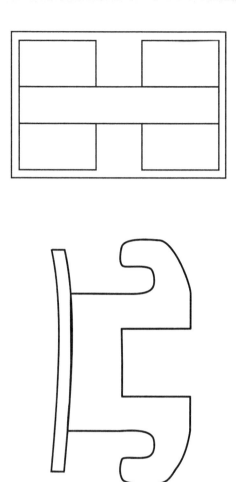

Fig. 18.5 Diagrammatic representation of an edgewise bracket.

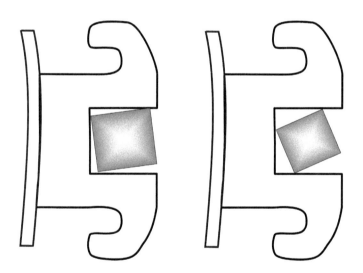

Fig. 18.4 When an archwire closely fits the dimensions of the bracket slot, there is less latitude before it binds and therefore interacts with the bracket. With a smaller rectangular archwire, more tilting and rotation can occur before it binds with the walls of the bracket slot. This latitude is known as 'slop' or 'play'.

modern orthodontics'. This was purely a horizontal slot cut into a rectangular block of metal which was attached to the tooth surface and allowed the insertion of an orthodontic wire (Fig. 18.5). The clinician then had to place individual bends into the wire which induced the desired tooth movements. There are three categories of bend that were placed into the orthodontic wire to correctly position each tooth. These are as follows:

- **First-order bend:** in/out bends to compensate for the varying thickness of the individual teeth.
- **Second-order bend:** angulation or tip bends placed in the vertical plane relative to the long axis of the tooth to allow better mesiodistal angulation/tilt.
- **Third-order bend:** inclination or torque bends relative to the true vertical and can only be produced with rectangular archwire. They are generated by twisting the plane of the wire where it inserts into the bracket slot, resulting in a buccolingual force on the root apex.

The placement of these three bends (Fig. 18.6) into the archwires for each individual tooth was extremely time-consuming and technically very challenging. To reduce the number of bends in the wire, brackets were subsequently manufactured so that the archwire slot was individualized for each tooth rather than having to place all the adjustments within the wire. In the 1970s, Lawrence Andrews was the first clinician

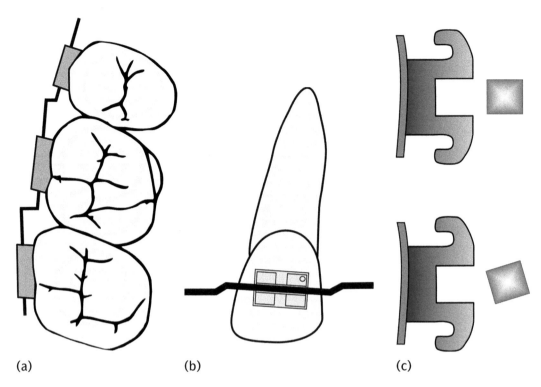

Fig. 18.6 (a) A first-order bend; (b) a second-order bend; (c) a third-order bend.

Box 18.1 Andrews' six keys to a normal occlusion

1. Molar relationship: the mesiodistal cusp of the upper first permanent molar falls within the groove between the mesial and middle cusps of the lower first permanent molar and the distal surface of the distobuccal cusp of the upper first permanent molar occludes with the mesial surface of the mesiobuccal cusp of the lower second molar.

2. Crown angulation: the mesiodistal tip of the crown. The gingival portion of the long axis of each crown is distal to the incisal portion.

3. Crown inclination: labiolingual inclination of the crown. The incisors have a labial crown inclination and the canines, premolars, and molars have a lingual crown inclination.

4. No rotations.

5. No spaces with tight contact points and no tooth size discrepancy.

6. Occlusal plane: varies from generally flat to a slight curve of Spee.

Reprinted from *American Journal of Orthodontics*, Volume 62, Issue 3, Lawrence F. Andrews, The six keys to normal occlusion, pp. 296–309, Copyright (1972), with permission from Elsevier.

---

to design a bracket which incorporated all three 'order bends' required to achieve his 'six keys to a normal occlusion' (Box 18.1) resulting in a 'pre-adjusted' edgewise appliance. The description of the modifications made to the individual brackets to accommodate the 'order bends' is known as the bracket prescription.

When the pre-adjusted edgewise brackets are placed onto the tooth in the ideal position, usually in the centre of the tooth on a point termed the facial axis of the clinical crown (FACC), then theoretically this allows for a straight wire to be placed into the bracket slots which would move the teeth into the ideal positions and eliminate the need for further adjustments to the wire (Fig. 18.7). This is the origin of the term 'straight wire appliance'.

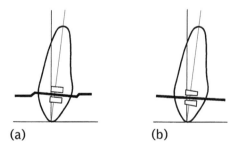

(a) (b)

Fig. 18.7 Diagrams to show (a) an edgewise bracket with a second-order bend placed in the archwire to achieve the desired amount of tip and (b) a pre-adjusted bracket with tip built into the bracket slot.

18.2 Indications for the use of fixed appliances

Fixed orthodontic appliances are often the treatment of choice as they can offer precise control of tooth movements in all three planes of space. However, while it is possible to achieve a more sophisticated range of tooth movement with fixed appliances when compared with removable appliances, the opportunity for problems to arise is also increased. Fixed appliances are more demanding of anchorage, and therefore adequate training should be obtained before embarking on treatment with fixed appliances.

Indications for the use of fixed appliances include:

* correction of mild to moderate skeletal discrepancies: as fixed appliances allow the maximum opportunity for achieving bodily movement, it is possible, within limits, to compensate for skeletal discrepancies and treat a greater range of malocclusions
* intrusion/extrusion of teeth: vertical movement of individual teeth, or tooth segments, requires some form of attachment onto the tooth surface on which the force can act
* correction of rotations
* overbite reduction by intrusion of incisors
* multiple tooth movements required within one arch

* active closure of extraction spaces, or spaces due to hypodontia. Fixed appliances can be used to achieve bodily space closure ensuring a good contact point between the teeth and parallel roots to reduce the risk of the space reopening after treatment.

However, it must be noted that fixed appliances are *not* as effective at moving blocks of teeth when compared to removable or functional appliances.

There are risks associated with fixed appliance treatment and their usage is only justified if the potential benefits outweigh the possible risks. Fixed appliances are only to be used in well-motivated individuals with excellent oral health and dietary control, and not as an alternative to poor cooperation with removable appliances. A successful orthodontic outcome will only be achieved by good teamwork between the orthodontist and a well-motivated patient. The patient has a responsibility to maintain a high level of oral hygiene and dietary control, avoiding hard and sticky foods which can break the orthodontic appliances and restricting sugar/acid-containing foods and drinks between meals to limit the risk of decalcification. The patient must be fully cooperative with adjuncts to treatment such as wearing headgear or inter-arch elastics and be able to attend regularly to enable the appliance to be adjusted.

18.3 Components of fixed appliances

Tooth movement with fixed appliances is achieved by the interaction between the attachment or bracket on the tooth surface and the arch-wire which is tied into the bracket. Brackets can be carried on a band which is cemented to the tooth or attached directly to the tooth surface by means of an adhesive (known colloquially as bonds).

18.3.1 Bands

An orthodontic band is a metal ring which encompasses the tooth onto which an orthodontic attachment is welded/soldered (Fig. 18.8). Historically, this was the only method of adhering an orthodontic attachment to a tooth, hence the term 'multiband appliance'. However, with the advent of modern bonding techniques 40 years ago, orthodontic bands have largely been superseded with bonded attachments, as they are more aesthetic and easier to keep clean. Bands are now only routinely used on molars when the bond strength of direct attachments is insufficient for the planned forces to be applied or where additional customized laboratory made components need to be utilized.

Bands can be used on teeth other than molars, most commonly following the repeated failure of a bonded attachment, on heavily restored or crowned teeth, or for use with rapid maxillary expansion devices (see Chapter 13, Section 13.4.6).

Prior to placement of a band it may be necessary to separate the adjacent tooth contacts. The most widely used method involves placing a small elastic doughnut or 'separator' around the contact point (Fig. 18.9), which is left *in situ* for 5–7 days and removed prior to band placement. These separating elastics are inserted by being stretched, with either special pliers, mosquito forceps, or floss (Fig. 18.10), and working one

side through the contact point. If an elastic separator cannot be placed due to the tightness of the contact point or due to restored nature of the teeth, then metal separators, often called Kesling separators, can be utilized (Fig. 18.11).

Band selection is aided by using the patient's study model to provide a guide to the approximate size of the tooth. A snug fit is essential to help prevent the band from becoming loose during treatment. The edges of the band should be flush with the marginal ridges of the tooth and the bracket should be positioned in the midpoint of the clinical

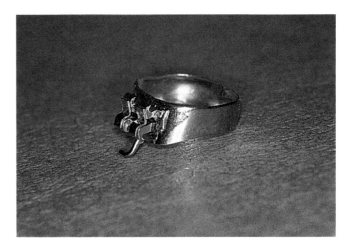

Fig. 18.8 A lower first permanent molar band. Note the gingivally positioned hook, which is useful for applying elastic traction.

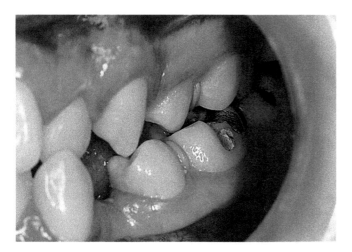

Fig. 18.9 Separating elastics have been placed between the contact points of the second premolars and first permanent molars prior to placement of bands on the latter.

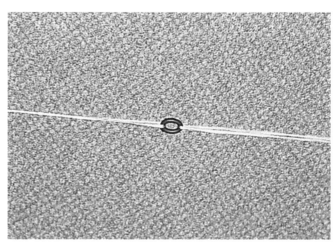

Fig. 18.10 A separating elastic being stretched between two pieces of floss. One side of the elastic is then worked through the contact point so that it encircles the contact point.

crown at 90° to the long axis of the tooth (or crown, depending upon the type of attachment). Most orthodontists use glass ionomer cement for band cementation.

18.3.2 Bonds

These are orthodontic components which are attached directly to the tooth surface utilizing acid-etch adhesive technology (see Fig. 18.12 and Section 18.3.3). The usual components are either brackets or tubes, which have a built-in prescription, which allow for the majority of desired tooth movements. Other components which can be utilized as auxiliaries to the main components are buttons, cleats, and gold chains (see Section 18.3.4). Adhesion to the metal base is achieved by mechanical interlocking (Fig. 18.13). The ability to place bonded attachments directly onto the enamel surface allows for a more aesthetic appearance as well as improved positional accuracy. The brackets are typically described by the height of the bracket slot, usually 0.018 or 0.022 inches, and have a depth of between 0.025 and 0.032 inches. Measurements are provided in inches because fixed appliances originated in America. Variations in the size and shape of the bracket will

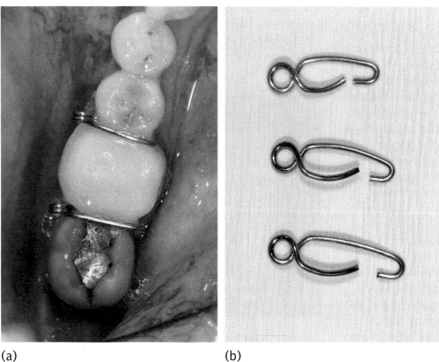

(a)   (b)

Fig. 18.11 Metal 'Kesling' separators: (a) Kesling separator placed on the mesial and distal aspects of a crowned tooth; (b) Kesling separators are available in a range of sizes to accommodate varying contact point widths.

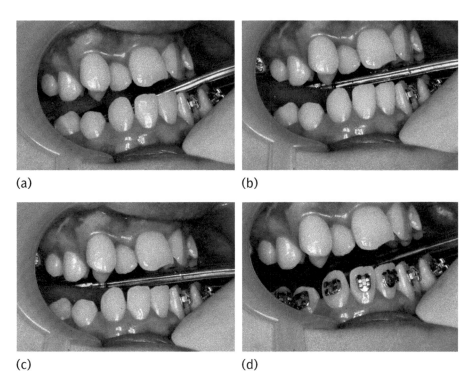

(a)　　　　　　　　　(b)

(c)　　　　　　　　　(d)

Fig. 18.12 Stages in the placement of bonded attachments: (a) isolation; (b) following etching for 15 seconds the teeth are washed and dried (note the frosted appearance of the etched enamel); (c) bonding adhesive is applied to the etched enamel prior to (d) placement of the pre-coated bonded attachments and light curing.

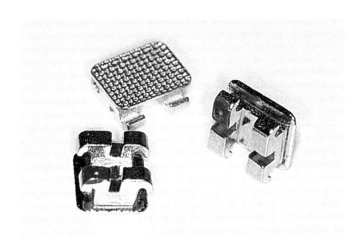

Fig. 18.13 Brackets for bonding showing a mesh base which increases the surface area for mechanical attachment of the composite.

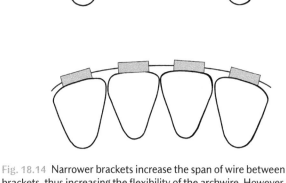

Fig. 18.14 Narrower brackets increase the span of wire between brackets, thus increasing the flexibility of the archwire. However, wider brackets allow greater rotational and mesiodistal control, as the force couple generated has a greater movement.

affect tooth movement, for example, narrow brackets result in a greater inter-bracket span which increases archwire flexibility but decreases the rotational control of a tooth (Fig. 18.14). A variety of approaches have been used to try and make fixed appliances more aesthetic (see Chapter 20) including the introduction of ceramic brackets (see Chapter 20, Fig. 20.5). Although these ceramic brackets lessen the visual impact of the orthodontic appliances, they are not without their problems (see Box 18.2 and Chapter 20).

Box 18.2 Problems with ceramic brackets

- Frictional resistance is high—limiting sliding mechanics.
- Brittle.
- Can cause tooth wear if opposing tooth in contact.
- Difficulties with their removal from the tooth.

18.3.3 Orthodontic adhesives

Adhesive technology for orthodontics has to be finely balanced between having sufficient strength to retain the appliance during the course of treatment, but also allowing its easy removal at the end. The most popular adhesive for cementing bands is glass ionomer, mainly because of its fluoride-releasing potential and affinity to both stainless steel and enamel. Glass ionomers can also be used for retaining bonded attachments, but the bracket failure rate with this material may not be clinically acceptable. Use of the acid-etch technique with a composite produces clinically acceptable bonded attachments with failure rates of the order of 5–10% for both self- and light-cured materials.

There are currently two basic techniques for bonding to enamel using either a separate etch and primer, or a self-etching primer (SEP) 'lollypop' system (Fig. 18.15), in which acidulated phosphoric ester effectively combines the etching and primer into one step and

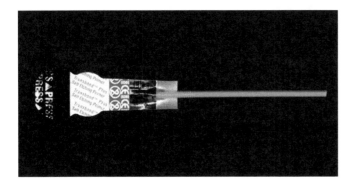

Fig. 18.15 Self-etching primer.

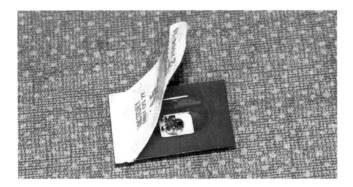

Fig. 18.16 Adhesive pre-coated bracket.

eliminates the need to wash away the etchant, thereby saving time. Research suggests that despite the slightly increased bond failure rates seen with SEPs, when compared with the conventional separate etch and prime technique, they are still clinically acceptable. However, this bond strength can be compromised if the manufacturer's instructions are not followed, for example, it is important to pumice the tooth surface to eliminate the acquired pellicle and any other debris, prior to bonding. For some orthodontic procedures, maximum bond strength is required and this will affect the clinician's chosen procedure. For example, for permanent retention with bonded retainers, some clinicians have advocated using conventional restorative materials to maximize the bond strength and the wear-resistant qualities to optimize the longevity of the attachment.

Brackets can be supplied with light-cure adhesive already applied to the base of the bracket, these are called adhesive pre-coated or APC brackets. The brackets are supplied in individual packages to prevent ambient light setting the adhesive (Fig. 18.16). It is claimed that this approach gives a more consistent bond, quicker application of the bracket, and more efficient stock control. Whatever material is used, any excess should be cleared from the perimeter of the bracket before the final set to reduce plaque retention around the bonded attachment. A recent innovation is a modification to the brackets used in the APC system which incorporates an internal well which 'sucks back' any excess composite to reduce the excess around the bracket itself.

18.3.4 Auxiliaries

Orthodontic auxiliaries are used to supplement the main components of bands, brackets, and archwires. There is a whole plethora of auxiliary components commercially available including archwire hooks and stops, cleats, buttons, coil springs, uprighting springs, power pins, elastomerics, elastics, separators, wire ligatures, quadhelix appliances, transpalatal arches, and headgear components.

Very small elastic bands, often described as elastomeric modules (Fig. 18.17), or wire ligatures (Fig. 18.18), are used to secure the archwire into the archwire slot (Fig. 18.19). Elastic modules are quicker to place and are usually more comfortable for the patient, but wire ligatures are still used selectively as they can be tightened to maximize contact between the wire and the bracket, or applied less tightly, reducing the friction to allow teeth to slide along the wire.

Intra-oral elastics used for traction (see Chapter 15) are commonly available in 2-, 3.5-, and 4.5-ounce strengths and a variety of sizes, ranging from 1/8 to 3/4 inch (Fig. 18.20). For most purposes, they should be changed daily and latex-free varieties are also now available.

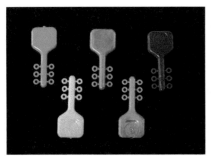

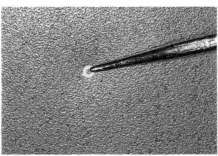

Fig. 18.17 Coloured elastomeric modules used to secure the archwire into the bracket slot.

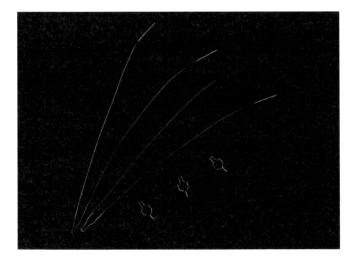

Fig. 18.18 Metal ligatures for securing the archwire into the bracket slot.

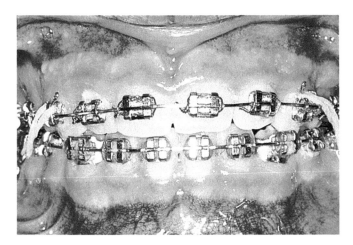

Fig. 18.19 This patient's archwire has been tied into place with wire ligatures in the upper arch and with elastomeric modules in the lower arch.

Palatal or lingual arches can be used to reinforce anchorage, to achieve expansion (the quadhelix appliance), or molar derotation. They can be made in the laboratory from an impression of the teeth

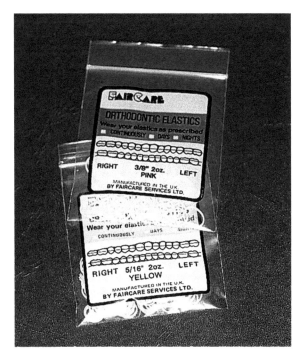

Fig. 18.20 Intra-oral elastics.

(Fig. 18.21). Proprietary forms of most of the commonly used designs are also available, and these have the additional advantage that they are removable, thus facilitating adjustment without removing the bands (Fig. 18.22).

18.3.5 Archwires

Orthodontic archwires and their interaction with the components attached to the teeth allow the clinician to generate tooth movement. This can be controlled by varying the cross-sectional diameter of the archwire and its material of construction (see Box 18.3). In the initial stages of treatment, a wire which is flexible with good resistance to permanent deformation is desirable, so that displaced teeth can be aligned without the application of excessive forces. In these early stages, the forces that move the teeth come from the wire itself, as it returns to its

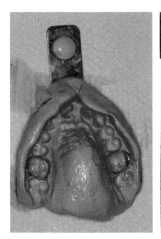
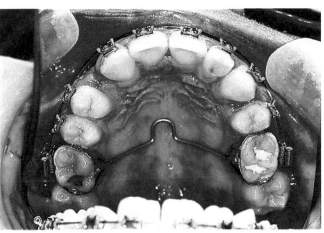

Fig. 18.21 A palatal arch, which is used to help provide additional anchorage in the upper arch by helping to resist forward movement of the maxillary molars. This arch has been constructed from an impression taken over the bands *in situ*. The bands are then removed and resited into the impression before disinfection and transfer to the laboratory for construction.

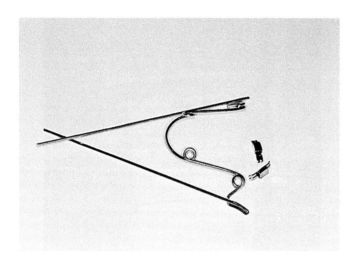

Fig. 18.22 A proprietary removable quadhelix. The distal aspect of the arms of the helix slot into the lingual sheaths (also shown) which are welded onto the palatal surface of bands on the upper molars.

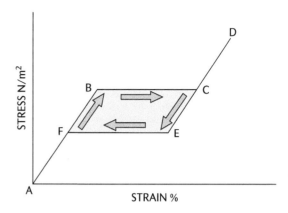

Fig. 18.23 Graph of stress (force) versus strain (wire deflection) of nickel titanium wires.

initial shape. In contrast, in the later stages of treatment, rigid archwires are required, as they act as a track along which the teeth are moved. The forces that move the teeth later in treatment are derived partly from the archwire, but predominantly from auxiliaries such as elastics, force closing springs, and powerchain.

The two most popular wires types which are used in orthodontic treatment are nickel titanium (NiTi) and stainless steel.

NiTi archwires demonstrate a 'shape memory effect'. This shape memory effect allows them to be distorted by tying the wire into the bracket slot, and the natural recoil of the wire returns the archwire to its original shape, aligning the tooth in the process. Their introduction greatly reduced the complexity of the wire bending required to achieve tooth alignment during the initial phases of orthodontic treatment. The original NiTi archwire was called 'Nitinol' which stood for Nickel Titanium Naval Ordnance Laboratories where the composition was first developed. There have been further modifications made to the composition to produce variations of the shape memory effect and to generate 'super/pseudoelasticity' caused by changes in temperature, or the amount of deflection. This leads to lower forces being placed onto the tooth, generating a more physiologically appropriate tooth movement. The graph in Fig. 18.23 demonstrates the special properties of NiTi that

allow it to deliver low forces (stress) even with larger deflections (strain), due to a change in the crystalline structure of the metal. By virtue of their flexibility, NiTi wires provide less control against the unwanted side effects of auxiliary forces.

This graph represents the ideal stress/strain curve for NiTi archwires. When the wire is loaded, the stress produces linear elastic behaviour (points A to B). As the wire continues to be stressed, the wire begins to undergo a change in its crystal structure. During this time, the stress with the wire remains the same, giving the plateau effect (point B to C). These changes are called *stress-induced phase transformations*. Once all the alloy's crystal structure has changed, then the wire begins to behave elastically again (point C to D). This occurs when the wire is tied into a bracket. Once the tooth begins to move, the stress in the wire begins to unload (point D to E) and eventually reaches the plateau phase (point E to F), which leads to a light continuous force being applied to the tooth (even though the tooth is moving and the deflection/strain is reducing). This will occur until the alloy has finished undergoing the reverse phase transformation, where upon the wire will behave linear elastically again (point F to A).

Stainless steel (often referred to as 18/8 stainless steel due to the 18% chromium and 8% nickel within its composition) is relatively inexpensive, easily formed, and exhibits good stiffness making it particularly useful during the later stages of treatment.

Other alloys which are less commonly used include titanium molybdenum alloy, known as TMA (Fig. 18.24).

Box 18.3 Physical properties of archwire materials

- Springback: this is the ability of a wire to return to its original shape after a force is applied. High values of springback mean that it is possible to tie in a displaced tooth without permanent distortion.

- Stiffness: the amount of force required to deflect or bend a wire. The greater the diameter of an archwire, the greater the stiffness.

- Formability: this is the ease with which a wire can be bent to the desired shape, for example, the placement of a coil in a spring, without fracture.

- Resilience: this is the stored energy available after deflection of an archwire without permanent deformation.

- Biocompatibility.

- Joinability: this is whether the material can be soldered or welded.

- Frictional characteristics: if tooth movement is to proceed quickly, a wire with low surface friction is preferable.

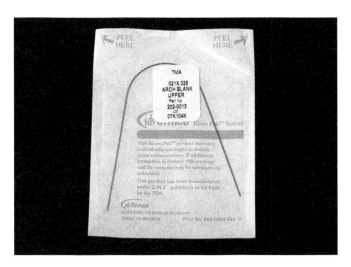

Fig. 18.24 TMA wire.

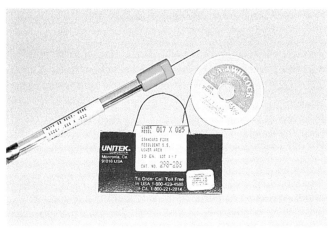

Fig. 18.25 The most popular archwire material is stainless steel which is available in straight lengths, as a coil on a spool, or preformed into archwires.

Archwires are described according to their dimensions. An archwire described as 0.016 inches (0.4 mm) is a round archwire with a diameter of 0.016 inches, and that described as 0.016 × 0.022 inches (0.4 × 0.55 mm), is a rectangular archwire.

Archwires are available in straight lengths, as coils, or as preformed archwires (see Fig. 18.25). The latter variant is more expensive but saves chairside time. There are a wide variety of archform shapes; however, regardless of what design is chosen, some adjustment of the archwire to match the pre-treatment archform of the patient will be required to maximize the post-treatment stability (see Section 18.4).

The force exerted by a particular archwire material is given by the formula:

$$F \propto \frac{dr^4}{l^3}$$

where d is the distance that the spring/wire is deflected, r is the radius of the wire, and l is the length of the wire.

Thus, it can be appreciated that increasing the diameter of the archwire will significantly affect the force applied to the teeth, and increasing the length or span of wire between the brackets will inversely affect the applied force. As mentioned earlier, the distance between the brackets can be increased by reducing the width of the brackets, but the inter-bracket span can also be increased by the placement of loops in the archwire. Prior to the introduction of the newer, more flexible alloys, multilooped stainless steel archwires were commonly used in the initial stages of treatment. Loops are still utilized in retraction archwires, but with the advent of the pre-adjusted appliance and sliding mechanics, they are not used routinely.

18.4 Treatment planning for fixed appliances

By virtue of their coverage of the palate, removable appliances inherently provide more anchorage than fixed appliances. It is important to remember that, with a fixed appliance, movement of one tooth or a segment of teeth in one direction will result in an equal but opposite force acting on the remaining teeth attached to the appliance. In addition, apical movement will place a greater strain on anchorage. For these reasons, it is necessary to pay particular attention to anchorage when planning treatment involving fixed appliances and, if necessary, this can be reinforced extra-orally, for example, with headgear or intra-orally, for example, with a palatal or lingual arch or temporary skeletal anchorage (see Chapter 15).

The importance of keeping the teeth within the zone of soft tissue balance has been discussed in Chapter 7. Care is therefore required to ensure that the archform, particularly of the lower arch, present at the beginning of treatment is largely preserved. It is wise to check the archform of any archwire against a model of the lower arch, taken before the start of treatment (Fig. 18.26), bearing in mind that the upper arch will by necessity be slightly broader.

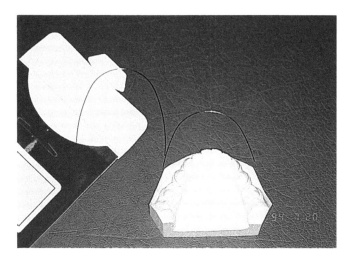

Fig. 18.26 The amount of adjustment required to a preformed lower archwire, as taken from the packet, to ensure that it conforms to the patient's pre-treatment archform and width.

18.5 Practical procedures

Accurate bracket placement is crucial to achieving success with fixed appliances. The 'correct' position of the bracket on the facial surface will depend upon the bracket system used. Most pre-adjusted systems require the bracket to be placed in the centre of the crown on the long/facial axis of the clinical crown (FACC). This can be quite difficult to judge, particularly if the tooth is worn. Bracket placement is particularly important with the pre-adjusted technique, as the values for tip and torque are calculated for the midpoint of the facial surface of the tooth. Incorrect bracket positioning will lead to the 'prescription' being improperly expressed resulting in incorrect tooth position and ultimately affecting the functional and aesthetic result. Errors in bracket placement should therefore be corrected as early as possible in the treatment. Alternatively, adjustments can be made to each archwire to compensate, but over the course of a treatment this can be time-consuming.

When a fixed appliance is first placed, a flexible archwire, such as a small diameter, round NiTi archwire, is advisable to achieve initial alignment. This avoids the application of excessive forces to any displaced teeth, which can be painful for the patient and result in bond failure.

It is important that full bracket engagement has been achieved to ensure complete alignment before progressing onto more rigid archwires. Correction of inter-arch relationships and space closure is usually best carried out using rectangular stainless steel wires for apical control. The exact archwire sequence will depend upon the dimensions of the archwire slot and operator preference.

Mesiodistal tooth movement can be achieved by one of the following:

1. Moving teeth with the archwire: this is achieved by incorporating loops into the archwire which, when activated, move a section of the archwire and the attached teeth as shown in Fig. 18.27.

2. Sliding teeth along the archwire either using elastic traction or (either opening or closing) coil springs (Fig. 18.28). This approach requires a greater force to overcome the friction between the bracket and the wire, and therefore places a greater strain on anchorage. This type of movement is known as 'sliding mechanics' and is applicable to pre-adjusted appliances where a straight archwire is used.

Fig. 18.29 shows the steps involved in the treatment of a maximum anchorage Class II division 2 malocclusion with fixed appliances.

Adjustments to the appliance need to be made on a regular basis, usually every 4–10 weeks. Once space closure is complete and incisor position corrected, some operators will place a more flexible full-sized

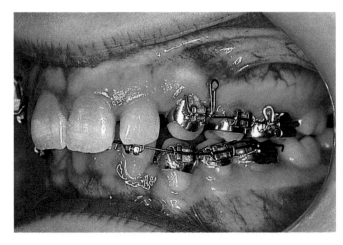

Fig. 18.27 A sectional archwire to retract the upper left canine.

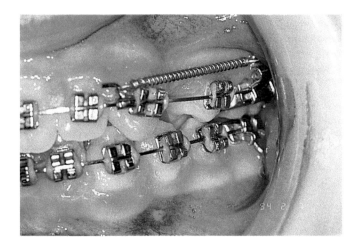

Fig. 18.28 Sliding teeth along the archwire using a nickel–titanium coil spring.

archwire, often in conjunction with vertical elastic traction, to help fully express the bracket prescription and 'sock-in' the buccal occlusion, or place 'artistic' bends in the more rigid wire to detail the final result (Fig. 18.30).

Following the attainment of the goals of treatment, it is important to retain the finished result. This is covered in detail in Chapter 16.

18.6 Fixed appliance systems

18.6.1 Pre-adjusted appliances

The in-built prescription of these appliances, which takes into account the first-, second-, and third-order bends, which historically would have had to be individually placed in the archwire for each tooth, has resulted in this type of appliance becoming the mainstay of contemporary orthodontic treatment. However, even with brackets containing a specific prescription being produced for each individual tooth type, there is still usually a need for additional adjustments to the archwire to achieve the optimal tooth position. This is because the prescription is based on average values and will not be able to take into account individual variations such as tooth size discrepancies or an underlying skeletal discrepancy.

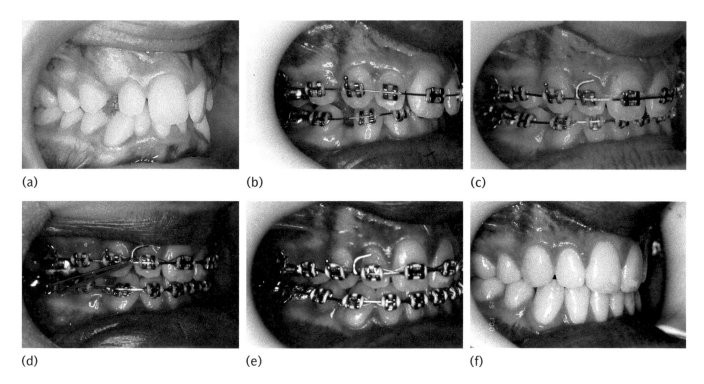

Fig. 18.29 The right buccal view of a 13-year-old with a Class II division 2 malocclusion treated by extraction of all four first premolars. (a) Pre-treatment; (b) flexible nickel–titanium archwires were used to achieve alignment; (c) showing rectangular stainless steel working archwires and elastic chain being used to close spaces between the upper incisors; (d) following overbite reduction Class II traction is used in conjunction with space closure to correct incisor and buccal segment relationships; (e) the final stage of treatment is to detail the occlusion; (f) finished result.

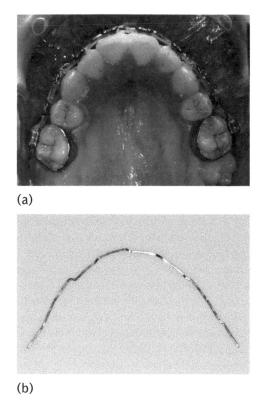

Fig. 18.30 (a, b) Finishing bends placed in the archwire to optimize the occlusion.

There are a large number of pre-adjusted systems on the market, each with their own individual prescription values. The most well known are the Andrew's prescription, the Roth system, and the MBT (McLaughlin, Bennett, and Trevisi) prescription (see Table 18.1). The actual prescription within a bracket, especially with regard to the third-order bends (torque) values, will usually not be fully realized due to the fact that the archwire is smaller than the slot size of the bracket which introduces 'play' or 'slop' between the archwire and bracket slot (Fig. 18.4). It is because of this fact that a number of systems on the market have increased the values of certain aspects of their prescription to maximize the opportunity to deliver the desired tooth movements without the clinician having to place additional adjustments into the archwire. The bracket position can be purposely adjusted away from the ideal, if the clinician wishes to manipulate the built-in prescription to alter the desired tooth movements or adjust the bracket shape to accommodate variations in tooth morphology (Fig. 18.31).

In practice, treatment using pre-adjusting systems comprises six main steps:

- Alignment
- Overbite reduction
- Overjet correction
- Space closure
- Finishing—this usually comprises placing small bends in the archwires to fine detail tooth position and occlusion
- Retention (Chapter 16).

Table 18.1 MBT prescription for tip and torque (at the midpoint of the facial surface)

	Torque (°)	Tip (°)
Maxilla		
Central incisor	17	4
Lateral incisor	10	8
Canine	−7	8
First premolar	−7	0
Second premolar	−7	0
First molar	−14	0
Second molar	−14	0
Mandible		
Central incisor	−6	0
Lateral incisor	−6	0
Canine	−6	3
First premolar	−12	2
Second premolar	−17	2
First molar	−20	0
Second molar	−10	0

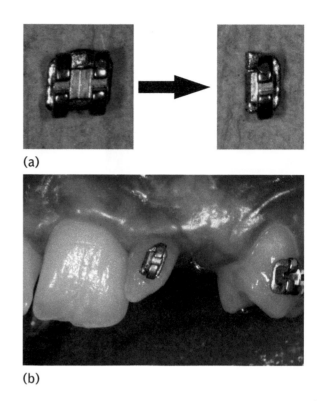

(a)

(b)

Fig. 18.31 (a, b) Sectioning of a bracket to allow an improved fit onto a diminutive lateral incisor while still maintaining the prescription values.

18.6.2 The Tip-Edge appliance

The Begg appliance (Fig. 18.32) was invented by Raymond Begg, an Australian orthodontist, in the 1930s. This appliance uses a vertical slot, round archwires, and light inter-arch elastics to tip the teeth and rapidly correct an increased overjet and close residual extraction space. Subsequent uprighting of the teeth is achieved with torqueing auxiliaries and complex wire bending which resulted in great difficulty in 'finishing' the cases and relied heavily on post-treatment

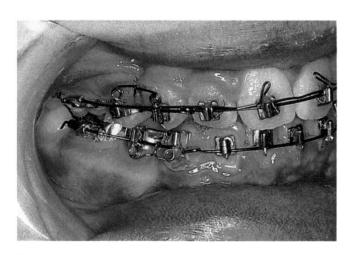

Fig. 18.32 The Begg appliance.

'settling' to improve the occlusal contacts. The Tip-Edge system was developed in an attempt to combine the perceived merits of the Begg and pre-adjusted edgewise appliances in an effort to produce quicker, less anchorage-demanding treatment, but with the ability to 'finish' the case to the optimum level. The technique focuses on three stages. Stage 1 primarily involved the molars, incisors, and canines and concentrates on achieving alignment with overjet and over-bite control utilizing tipping movements generated by adjustments to the stainless steel archwires and the use of light Class II elastics. During Stage 2, the clinician engages the premolar teeth and closes any residual space before progressing onto Stage 3 which involves the insertion of a full-dimension rectangular archwire and uprighting the teeth to fully express the 'prescription' of the appliance and generate the desired final tooth positions. Originally the uprighting tooth movement was generated by the use of uprighting springs or 'sidewinders', which could be technically challenging and time-consuming. To overcome this difficulty, the manufacturers have developed Tip-Edge Plus (Fig. 18.33), which utilizes an underarch wire, placed within an additional horizontal slot within the bracket base, to achieve the uprighting tooth movements, without the need for additional springs, making the appliance considerably more user friendly.

18.6.3 Self-ligating systems

The concept of reducing the friction between the bracket and archwire by using a bracket which did not require an elastomeric or wire ligature, but with a built mechanism to secure the archwire, is not new. A version

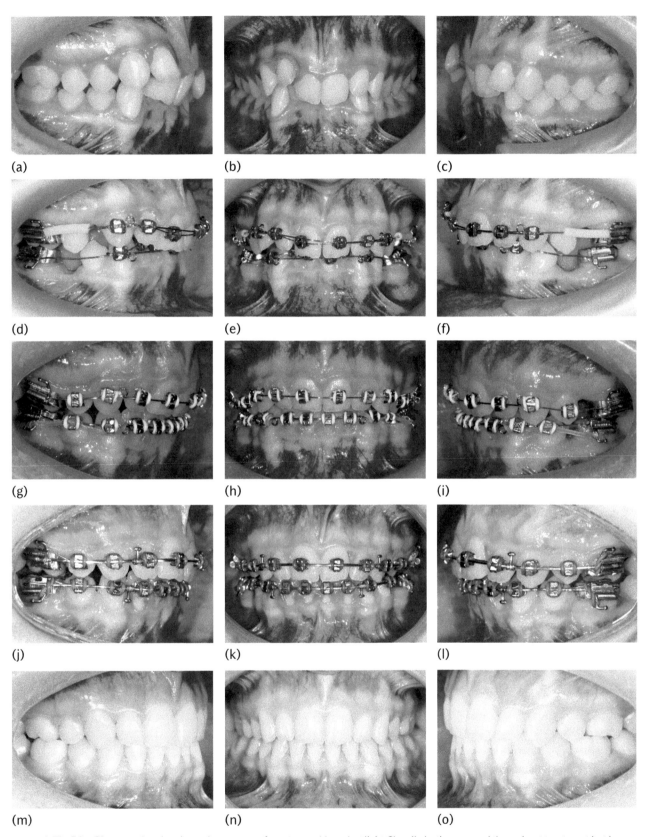

Fig. 18.33 A Tip-Edge Plus case showing the various stages of treatment. Note that light Class II elastics are used throughout treatment but have not been shown in the photographs so as not to obscure the tooth positions. (a–c) Initial presentation. (d–f) Stage I—incisors, canines, and first molars bonded and 0.016-inch stainless steel wires placed with Class II elastics to align and correct the overjet and overbite. (g–i) Stage II—pick up the premolars, align, and level the arches, closing any residual space aided with Class II elastics. (j–l) Stage III—correction of the torque and tip using a 0.0215-inch × 0.028-inch stainless steel with a 0.014-inch NiTi underarch within the deep tunnel, with Class II elastic support to maintain overjet correction while buccal segments establish a Class I relationship.

called the 'Russell Lock' was originally described by Stolzenberg back in 1935. However, the early designs did not achieve commercial success often due to the fragility of the mechanism or the costs involved in the manufacturing process. This changed in the 1990s and 2000s with the introduction of a number of bracket systems. These included Damon (Fig. 18.34), Innovation, and SmartClip, which were often associated with 'treatment philosophies', and supported by improved manufacturing techniques and marketing which made a number of claims about the superiority of these appliance types, especially relating to reduced overall treatment time and reducing the need to undertake orthodontic related extractions. Since the increase in the popularity of self-ligating appliances, many studies have been conducted which suggest that the use of these appliances does not necessarily achieve either of these aims. However, their ingenious designs mean that they still deliver many benefits including secure wire engagement, reduced friction between the bracket and archwire, and a reduction in chairside time. These appliances are subdivided into active or passive bracket designs depending upon whether or not closure of the clip or gate results in an active seating of the archwire in the bracket slot.

18.6.4 Lingual appliances

These have been developed to improve aesthetics during treatment by placing the attachments on the lingual surfaces of the teeth, thus reducing the visual impact of orthodontic treatment. This appliance system inevitably increases the challenges faced by the clinician due to reduced accessibility to the appliance as well as the complexity of bracket/component and wire manufacturing (see Chapter 20).

18.6.5 Future developments

Possible future developments in the field of fixed appliances include the following:

Individualized appliances

The current evidence base suggests that there is little benefit of one appliance type over another when it comes to reducing overall length of treatment. The choice of appliance used is more often determined by the clinician's preference while also taking into account patient choice, cost, and the treatment mechanics which are to be utilized.

However, with the introduction of both aligner treatment (see Chapter 21) and some lingual appliances (see Chapter 20), the concept of fully customized appliances has become a reality. These are appliances that are manufactured to the specific requirements of an individual patient. With lingual appliances, the bracket design is tailored to the morphological variations of each tooth plus the archwires are created with any adjustments already built-in to achieve the desired tooth movements. These systems rely on absolute precision during bracket placement and as such are more suitable for the indirect bonding technique. These fully customized systems offer the potential to achieve quicker and more predictable treatment. However, due to the significantly increased manufacturing

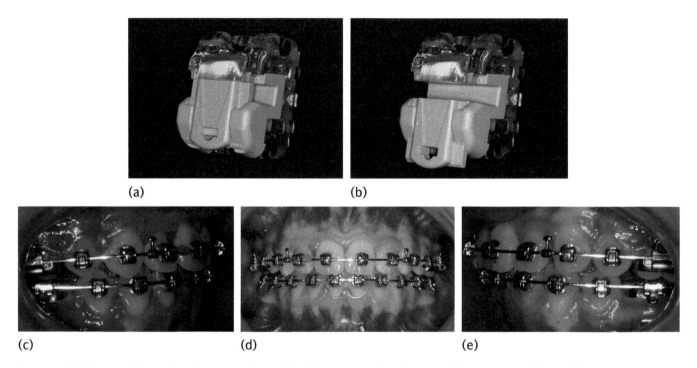

(a)　　　　　　　　　　　　　(b)

(c)　　　　　　　　(d)　　　　　　　　(e)

Fig. 18.34 The Damon self-ligating bracket system. (a) A model of a Damon 3 bracket with the archwire slot closed; (b) a model Damon 3 bracket with the archwire slot open; (c–e) a patient being treated with a Damon Q appliance (a newer modification of the Damon bracket).

costs, they are not currently a cost-effective treatment option for the majority of patients. This situation may change with further advances in manufacturing and computer-assisted design and manufacture technology.

Accelerated tooth movement

Orthodontic tooth movement is reliant on the activity of the bone cells (osteoclasts and osteoblasts) which are responsible for the bone resorption and deposition. It is hypothesized that if these cells can be stimulated further, then tooth movement may be accelerated; and as such, overall treatment time reduced, along with a potential reduction in some of the risks associated with orthodontic treatment.

Three approaches are currently being considered:

Non-surgical adjunctive interventions for accelerating tooth movement

Interventions such as low-energy laser radiation to the mucosa of the targeted teeth, intermittent vibration of the teeth using an electrical appliance, pulsed electromagnetic waves, and utilization of muscle exercises as methods to accelerate tooth movement are currently being investigated. At the present time, there is no high-quality evidence to support the claims that these approaches consistently accelerate treatment.

Surgical adjunctive interventions for accelerating tooth movement

A number of methods have been proposed including surgical procedures to the interseptal bone to reduce the resistance to tooth movement; alveolar decortication, where a series of small holes are drilled into the alveolar bone; and corticision where the cortices are divided transmucosally without the need to raise a flap.

These procedures may reduce the bone density, and thus the resistance to tooth movement as well as increasing the body's inflammatory response (a process known as RAP or regional acceleratory phenomenon). Research is currently ongoing looking at the efficacy and cost-effectiveness of these adjuncts as well as the acceptability from a patient perspective.

Pharmacological interventions for accelerating tooth movement

Pharmacological agents have the potential to interfere with the biological processes involved in tooth movement, and therefore may have the potential to both accelerate and retard tooth movement which could be advantageous during active tooth movement and also when patients are in retention. This is still experimental at the current time. Alternative methods of delivery are also being investigated to allow the areas of interest to be targeted and to limit unwanted local and systemic side effects.

18.7 Demineralization and fixed appliances

Placement of a fixed attachment upon a tooth surface increases the risk of plaque accumulation. In addition, if a diet rich in sugar and acid is consumed, this results in demineralization of the enamel surrounding the bracket and occasionally frank cavitation. The incidence of demineralization (Fig. 18.35) with fixed appliances has been variously reported as between 15% and 85%. As any decalcification is undesirable, considerable interest has focused on ways of reducing this problem. The main approaches that have been used are as follows:

1. Careful patient selection. It is unwise to embark upon treatment in a patient with a high caries rate or poor levels of plaque control.

2. Fluoride mouth rinses for the duration of treatment. The problem with this approach is that the individuals most at risk of demineralization are those least likely to comply fully with an additional rinsing regimen.

3. Local fluoride release from fluoride-containing cements and bonding adhesives. Variable results have been reported for those bonding composites which have been marketed for their fluoride-releasing potential. Glass ionomer cements have been shown to be effective at reducing the incidence of demineralization around bands, while achieving equal or better retention results than conventional cements. Although glass ionomer cements appear effective at reducing demineralization around bonded attachments, this is at the expense of higher failure rates (see Section 18.3.3).

4. Dietary advice. This important aspect of preventive advice should not be forgotten. Patients are often advised to avoid chewy sweets during treatment, but the importance of avoiding sugared beverages and fizzy drinks, particularly between meals, should not be overlooked.

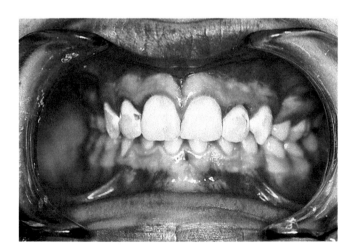

Fig. 18.35 Picture showing severe decalcification following fixed appliance treatment (naturally this patient was not treated by the author!).

18.8 Starting with fixed appliances

Some orthodontic supply companies offer the practitioner a kit containing brackets, bands, and a few archwires in return for an impression and a fee. Of course, this is an expensive alternative and, in addition, bands selected remotely from the patient using an impression are unlikely to be a good fit. However, it is extremely unwise, and arguably unethical, to embark on treatment with fixed appliances without first gaining adequate expertise in their use. This is best achieved by a longitudinal course in the form of an apprenticeship with a skilled operator. It is mandatory that this is supplemented by a thorough appreciation of orthodontic diagnosis and treatment planning, which is the most difficult aspect of orthodontics.

Key points

- Fixed appliances are capable of producing tooth movement in all three planes of space.
- Fixed appliances are more demanding of anchorage so this must be planned and monitored carefully.
- Training is required as fixed appliances have the potential to cause problems in all three planes of space.
- A cooperative patient with good dental health is a prerequisite for success.

Relevant Cochrane reviews

Millet, D. T., Mandall, N. A., Mattick, R. C., Hickman, J., and Glenny, A. M. (2017). Adhesives for bonded molar tubes during fixed brace treatment. *Cochrane Database of Systematic Reviews*, Issue 2. Art. No.: CD008236. DOI: 10.1002/14651858.CD008236.pub3 https://www.cochranelibrary.com/cdsr/doi/10.1002/14651858.CD008236.pub3/full
Only two studies satisfied the inclusion criteria and these both compared bonded molar tubes with molar bands. The studies had a low risk of bias and concluded that bonded molar tubes are associated with a higher failure rate (2–6×) than molar bands. Interestingly, one study found a decreased incidence of decalcification with molar bands.

Millet, D.T., Glenny, A. M., Mattick, R. C., Hickman, J., and Mandall, N. A. (2016). Adhesives for fixed orthodontic bands. *Cochrane Database of Systematic Reviews*, Issue 10. Art. No.: CD004485. DOI: 10.1002/14651858.CD004485.pub4 https://www.cochranelibrary.com/cdsr/doi/10.1002/14651858.CD004485.pub4/full
Five randomized controlled trials and three controlled clinical trials, which were all of a split-mouth design, were included within the review. The majority of orthodontists use glass ionomer-based adhesives when cementing orthodontic bands due to their ease of use and potential caries-preventing qualities. There were varying failure rates for all cement types included within the review with the more recent studies reporting much lower failure rates; however, there was insufficient evidence to determine the most effective adhesive for attaching orthodontic bands to molar teeth in patients with full arch fixed orthodontic appliances and the authors felt that due to inherent bias in most of the study designs the information included within the review should be interpreted with great caution.

Mandall, N. A., Hickman, J., Macfarlane, T. V., Mattick, R. C. R., Millett, D.T., and Worthington, H. V. (2018). Adhesives for fixed orthodontic brackets. *Cochrane Database of Systematic Reviews*, Issue 4, Art. No.: CD002282. DOI: 10.1002/14651858.CD002282.Pub2 https://www.cochranelibrary.com/cdsr/doi/10.1002/14651858.CD002282.pub2/full
Three trials satisfied the inclusion criteria. The authors were unable to draw any conclusions from this review as there was only weak, unreliable evidence that one adhesive may possibly have more failures associated with it and another adhesive may be more protective against early decay.

Benson, P. E., Parkin, N., Dyer, F., Millett, D. T., Furness, S., and Germain, P. (2013). Fluorides for the prevention of early tooth decay (demineralised white lesions) during fixed brace treatment. *Cochrane Database of Systematic Reviews*, Issue 12. Art. No.: CD003809. DOI: 10.1002/14651858.CD003809.pub3 https://www.cochranelibrary.com/cdsr/doi/10.1002/14651858.CD003809.pub3/full
Three studies which satisfied the new inclusion criteria were analysed in this updated review. This review found some moderate evidence that fluoride varnish applied every 6 weeks at the time of orthodontic review during treatment is effective at reducing the incidence of white spot lesions. However, further high-quality trials are required to determine the best means of preventing demineralized white lesions in patients undergoing orthodontic treatment. Based on current best practice in other areas of dentistry, for which there is evidence, we recommend that patients with fixed appliances rinse daily with a 0.05% sodium fluoride mouth rinse.

Wang, Y., Llu, C., Jlan, F., McIntyre, G. T., Millett, D. T., Hickman, J., et al. (2018). Initial arch wires used in orthodontic treatment with fixed appliances. *Cochrane Database of Systematic Reviews*, Issue 7, Art No.: CD007859. DOI: 10.1002/14651858.CD007859.pub 4. https://www.cochranelibrary.com/cdsr/doi/10.1002/14651858.CD007859.pub4/full
Twelve randomized controlled trials were included in this review. The authors concluded that there was some evidence to indicate that coaxial superelastic nickel-titanium (NiTi) archwires can produce greater tooth movement over 12 weeks than archwires made of single-stranded superelastic NiTi. They also felt that there was insufficient evidence to determine whether any particular archwire material is superior to any other in terms of alignment rate, time to alignment, pain, and root resorption.

Hu, H., Li, C., Li, F., Chen, J., Sun, J., Zou, S., et al. (2013). Enamel etching for bonding fixed orthodontic braces. *Cochrane Database of Systematic Reviews*, Issue 11. Art. No.: CD005516. DOI: 10.1002/14651858.CD005516.pub2 https://www.cochranelibrary.com/cdsr/doi/10.1002/14651858.CD005516.pub2/full

This review included 13 studies. There is currently insufficient high-quality evidence to determine if there is a difference in the bond failure rate between SEPs and conventional etching systems or with regard to decalcification, participant satisfaction, and cost effectiveness.

El-Angbawi, A., McIntyre, G. T., Fleming, P. S., and Bearn, D. R. (2015). Non-surgical adjunctive interventions for accelerating tooth movement in patients undergoing fixed orthodontic treatment. *Cochrane Database of Systematic Reviews*, Issue 11. Art. No.: CD010887. DOI: 10.1002/14651858.CD010887. pub2 https://www.cochranelibrary.com/cdsr/doi/10.1002/14651858. CD010887.pub2/full
There is currently very little clinical research regarding the effectiveness of non-surgical interventions to accelerate orthodontic treatment. The

claims about the potential positive effects of light vibrational forces are not currently supported by the evidence base.

Fleming, P. S., Fedorowicz, Z., Johal, A., El-Angbawi, A., and Pandis, N. (2015). Surgical adjunctive procedures for accelerating orthodontic treatment. *Cochrane Database of Systematic Reviews*, Issue 6. Art. No.: CD010572. DOI: 10.1002/14651858.CD010572.pub2 https://www.cochranelibrary.com/cdsr/doi/10.1002/14651858.CD010572.pub2/full
The four studies included within the review undertook corticotomies to facilitate tooth movement. It concluded that this technique does potentially accelerate orthodontic tooth movement; however, further high-quality trials are required to confirm any possible benefits.

Principal sources and further reading

Andrews, L. F. (1972). The six keys to normal occlusion. *American Journal of Orthodontics*, **62**, 296–309. [DOI: 10.1016/S0002-9416(72)90268-0] [PubMed: 4505873]
The classic paper by the developer of the straight wire appliance.

Archambault, A., Lacoursiere, R., Badawi, H., Mahor, P. W., and Flores-Mir, C. (2010). Torque expression in stainless steel orthodontic brackets. A systematic review. *Angle Orthodontist*, **80**, 201–10. [DOI: 10.2319/080508-352.1] [PubMed: 19852662].

Dehbi, H., Azaroual, M. F., Zaoui, F., Halimi, A., and Benyahia, H. (2017). Therapeutic efficacy of self-ligating brackets: a systematic review. *International Orthodontics*, **15**, 297–311. [DOI: 10.1016/j.ortho.2017.06.009] [PubMed: 28778722]
The authors included 20 randomized controlled trials and concluded that there were no significant differences between self-ligating and conventional bracket systems.

DiBiase, A. T., Woodhouse, N. R., Papageorgiou, S. N., Johnson, N., Slipper, C., Grant, J., et al. (2018). Effects of supplemental vibrational force on space closure, treatment duration, and occlusal outcome: a multicentre randomised clinical trial. *American Journal of Orthodontics and Dentofacial Orthopedics*, **153**, 469–80. [DOI: 10.1016/j.ajodo.2017.10.021] [PubMed: 29602338]
The results indicate that the application of a supplemental vibrational force did not affect space closure, treatment duration, total number of visits, or final occlusal outcome.

Gange, P. (2015). The evolution of bonding in orthodontics. *American Journal of Orthodontics and Dentofacial Orthopedics*, **147**, S56–63. [DOI: 10.1016/j.ajodo.2015.01.011] [PubMed: 25836345]

Höchli, D., Hersberger-Zurfluh, M., Papageorgiou, S. N., and Eliades, T. (2017). Interventions for orthodontically induced white spot lesions: a systematic review and meta-analysis. *European Journal of Orthodontics*, **39**, 122–33. [DOI: 10.1093/ejo/cjw065] [PubMed: 27907894]

Hoffman, S., Papadopoulos, N., Visel, D., Visel, T., Jost-Brinkmann, P. G., and Präger, T. M. (2017). Influence of piezotomy and osteoperforation of the alveolar process on the rate of orthodontic tooth movement: a systematic review. *Journal of Orofacial Orthopedics*, **78**, 301–11. [DOI: 10.1007/s00056-017-0085-1] [PubMed: 28321457]

Kapila, S. and Sachdeva, R. (1989). Mechanical properties and clinical applications of orthodontic wires. *American Journal of Orthodontics and Dentofacial Orthopedics*, **96**, 100–9. [DOI: 10.1016/0889-5406(89)90251-5] [PubMed: 2667330].
An excellent, and readable, account of archwire materials.

Kouskoura, T., Katsaros, C., and von Gunten, S. (2017). The potential use of pharmacological agents to modulate orthodontic tooth movement (OTM). *Frontiers in Physiology*, **8**, 67. [DOI: 10.3389/fphys.2017.00067] [PubMed: 28228735]
This paper includes a detailed description of the biology of tooth movement as well as the current areas of investigation for pharmacologically influencing orthodontic tooth movement.

Kusy, R. P. (1997). A review of contemporary archwires: their properties and characteristics. *Angle Orthodontist*, **67**, 197–207. [DOI: 10.1043/0003-3219(1997)067<0197:AROCAT>2.3.CO;2] PubMed:9188964].

McLaughlin, R. P., Bennett, J., and Trevisi, H. J. (2001). *Systemised Orthodontic Treatment Mechanics*. Edinburgh: Mosby.
A clearly written and beautifully illustrated book, which should be read by anyone using fixed appliances.

Millett, D. T. and Gordon, P. H. (1994). A 5-year clinical review of bond failure with a no-mix adhesive (Right-on). *European Journal of Orthodontics*, **16**, 203–11. [DOI: 10.1093/ejo/16.3.203] [PubMed: 8062860]

O'Higgins, E. A., Kirschen, R. H., and Lee, R. T. (1999). The influence of maxillary incisor inclination on arch length. *British Journal of Orthodontics*, **26**, 97–102. [DOI: 10.1093/ortho/26.2.97] [PubMed: 10420243]
A fascinating article—a 'must read' for those practitioners using fixed appliances.

Rogers, S., Chadwick, B., and Treasure, E. (2010). Fluoride-containing orthodontic adhesives and decalcification in patients with fixed appliances: a systematic review. *American Journal of Orthodontics and Dentofacial Orthopedics*, **138**, 390e. [DOI: 10.1016/j.ajodo.2010.05.002] [PubMed: 20889037]

Russell, J. (2005). Aesthetic orthodontic brackets. *Journal of Orthodontics*, **32**, 146–63. [DOI: 10.1179/146531205225021024] [PubMed: 15994990]
An easy-to-read résumé of currently available aesthetic brackets and their limitations.

Wright, N., Modarai, F., and Cobourne, M. (2011). Do you do Damon? What is the current evidence base underlying the philosophy of this appliance system? *Journal of Orthodontics*, **38**, 222–30. [DOI: 10.1179/14653121141479] [PubMed: 21875995].
As the title suggests!

Woodhouse, N. R., DiBiase, A. T., Johnson, N., Slipper, C., Grant, J., Alsaleh, M., et al. (2015). Supplemental vibrational force during orthodontic alignment: a randomized trial. *Journal of Dental Research*, **94**, 682–9. [DOI: 10.1177/0022034515576195] [PubMed: 25758457]
The results indicate that the application of a supplemental vibrational force did not significantly increase the rate of tooth alignment or reduce the rate of orthodontically induced inflammatory root resorption to the central incisors during the alignment phase of fixed appliance therapy.

Yang X., He, Y., Chen, T., Zhao, M., Yan, Y., Wang, H, et al. (2017). Differences between active and passive self-ligating brackets for orthodontic treatment: systematic review and meta-analysis based on randomized clinical trials. *Journal of Orofacial Orthopedics*, **78**, 121–8. [DOI: 10.1007/s00056-016-0059-8] [PubMed: 28224175]

References for this chapter can also be found at: **www.oup.com/uk/orthodontics5e**. Where possible, these are presented as active links which direct you to the electronic version of the work, to help facilitate onward study. If you are a subscriber to that work (either individually or through an institution), and depending on your level of access, you may be able to peruse an abstract or the full article if available.

19

Functional appliances

S. J. Littlewood

Chapter contents

19.1 Definition

Functional appliances utilize, eliminate, or guide the forces of muscles of mastication, tooth eruption, and growth to correct a malocclusion.

19.2 History

The term 'functional appliance' is used, because it was once believed that these appliances corrected abnormal function around the dentition, leading to a change in growth response. Although we now believe that function probably has little to do with the treatment effect, the term has remained.

The initial idea for functional appliances was derived from the monobloc, developed by Pierre Robin. This appliance postured the mandible forward in babies born with severely retrognathic mandibles. This posturing opened compromised airways. Andresen in the 1920s used this principle of forward posturing of the mandible to treat malocclusions with his activator appliance, the first functional appliance.

19.3 Overview

There are many different types of functional appliances, but most work by the principle of posturing the mandible forwards in growing patients. They are most effective at changing the anteroposterior occlusion between the upper and lower arches, usually in patients with a mild to moderate Class II skeletal discrepancy. They are not as effective at correcting tooth irregularities and improving arch alignment, so treatment

often involves a phase of fixed appliances. There are many areas of controversy surrounding functional appliances, in particular treatment timing and mode of action. These areas will be addressed later in this chapter.

A typical functional appliance case is shown in Section 19.4 and Fig. 19.1. This case study gives an overview of the appliance in clinical use.

19.4 Case study: functional appliance

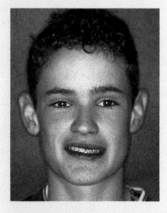 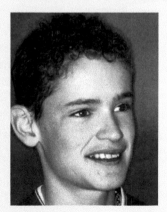 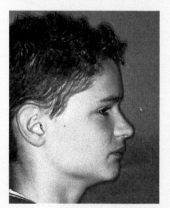 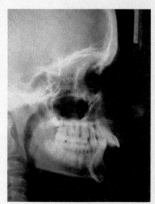

Fig. 19.1 (a) Extra-oral start records. Patient OP is 12 years old and complains of his prominent upper incisors. His clinical and radiographic records show he has a Class II division 1 incisor relationship on a Class II skeletal base. His principal problems are an increased overjet of 12 mm, due to proclined and spaced upper incisors and a retrognathic mandible.

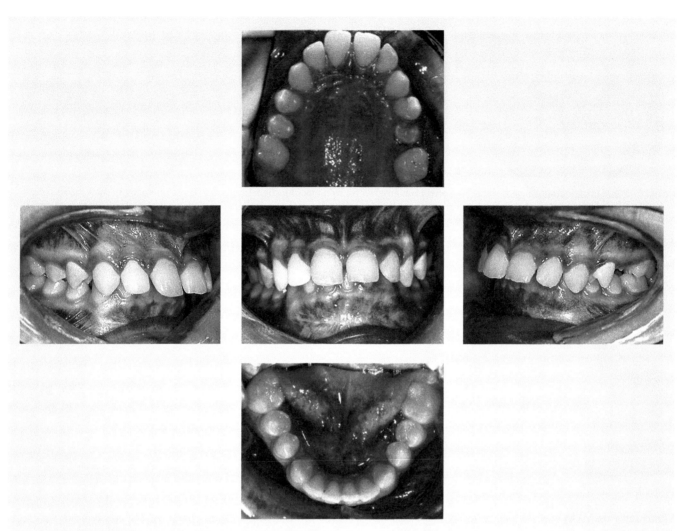

Fig. 19.1 (b) Intra-oral start records for OP.

Aims of treatment	Treatment plan
1. Growth modification to improve skeletal pattern	1. Growth modification with a functional appliance (twin-block)
2. Camouflage any remaining skeletal discrepancy with fixed appliances	2. Towards end of functional appliance begin anterior alignment with fixed appliances
3. Align the teeth and close the spaces	3. Reassess case at end of functional appliance
	4. Upper and lower fixed appliances
	5. Retention

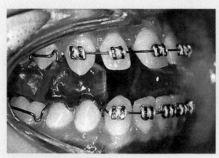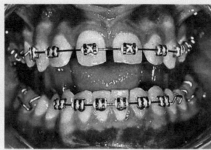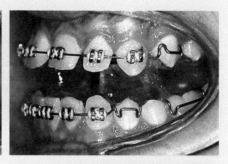

Fig. 19.1 (c) Functional appliance in place. The patient was fitted with a twin-block functional appliance. These photographs show the end of the functional appliance treatment, with fixed appliances on the labial segment. This is the beginning of the alignment of the teeth in preparation for transition to the fixed appliance phase of treatment.

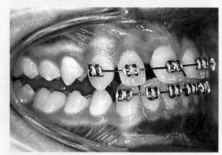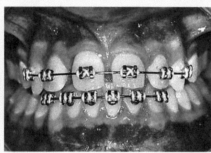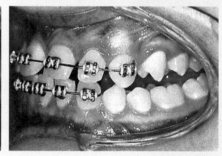

Fig. 19.1 (d) End of functional stage. After 10 months of the functional appliance the anteroposterior discrepancy has been corrected. Note that although there is still a small residual overjet, the buccal segments have been overcorrected to a Class III relationship. This overcorrection allows for the risk of relapse in the second phase of treatment. At this stage, full records are taken again to reassess the case, principally to see if any extractions are required before the second phase (extractions were not needed in this case). The posterior lateral open bites are a typical feature at this stage of a case treated with a twin-block appliance.

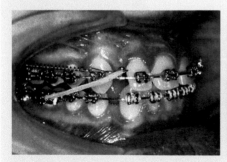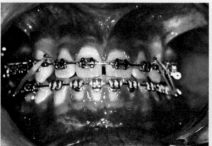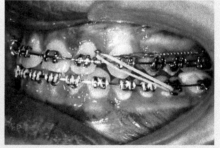

Fig. 19.1 (e) Fixed appliances in the second phase of treatment, with Class II elastics to maintain the changes achieved in the first phase of treatment. The fixed appliances were worn for 16 months.

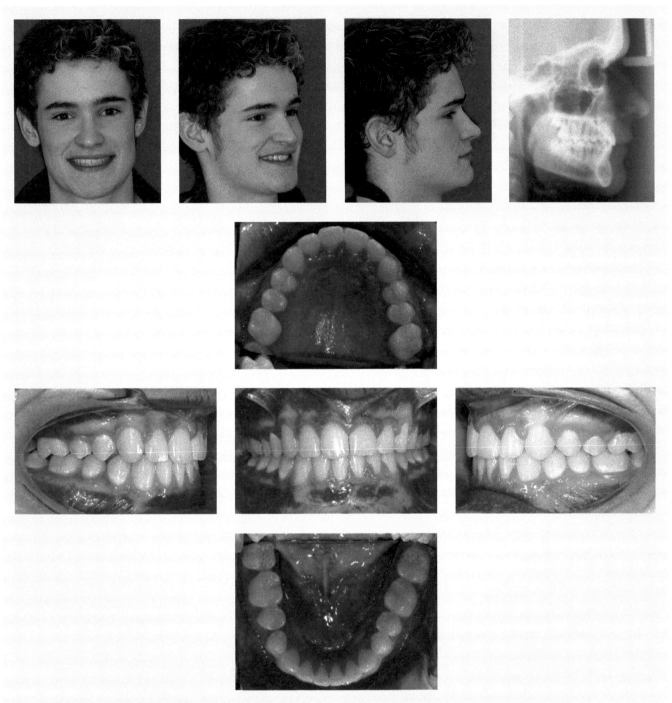

Fig. 19.1 (f) End of treatment records.

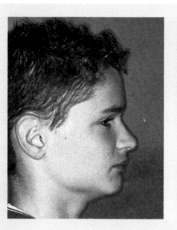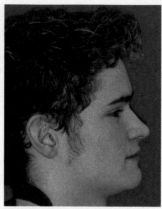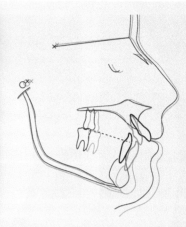

Fig. 19.1 (g) Effects of treatment. The treatment has been successful due to good patient compliance, an appropriate treatment plan, and favourable growth. The growth response to functional appliances is variable, and the growth shown here is better than average. As a result, in this case the skeletal discrepancy was corrected by the growth modification phase of the twin-block appliance. If growth had not been so favourable, then the residual skeletal discrepancy would have had to have been corrected either by orthodontic camouflage, or combined orthodontics and orthognathic surgery when the patient was older.

19.5 Timing of treatment

Functional appliances are most effective when the patient is growing. As girls complete their growth slightly earlier than boys, functional appliances can be used a little later in boys. It has been suggested that treatment should, if possible, coincide with the pubertal growth spurt. There have been various attempts to predict this growth spurt, including taking multiple height measurements of the patient, as rapid changes in height coincide closely with the peak changes in the maxilla and mandible. However, this does require multiple height measurements spread over a period of time. An alternative approach uses maturation changes seen on the cervical vertebrae visible on lateral skull radiographs. During the period of maximum mandibular growth, characteristic maturation changes are visible on cervical vertebrae C3 and C4. Further details about this are provided in the section on 'Principal sources and further reading' at the end of this chapter. However, whichever technique is used it can be difficult to predict the pubertal growth spurt accurately. Fortunately, studies have shown that favourable changes with functional appliances can occur outside this growth spurt. The key factor is that the patient is still actively growing.

While it is widely acknowledged that functional appliances must be used in growing patients, one area of controversy is whether to provide early treatment (in the early mixed dentition when the patient is under 10 years old) or wait until the late mixed dentition. Early treatment usually involves two phases of treatment: an initial phase with the functional appliance, followed by a pause while the adult dentition erupts, and then a second phase of fixed appliances. In contrast to this, if functional appliance treatment is started in the late mixed dentition, then by the end of the functional stage of treatment the adult dentition is usually erupted sufficiently to proceed straight onto the fixed appliances.

High-quality research has shown that both approaches successfully corrected the increased overjet, and there was no difference in the amount of skeletal change achieved, the need for extractions, or the quality of the final occlusal alignment. Early treatment does, however, provide a transient improvement in self-esteem and there is some evidence that it reduces the risk of incisal trauma by up to 40%. However, when patients had their functional appliance fitted earlier, their treatment lasted longer and they needed to attend more appointments. This means that early treatment is more expensive and more importantly, the treatment burden is greater for the patient.

Early treatment should therefore be restricted to patients where there is thought to be a particular risk of trauma to the teeth, or if they are experiencing bullying or teasing about their malocclusion.

19.6 Types of malocclusion treated with functional appliances

Although functional appliances have been used to treat a whole variety of malocclusions, they are usually used for the treatment of Class II malocclusions. They are typically used for treatment of Class II division 1, but with minor alterations can be used for the treatment of Class II division 2 (see Fig. 19.2). Some functional appliances, such as modified twin-block and FR3 Frankel appliances, have been described for the treatment of Class III malocclusions, but there is no evidence of any skeletal correction. These Class III malocclusions are often more simply treated by orthodontic camouflage using fixed appliances, so functionals are less frequently used for the treatment of Class III malocclusions.

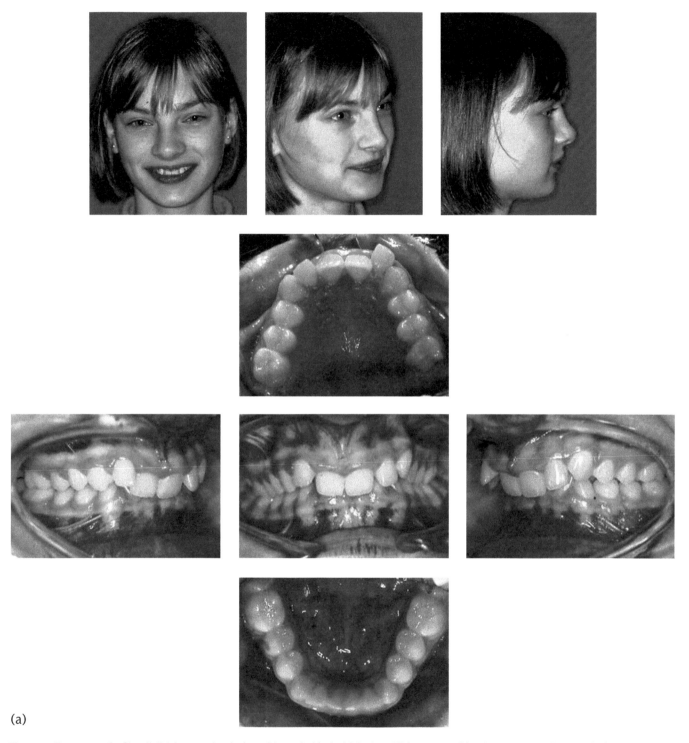

(a)

Fig. 19.2 Treatment of a Class II division 2 malocclusion with a twin-block. (a) Patient AD is 12 years old and complained of her crooked upper teeth. She presented with a Class II division 2 incisor relationship on a Class II skeletal base. Her principal problems were retroclined upper central incisors, an increased overbite, and a retrognathic mandible. The treatment plan was to correct the anteroposterior discrepancy and procline the upper central incisors using a modified twin-block appliance. The functional appliance was then followed by a phase of fixed appliances and then retainers.

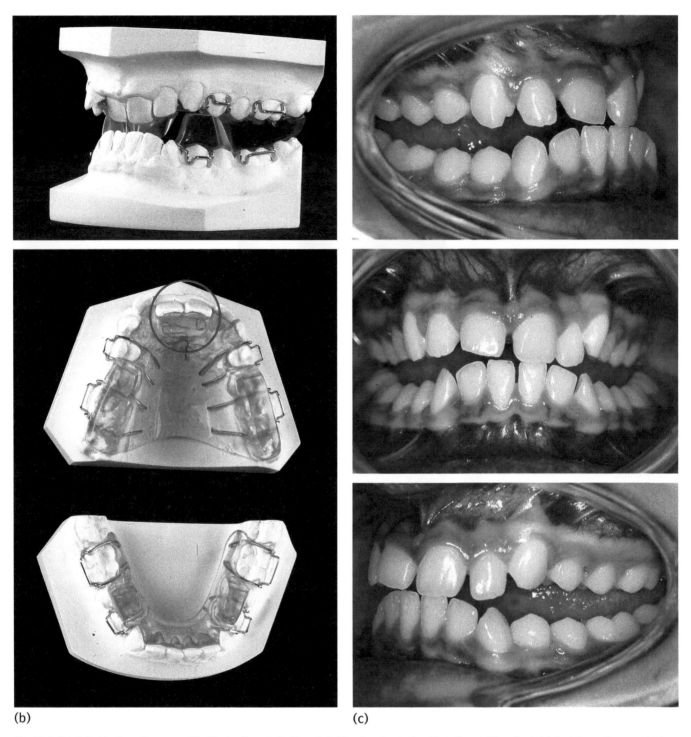

(b)

(c)

Fig. 19.2 (b) Twin-block appliance modified for treatment of a Class II division 2 malocclusion. Note the additional palatal double-cantilever spring (highlighted in red circle) in the upper arch, which is used to procline the central incisors. An alternative approach would be to place a sectional fixed appliance on the upper 6 labial segment teeth. (c) End of functional stage. The anteroposterior discrepancy has been corrected and the retroclined upper central incisors proclined to normal inclinations. Note the posterior lateral open bites, which were closed in the second phase of fixed appliances.

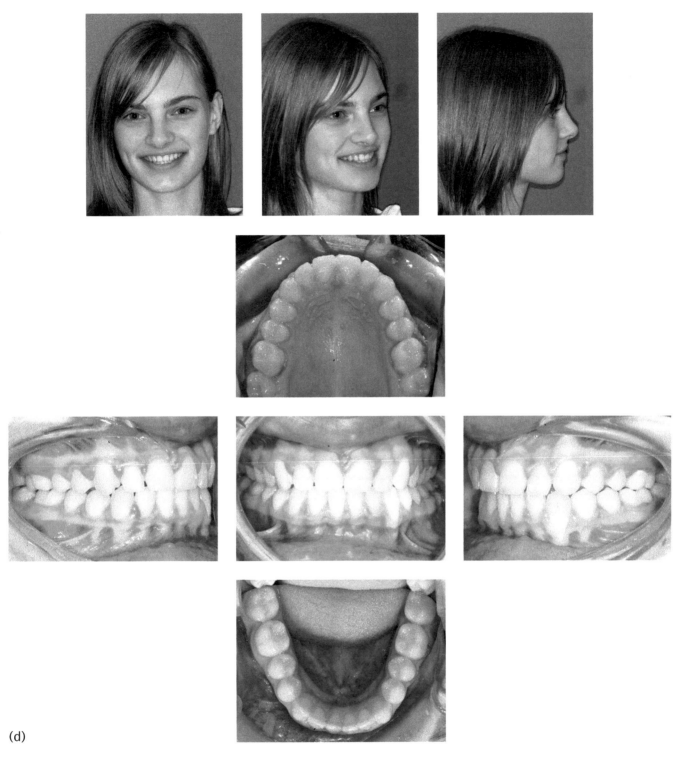

(d)

Fig. 19.2 (d) End of treatment.

19.6.1 Treatment of Class II division 1 malocclusions

Functional appliances are most commonly used for the treatment of Class II division 1 malocclusions. If the arches are well aligned at the start of treatment, and the only problem is an anteroposterior discrepancy between the arches, then the functional appliance alone may be sufficient. In these cases, it is wise to slightly overcorrect the malocclusion to allow for some relapse and ask the patient to wear the appliance at night until the end of their growth period.

Functional appliances are often used as a first phase of treatment, followed by a second phase of fixed appliances. The functional appliance corrects, or at least reduces, the skeletal discrepancy in a process known as growth modification or dentofacial orthopaedics. By correcting the anteroposterior problems with the functional appliance, the amount of anchorage required during the fixed appliance stage is reduced. However, since functional appliances also cause some tilting of the teeth, a significant part of the correction caused by a functional appliance is probably orthodontic camouflage.

Following the functional phase the patient is reassessed with regard to the need for possible extractions and fixed appliances to align the arches.

19.6.2 Treatment of Class II division 2 malocclusions

Class II division 2 malocclusions can also be treated using functional appliances. As mentioned in Chapter 10, this type of malocclusion can be difficult to treat, partly due to the increased overbite. The use of a functional appliance, before fixed appliances, may provide a more efficient alternative to treating these malocclusions with fixed appliances alone.

The approach to treatment is simple. The Class II division 2 incisor relationship is converted to a Class II division 1 relationship and then treated with a functional appliance. The retroclined upper incisors can be proclined forward using a pre-functional removable appliance, or a sectional fixed appliance on the upper labial segment. Alternatively, some functional appliances can be modified to procline the upper incisors as part of the functional appliance phase of treatment. Fig. 19.2 shows a Class II division 2 case treated with a modified twin-block appliance.

19.7 Types of functional appliance

There are many types of functional appliance, but most share the common feature of holding the mandible in a postured position. Functional appliances can be tissue borne or tooth borne, and may be removable or fixed. Some are also worn with headgear that may enhance the Class II correction. The use of headgear attached to a functional appliance attempts to restrict the anterior and vertical development of the maxilla. This can particularly helpful in cases where there is excess incisor show and a so-called gummy smile. The disadvantage of using the additional headgear is that it is an extra burden for the patient, which may adversely affect overall compliance.

Five popular designs of functional appliances will be described here. There is no such thing as a standard functional appliance design, as every appliance should be individually tailored to the patient and their malocclusion.

19.7.1 Twin-block appliance

The twin-block appliance (Fig. 19.3) is the most popular functional appliance in the UK. The reason for its popularity is that it is well tolerated by patients as it is constructed in two parts. The upper and lower parts fit together using posterior bite blocks with interlocking bite-planes, which posture the mandible forwards. The blocks need to be at least 5 mm high, which prevents the patient from biting one block on top of the other. Instead the patient is encouraged to posture the mandible forwards, so that the lower block occludes in front of the upper block. The appliance can be worn full time, including during eating in some cases, which means that rapid correction is possible. It is also possible to modify the appliance to allow expansion of the upper arch during the functional appliance phase. An alternative modification to allow correction of Class II division 2 malocclusions is shown in Fig. 19.2.

It is also easy to reactivate the twin-block appliance (Fig. 19.4). This means that during treatment if further advancement of the mandible is required, it is possible to modify the existing appliance rather than having to construct a new appliance.

One of the side effects of the twin-block appliance is the residual posterior lateral open bites at the end of the functional phase (see Fig. 19.2c). This is seen particularly in cases initially presenting with a deep overbite. The posterior teeth are prevented from erupting by the occlusal coverage of the bite blocks. Some clinicians will trim the acrylic away from the occlusal surfaces of the upper block to allow the lower molars to erupt. Any remaining lateral open bites are closed down in the fixed appliance phase of treatment.

19.7.2 Herbst appliance

The Herbst appliance (Figs 19.5 and 19.10) is a fixed functional appliance. There is a section attached to the upper buccal segment teeth and a section attached to the lower buccal segment teeth. These sections are joined by a rigid arm that postures the mandible forwards. As it is a fixed appliance, it removes some (but not all) compliance factors. It is as successful at reducing overjets as the twin-block appliance. It is, however, slightly better tolerated than the bulkier twin-block appliance, with patients finding it easier to eat and talk with it in place. The principal disadvantages are the increased breakages and higher cost of the Herbst appliance.

19.7.3 Medium opening activator (MOA)

This is a one-piece functional appliance, with minimal acrylic to improve patient comfort (Fig. 19.6). The lower acrylic extends lingual to the lower labial segment only, and the upper and lower parts are joined

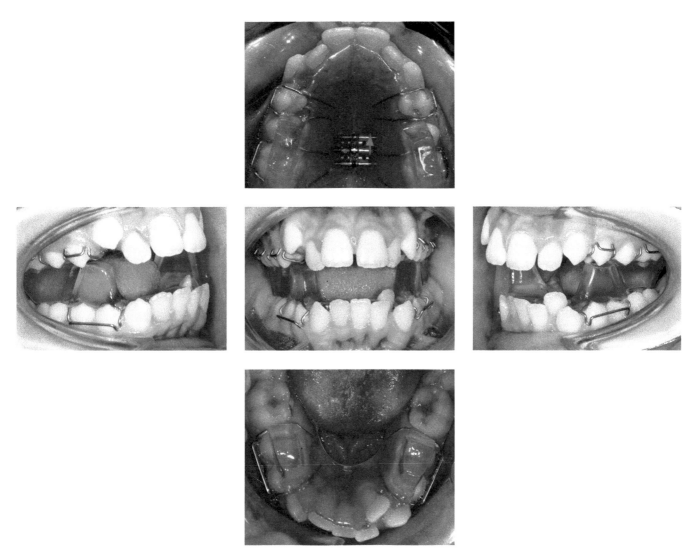

Fig. 19.3 Twin-block appliance. This twin-block also has an upper midline screw to permit expansion of the upper arch.

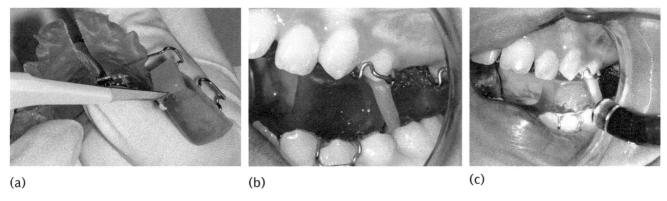

(a)   (b)   (c)

Fig. 19.4 Reactivation of the twin-block appliance. The twin-block can be reactivated during treatment to posture the mandible further forwards. This particular technique involves adding light-cured acrylic to the inclined bite-plane on the upper block. (a) Trimming the uncured acrylic to fit the left inclined bite-plane of the upper block. (b) The light-cured acrylic is placed on the upper block, forcing the lower block, and therefore the mandible, further anteriorly. (c) Light-curing the acrylic.

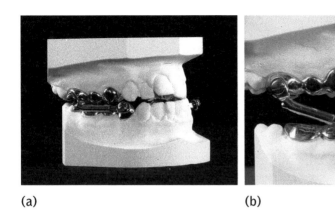

(a)   (b)

Fig. 19.5 Herbst appliance. (a) Closed; (b) open.

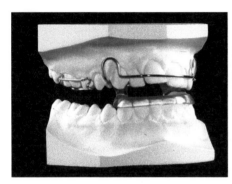

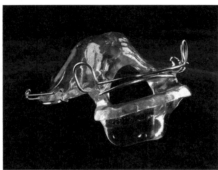

Fig. 19.6 Medium opening activator (MOA).

by two rigid acrylic posts, leaving a breathing hole anteriorly. As there is no molar capping on the lower posterior teeth, these teeth are free to erupt. The MOA is therefore useful when trying to reduce a deep overbite.

19.7.4 Bionator

The bionator (Fig. 19.7) was originally designed to modify tongue behaviour, using a heavy wire loop in the palate. We now know that the tongue is unlikely to be the cause of the increased overjet, but the lack of acrylic in the palate makes it easy to wear. A buccal extension of the labial bow holds the cheeks out of contact with the buccal segment teeth, allowing some arch expansion.

19.7.5 Frankel appliance

The Frankel appliance (Fig. 19.8) is the only completely tissue-borne appliance. It is named after the inventor, who originally called it the function regulator (or FR). There are different versions designed to treat different types of malocclusions. Like other functional appliances, it postures the mandible forwards. It also has buccal shields to hold the cheeks away from the teeth and stretch the periosteum, allegedly to cause bone formation, although this has never been proved. It can be difficult to wear, is expensive to make, and is troublesome to repair. As a result, it is now used less frequently.

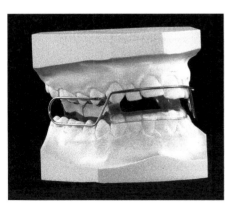

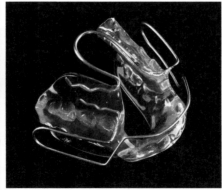

Fig. 19.7 Bionator.

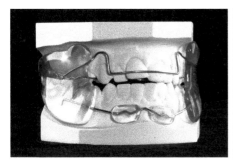
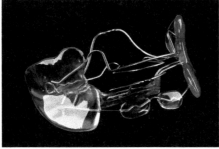

Fig. 19.8 Frankel appliance (FR1).

19.8 Clinical management of functional appliances

19.8.1 Preparing for the functional appliance

Well-extended upper and lower alginate impressions are required along with a recording of the postured bite. The bite recording should prescribe to the laboratory the exact position of the postured mandible in all three dimensions—anteroposteriorly, vertically, and transversely. Fig. 19.9 shows a wax bite recording for a functional appliance patient.

The degree of protrusion will depend on the size of the overjet and the comfort of the patient. For patients with a large overjet, protruding the patient's mandible more than 75% of their maximum protrusion can make the appliance difficult to tolerate. It is relatively easy to reactivate some functional appliances during treatment if further protrusion is required (Fig. 19.4).

Research would suggest that it makes no difference to the final result whether we activate the appliance to the maximum advancement initially, or in increments of a few millimetres at a time during treatment. The decision of whether to protrude the patient to the maximum amount initially, or advance incrementally during treatment, should be based on patient comfort. For some patients, incremental advancement of the mandible during treatment may make it easier to tolerate, improving compliance.

19.8.2 Fitting the functional appliance

The patient should be made aware that although the functional appliance will not be painful, it can be difficult to get used to initially. Good motivation is important in all aspects of orthodontics, but this is particularly true with functional appliances. They can be demanding appliances to wear at first, but children will adapt to them very quickly provided they are worn sufficiently. The number of hours the appliance needs to be worn each day depends on the type of appliance. Functional appliances such as the twin-block and Herbst that can be worn full time often allow the patient to adapt more quickly.

19.8.3 Reviewing the functional appliance

It is advisable to see the patient 2–3 weeks after fitting. At every review appointment, motivation of the patient is vital, as well as checking the fit of the appliance and treatment progress. Once the clinician is confident

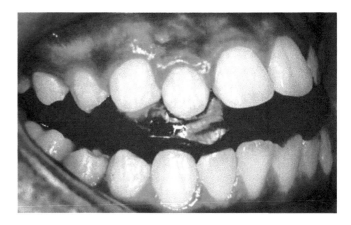

Fig. 19.9 Wax bite used to record the position of the mandible anteroposteriorly, vertically, and transversely.

that the patient is wearing the appliance as instructed, the review appointments can be made at 6–10-week intervals.

If there is no progress, this could be due to a number of factors:

- Poor compliance
- Lack of growth or an unfavourable growth rotation
- Problems with the design or fit of the appliance.

Poor compliance is the most common potential problem with these appliances. Compliance tends to be better with the younger patients and those wearing fixed functionals, such as the Herbst appliance.

19.8.4 End of functional appliance treatment

At the end of the functional appliance treatment it is sensible to slightly overcorrect the overjet reduction to edge-to-edge, due to the risk of relapse. Most functional appliances are followed by fixed appliances. With some functional appliances the functional and fixed appliance stages overlap (see Fig. 19.10). Fixed Class II correctors are used simultaneously with the fixed appliances (see Fig. 19.11).

If the arches were initially well aligned, and a second phase of fixed appliances is not required, then the patient is asked to wear the functional appliance at night for a period until growth is complete.

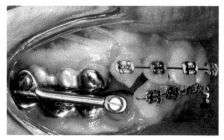
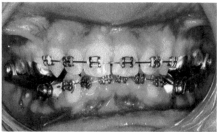
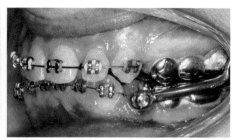

Fig. 19.10 Herbst appliance with sectional labial fixed appliances. Most functional appliances are followed by a stage of fixed appliances. The transition to fixed appliances can be complex. Some functionals, for example, the Herbst appliance shown here, allow alignment of the upper and lower labial segments using fixed appliances, during the functional stage of treatment.

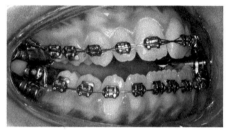
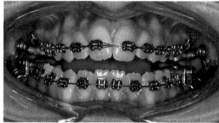
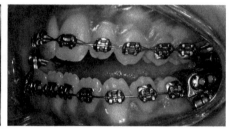

Fig. 19.11 Fixed Class II corrector (AdvanSync™). This appliance has a molar to molar attachment to protrude the mandible, allowing fixed appliances to be placed on the premolars and incisors at the same time.

19.9 How functional appliances work

The mode of action of functional appliances is one of the most controversial areas in orthodontics. There seems to be little doubt that in compliant patients who are growing, a favourable improvement in the occlusion can be achieved in most cases. When the mandible is postured, pressures are created by stretching of the muscles and soft tissues. These pressures are then transmitted to the dental arches and skeletal structures. However, it is not clear what proportion of the treatment effects are due to dental changes and what proportion are due to skeletal changes.

Early animal experiments seemed to suggest that substantial changes in the skeletal structure, including condylar growth, remodelling of the glenoid fossa, mandibular growth, and maxillary restraint, could be achieved with functional appliances. However, these results should be interpreted with caution. Animals have different facial morphologies to humans and rarely have facial skeletal discrepancies and malocclusions. In addition, the functional appliances used in the animal experiments are fixed and posture the mandible in more extreme positions than would be realistic for human usage.

Randomized controlled clinical trials show that changes caused by functional appliances are principally dento-alveolar. This means there is distal movement of the upper dentition and mesial movement of the lower dentition, with tipping of the upper incisors palatally and the lower incisors labially. There are some minor skeletal changes, with some degree of maxillary restraint as well as mandibular growth. These changes, although clinically welcome, are on average too small

(1–2 mm) to predictably replace the need for orthognathic surgery in severe skeletal discrepancies. The results of trials have also shown a large variability of response between individuals, with some patients showing more extensive skeletal changes (Fig. 19.1). This may explain why some cases seem to progress extremely well with obvious facial changes, while others show limited facial improvement. In some cases, even with minimal skeletal change, the patient's facial appearance can be improved. This is because the patient's incisor relationship has been corrected, often allowing the patient to comfortably obtain competent lips at rest.

Functional appliances have often been prescribed to cause 'growth modification'. The results of high-quality studies suggest that on average, growth changes achieved are smaller than was once initially hoped. This does not mean that total correction is impossible, but total correction of a severe deformity with growth modification alone rarely occurs. It is more likely that functional appliances improve the malocclusion, in many cases perhaps to a point where orthodontic camouflage rather than orthognathic surgery can be used to complete the treatment.

One area of difficulty for the clinician is whether to attempt growth modification for a child with a severe mandibular deficiency. The severity of the mandibular discrepancy is not a good indicator of the chance of a successful outcome. However, if the child, parents, and clinician understand that the chance of major improvement is only about 20–30% then the treatment can be undertaken. If the growth modification fails, or is insufficient to fully correct the problem, then camouflage or orthognathic surgery when the patient is older may need to be considered.

19.10 How successful are functional appliances?

This chapter has shown that functional appliances can be effective at reducing increased overjets and helping to treat Class II malocclusions in growing patients, but how successful are functional appliances?

The average failure rate for functional appliances is about 20–30%. This needs to be explained to the patient and parents at the start of the treatment. The commonest reason for failure is lack of compliance, with the patient failing to wear the functional appliance as prescribed. It is therefore vital that treatment with functional appliances is focused on improving the compliance rate by motivating the patient, and making the appliance as comfortable as possible.

Key points about functional appliances

- Functional appliances posture the mandible and are used in growing patients.
- They are usually used for correction of mild to moderate Class II skeletal problems.
- In most cases, they are followed by a second phase of fixed appliances.
- They can be used alone to treat Class II division 1 malocclusions if the arches are well aligned.
- They are used in the late mixed dentition, provided the patient is still growing.
- They can be used earlier for psychological reasons if the patient is being teased, or to reduce the risk of trauma, but this means more appointments and increased overall treatment time.
- They produce predominantly dento-alveolar effects, with small skeletal changes.
- Individual patient response to functional appliances is variable.
- They can be difficult to wear initially and require encouragement and motivation from the clinician.
- They are successful in approximately 70–80% of cases—failure is usually due to problems of patient compliance.

Relevant Cochrane review

Batista, K. B., Thiruvenkatachari, B., Harrison, J. E., and O'Brien, K. D. (2018). Orthodontic treatment for prominent upper front teeth (Class II malocclusion) in children. *Cochrane Database of Systematic Reviews*, Issue 3, Art. No.: CD003452. DOI: 10.1002/14651858.CD003452.pub4 https://www.cochranelibrary.com/cdsr/doi/10.1002/14651858.CD003452.pub4/full
This systematic review discusses the evidence behind the treatment of patients with increased overjets, and includes summaries of the best quality studies using functional appliances.

Principal sources and further reading

Dolce, C., McGorray, S. P., Brazeau, L., King, G. J., and Wheeler, T. T. (2007). Timing of Class II treatment: skeletal changes comparing 1-phase and 2-phase treatment. *American Journal of Orthodontics and Dentofacial Orthopedics*, **132**, 481–9. [DOI: 10.1016/j.ajodo.2005.08.046] [PubMed: 17920501]

O'Brien, K. D., Wright, J., Conboy, F., Appelbe, P., Davies, L., Connolly, I., et al. (2009). Early treatment for Class II division 1 malocclusion with the twin-block appliance: a multi-center, randomized, controlled trial. *American Journal of Orthodontics and Dentofacial Orthopedics*, **135**, 573–9. [DOI: 10.1016/j.ajodo.2007.10.042] [PubMed: 19409339]

O'Brien, K. D., Wright, J., Conboy, F., Sanjie, Y., Mandall, N., Chadwick, S., et al. (2003). Effectiveness of treatment for Class II malocclusion with the Herbst or twin-block appliances: a randomised controlled trial. *American Journal of Orthodontics and Dentofacial Orthopedics*, **124**, 128–37. [DOI: 10.1016/S0889-5406(03)00345-7] [PubMed: 12923506]

Tulloch, J. F. C., Proffit, W. R., and Phillips, C. (2004). Outcomes in a 2-phase randomized clinical trial of early class II treatment. *American Journal of Orthodontics and Dentofacial Orthopedics*, **125**, 657–67. [DOI: 10.1016/j.ajodo.2004.02.008] [PubMed: 15179390]
These four papers describe randomized controlled clinical trials involving functional appliances and are well worth reading.

Franchi, L., Bacetti, T., and McNamara, J. A. (2000). Mandibular growth as related to cervical vertebral maturation and body height. *American Journal of Orthodontics and Dentofacial Orthopedics*, **118**, 335–40. [DOI: 10.1067/mod.2000.107009] [PubMed: 10982936]

This paper describes how to determine the peak stage of growth of the mandible by looking at the development and maturation of the cervical vertebrae visible on lateral skull radiographs.

References for this chapter can also be found at: **www.oup.com/uk/orthodontics5e**. Where possible, these are presented as active links which direct you to the electronic version of the work, to help facilitate onward study. If you are a subscriber to that work (either individually or through an institution), and depending on your level of access, you may be able to peruse an abstract or the full article if available.

20
Adult orthodontics

S. J. Littlewood

Chapter contents

20.1 Introduction

The demand for adult orthodontics is increasing. This is due to an increased desire for improved smile aesthetics and better social acceptance of orthodontic appliances, resulting in more adults willing to wear appliances. Adult patients may request orthodontic treatment for a number of reasons:

- To achieve better dental and smile aesthetics.
- To improve function.

- Re-treatment of previous treatment that has either relapsed or was unsuccessful.
- As an adjunct to other dental treatment (e.g. periodontal or restorative).
- To allow correction of jaw discrepancy in association with orthognathic surgery (see Chapter 22).

Adult patients may also seek treatment from an orthodontist as part of non-surgical treatment of obstructive sleep apnoea (OSA), using a mandibular advancement splint (see Section 20.7)

20.2 Comprehensive, adjunctive, or limited treatment orthodontics

Some adult patients will seek comprehensive orthodontic treatment to definitively treat the whole malocclusion (the approach usually used to treat children and adolescents). Another group of adults may only be seeking orthodontic treatment as an adjunct to other dental treatment, for example, to facilitate periodontal treatment (see Section 20.4) or as an adjunct to restorative treatment (see Section 20.5).

Many adults may only wish to address certain aspects of their malocclusion, often related to aesthetics, while accepting other areas (see Fig. 20.1). This is sometimes referred to as limited treatment orthodontics, with limited aims and objectives. Before treatment begins, it is very important that the patient understands and agrees with the limited aims and objectives of treatment, accepting any compromises that will occur. This is discussed in more detail in Chapter 7, Section 7.8.3.

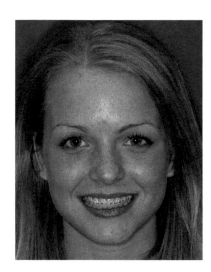

Fig. 20.1 Adult wearing ceramic brackets as part of limited objectives orthodontic treatment. The patient is seeking improvement in the appearance of the upper teeth only, to improve the smile aesthetics. She has consented to the fact that there will be no change in the slight upper centreline discrepancy or the lower arch.

20.3 Specific challenges in adult orthodontic treatment

In many ways the approach to treatment in adult patients follows the same process as that for children. There are, however, some differences that are specific to adult patients:

- Lack of growth
- Periodontal disease
- Missing or heavily restored teeth
- Physiological factors affecting tooth movement
- Motivation for treatment
- Previous orthodontic treatment
- Request for more aesthetic appliances.

20.3.1 Lack of growth

Although growth continues at a very slow rate throughout adulthood, the majority of growth changes have occurred by the end of puberty. This means that there is no scope for growth modification, so skeletal discrepancies can only be treated with either orthodontic camouflage, or combined orthodontics and orthognathic surgery.

It can also be more difficult to reduce overbites without the benefit of growth. Where possible, overbite reduction should be achieved by intrusion of the incisors, rather than the more common method of extruding the molars (provided this does not compromise the smile aesthetics). This is because extrusion of posterior teeth is more prone to relapse in adults.

The mid-palatal suture is fused in adulthood, so the skeletal expansion that is possible in adolescents using rapid maxillary expansion (see Chapter 13, Section 13.4.6) is only possible with additional surgery in adults.

20.3.2 Periodontal disease

Adult patients are more likely to be suffering, or have suffered, from periodontal disease. A reduced periodontium is not a contraindication to orthodontic treatment, but it is vital that any active periodontal disease is treated and stabilized before orthodontic treatment can begin. This is discussed in more detail in Section 20.4.

20.3.3 Missing or heavily restored teeth

Tooth loss may lead to drifting and/or tilting of adjacent teeth and over-eruption of opposing teeth into the space. In addition, atrophy of the alveolar bone can occur, leading to a narrowing or 'necking' in the site of the missing tooth or teeth (Fig. 20.2). This can make tooth movement into these areas more difficult.

Heavily restored teeth are more common in adults and may complicate the orthodontic treatment. The choice of extractions may be determined by the prognosis of restored teeth, and bonding to certain restorative materials is more difficult than bonding directly to enamel. Specialist techniques and materials are needed when bonding fixed

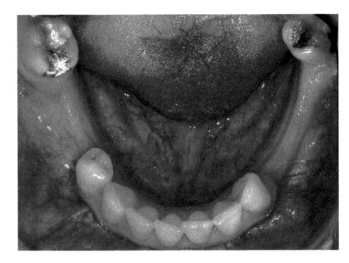

Fig. 20.2 **Atrophy of alveolus after tooth loss.**

appliances to gold, amalgam, and porcelain, and the patient needs to be warned that the restoration may be damaged when removing the fixed appliance. For this reason, if possible, it is best to leave any definitive restorations until after the orthodontic treatment.

20.3.4 Physiological factors affecting tooth movement

There is a reduced tissue blood supply and decreased cell turnover in adults, which can mean that initial tooth movement is slower in adults, and may be more painful. Lighter initial forces are therefore advisable.

20.3.5 Motivation for treatment

Adults have the potential to be excellent, well-motivated patients. Physiological factors might suggest that adult treatment should take longer than it does in children; however, this is not always the case. It has been suggested that the increased cooperation may compensate for slower initial tooth movement.

20.3.6 Previous orthodontic treatment

Some adults seeking orthodontic treatment have previously had orthodontic treatment and are now unhappy with the appearance of their teeth. This may be due to the fact that they didn't comply with the initial treatment, or it has relapsed as a result of inadequate retention (see Chapter 16), or the initial treatment was unsuccessful. It is important to determine the underlying cause, to ensure the same problem does not arise again. It is also important to assess the degree of any previous root resorption, to determine whether it is safe to proceed with another course of orthodontic treatment.

20.3.7 Request for more aesthetic appliances

Adults tend to be more conscious of the appearance of orthodontic appliances, so there has been a drive towards more aesthetic orthodontic appliances (see Section 20.6). Although distal movement of the upper molars with headgear is technically feasible, adults are more reluctant to wear extra-oral appliances. Alternative sources of anchorage are therefore more commonly used in adult patients, such as temporary anchorage devices (see Chapter 15, Section 15.4.8). Box 20.1 describes the hierarchy of aesthetics for different orthodontic appliances.

> **Box 20.1 Hierarchy of aesthetics of orthodontic appliances**
>
> (From most aesthetic to least aesthetic.)
> - Lingual orthodontic appliances
> - Clear plastic orthodontic aligners
> - Labial ceramic brackets and aesthetic wires
> - Metal labial appliances.

20.4 Orthodontics and periodontal disease

Periodontal disease is more common in adults, and is therefore an important factor that must be considered in all adult orthodontic patients. It is wise to undertake a full periodontal examination in all adult patients to exclude the presence of active periodontal disease. Periodontal attachment loss is not a contraindication to orthodontic treatment, but active periodontal disease must be treated and stabilized before treatment begins. The presence of plaque is the most important factor in the initiation, progression, and recurrence of periodontal disease. Teeth with reduced periodontal support can be safely moved provided there is adequate plaque control and an absence of inflammation.

20.4.1 Malalignment problems caused by periodontal disease

Loss of periodontal support can lead to pathological tooth migration of a single tooth or a group of teeth. The commonest presentation of periodontal attachment loss is labial migration and spacing of the incisors (Fig. 20.3). The teeth lie in an area of balance between the tongue lingually and the lips and cheeks buccally. The forces from the tongue are higher than those exerted by the lips and cheeks, but a normal healthy periodontium resists these proclining forces from the tongue. If, however, periodontal attachment is lost as a result of disease, then the teeth will be proclined forwards. In addition, if posterior teeth are lost then this lack of posterior support produces more pressures on the labial segment, leading to further proclination of the incisors.

20.4.2 Orthodontic management of patients with periodontal disease

Once the periodontal disease has been fully stabilized, and the patient is able to maintain a good standard of oral hygiene, treatment can begin (Fig. 20.4). Lighter forces are required, due to the reduced periodontal support, and ideally bonds rather than bands should be used on the molars to aid oral hygiene. Removal of excess adhesive will also help to reduce plaque retention. It has also been suggested that clear aligners may be useful in these cases as they can be removed to aid oral hygiene (see Chapter 21). Due to the reduced alveolar bone support, the centre of resistance of the tooth moves apically. This means there is a greater tendency for teeth to tip excessively, so this must be carefully controlled with appropriate treatment mechanics.

One feature that patients with previous periodontal disease often notice at the end of treatment is the so-called black triangles between the contact points and the gingival margins, located in the

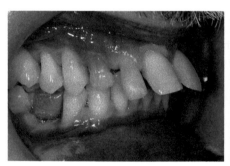 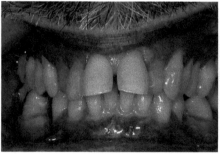 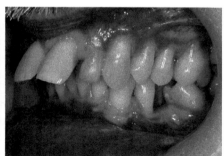

Fig. 20.3 Proclination and spacing of incisors secondary to periodontal attachment loss. This patient initially presented with a Class II division 1 incisor relationship with an overjet of 6 mm. However, due to periodontal disease and the subsequent loss of periodontal attachment around the upper labial segment, these upper incisors have flared forward, and become spaced.

interproximal regions of the anterior teeth. This can be due to api-cal migration of the gingivae. The appearance can be improved by appropriate interproximal reduction and some restorative camou-flage. However, having black triangles at the end of orthodontic treat-ment is a common risk for all adult orthodontic patients, even those without previous periodontal disease. It is therefore advisable, as part of the consent process, to warn all adult patients of the risk of black triangles at the end of treatment.

Retention at the end of treatment needs to be carefully considered. Even when the teeth are aligned and the periodontium is healthy, the problem of reduced periodontal support remains. With reduced peri-odontal attachment there will always be a tendency for the forces of the tongue to procline the incisors. These cases require permanent reten-tion, often in the form of bonded retainers, and the patient must be taught how to maintain excellent oral hygiene around these retainers (see Chapter 16).

20.5 Orthodontic treatment as an adjunct to restorative work

With an increasing number of patients keeping their teeth for longer, there is a greater need for interdisciplinary treatment of patients with complex dental problems. Where collaboration is needed between the orthodontist and the restorative dentist, it is helpful to see the patients jointly to formulate a coordinated and appropriate treatment plan. Orthodontic treatment in these cases does not necessarily require com-prehensive correction aiming for an ideal occlusion. The aims of adjunc-tive orthodontic treatment are to:

- facilitate restorative work by appropriate positioning of teeth
- improve the periodontal health by reducing areas that harbour plaque, and making it simpler for the patient to maintain good oral hygiene
- position the teeth so that occlusal forces are transmitted along the long axis of the tooth, and tooth wear is more evenly distributed throughout the arch.

The following are examples of problems that benefit from a joint approach between the orthodontist and the restorative dentist:

- *Uprighting of abutment teeth*: following tooth loss adjacent teeth may drift into the space. Uprighting these abutment teeth can facili-tate the placement of replacement prosthetic teeth (Fig. 20.4).
- *Redistribution or closure of spaces*: following tooth loss it may be possible to close the remaining space, or move a proposed abut-ment tooth into the middle of an edentulous span, in order to aid construction of a more robust prosthesis. If implants are required then the roots may need to be repositioned to permit surgical placement.
- *Intrusion of over-erupted teeth*: one of the side effects of tooth loss is over-eruption of the opposing tooth. This can interfere with restora-tion of the space, so the over-erupted tooth can be intruded using orthodontics.
- *Extrusion of fractured teeth*: sometimes it is necessary to extrude a fractured tooth, to bring the fracture line supragingivally to allow placement of a crown or restoration. There is a limit to this, as excess extrusion will reduce the amount of tooth supported by bone, reduc-ing the crown-to-root ratio.

20.6 Aesthetic orthodontic appliances

Although aesthetic orthodontic appliances are not restricted to adult patients, the drive for less visible appliances has come from adults. This demand has led to the development of a number of orthodontic appli-ances with improved aesthetics (see Box 20.1).

20.6.1 Aesthetic orthodontic brackets and wires

Aesthetic orthodontic brackets (Fig. 20.1) are made of clear or tooth-coloured material. Although not invisible, they can significantly reduce the appearance of fixed appliances. They can either be made of ceramic materials (monocrystalline, polycrystalline, or zirconia) or plastic materi-als (polycarbonate, polyurethane, or polyoxymethylene). Original plas-tic brackets showed problems with staining and a lack of stiffness, which led to deformation of the bracket when trying to apply torque. Although

improvements to plastic brackets have been made, by the addition of metal slots or the addition of ceramic particles, they still have a problem with loss of torque and this lack of control means that at the present time ceramic brackets are preferred. Zirconia brackets had poorer aesthet-ics, so their popularity has rapidly decreased. So most aesthetic brack-ets are now ceramics made of aluminium oxide in a polycrystalline or monocrystalline form (depending on their method of fabrication).

Despite their undoubted aesthetic advantages, ceramic brackets do have some potential disadvantages:

- *Bonding and bond strength*. Ceramic brackets cannot bond chemi-cally with composite resin, because the aluminium oxide is inert. In an attempt to address this, early ceramic brackets were coated with a silane bonding agent, but this produced bonds that were

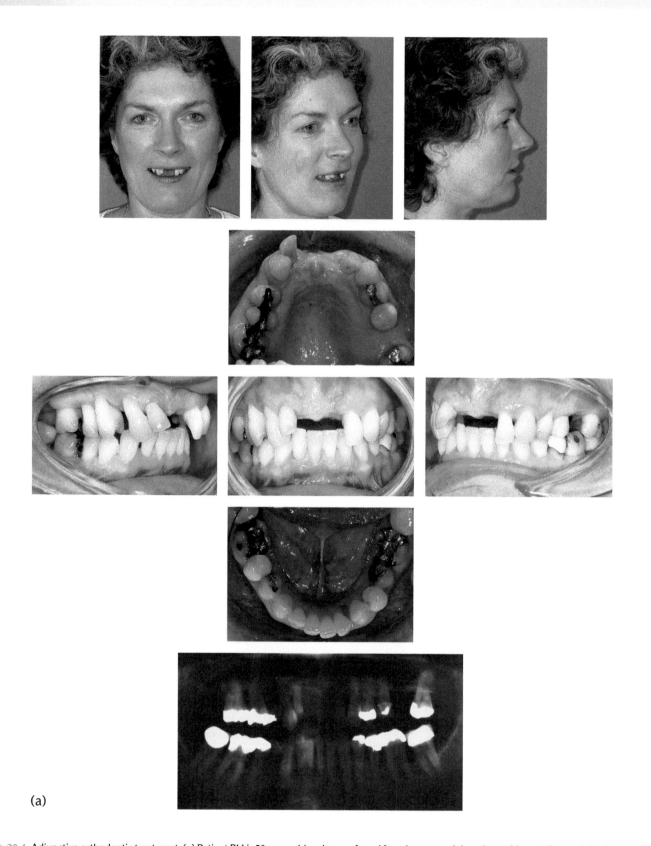

(a)

Fig. 20.4 Adjunctive orthodontic treatment. (a) Patient PM is 50 years old and was referred from her general dental practitioner with combined restorative and orthodontic problems. She had initially presented with moderate chronic periodontitis, with extensive bone loss (see DPT radiograph). This had led to migration of the teeth, particularly the upper right lateral incisor and upper right canine, which had both drifted and extruded. Following treatment and stabilization of the periodontal disease, restoration of the upper central incisor space was complicated by the position of these two teeth. The treat-

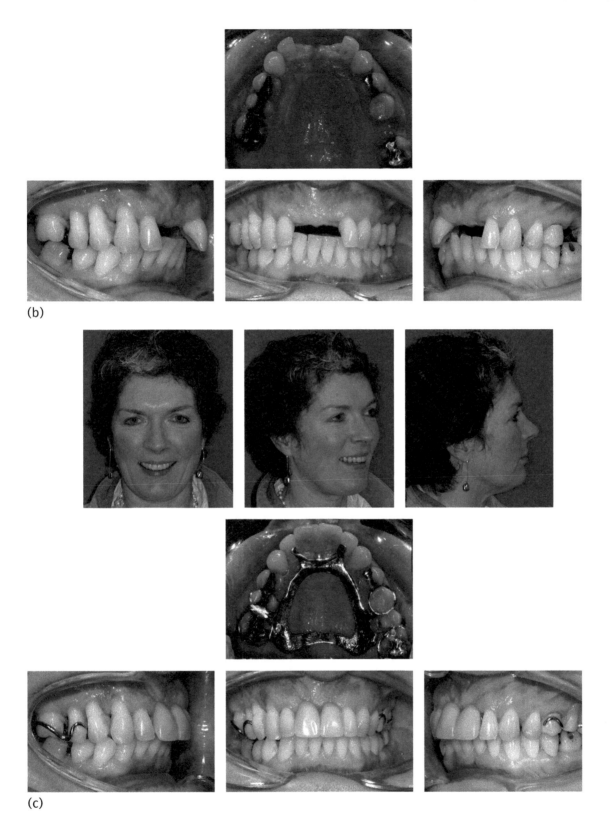

ment plan was adjunctive fixed appliance treatment to reposition these teeth, align the upper arch, and allow provision of an upper removable prosthesis. (b) Following 8 months of upper fixed appliance treatment, the upper arch was aligned and appropriate space made for the prosthesis. No attempt was made at comprehensive orthodontic correction, with no treatment in the lower arch and no reduction in overjet. (c) A removable partial denture was made. A well-fitting aesthetic prosthesis was made possible by the adjunctive orthodontic treatment.

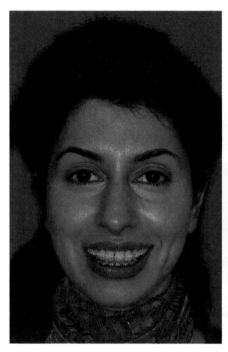
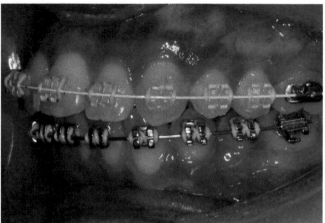

Fig. 20.5 Patient wearing upper ceramic brackets and lower metal brackets. Note the aesthetic wire in the upper arch.

too strong, resulting in enamel fractures at debond. Most current ceramic brackets therefore bond by mechanical retention using a variety of ingenious designs.

- *Frictional resistance.* Ceramic brackets offer more friction to sliding of the archwire, than standard metal brackets, which may increase the treatment time.
- *Bracket breakage.* Bracket breakage, particularly of the tie-wings, is more common with ceramic brackets, but improvements in the bracket morphology as well as refining of the manufacturing process have helped to reduce the number of breakages.
- *Iatrogenic enamel damage.* Ceramic brackets are up to nine times harder than enamel, so if these brackets are in occlusal contact with the opposing teeth there is a significant risk of enamel wear. Consequently, if occlusal contact between ceramic brackets and enamel is possible, bite-opening material needs to be placed on the occlusal surfaces posteriorly or palatally on the upper labial segment. In some cases, it may be advisable to avoid ceramic brackets in the lower arch if there is a possibility of heavy occlusal contacts. Many patients will accept metal brackets on the lower arch, as they will be barely visible in many patients (Fig. 20.5).
- *Debonding.* Removing metal brackets at the end of treatment is not usually a problem, as they are relatively pliable and the base can be easily distorted. Ceramic brackets are more rigid and the sudden force used to debond brackets can shatter the bracket, or on occasion, may cause enamel fractures. It is recommended that excess adhesive flash is removed from around the bracket before debonding. It is also vital to follow the bracket manufacturer's instructions, as different brands of brackets are designed to be removed in different ways, often using specific recommended instruments.

Attempts to make orthodontic wires more aesthetic have proved more challenging. Two approaches have been attempted to produce aesthetic orthodontic wires:

- Coated metallic wires (Fig. 20.6)
- Non-metallic aesthetic wires.

Both stainless steel and nickel titanium wires are available coated with white epoxy or Teflon®. Unfortunately, in both cases the coating can become discoloured and wear off during clinical use. An alternative that has been tried is rhodium coating, which reduces the reflectivity of the wire, giving it a matt white or frosted appearance, which

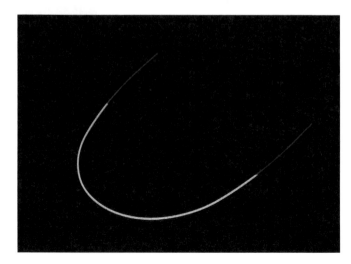

Fig. 20.6 Coated metallic aesthetic archwire.

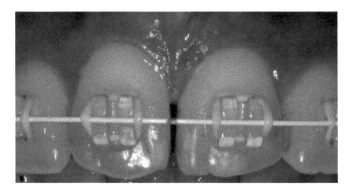

Fig. 20.7 Tooth-coloured modules on brackets using conventional ligation. The photograph shows the appearance when they are first placed. However, with time the elastomeric modules often discolour, compromising the aesthetic appearance of the appliance.

although not tooth coloured is more aesthetic than the normal metallic wire appearance.

Attempts to make non-metallic aesthetic wires have so far been unsuccessful, as the wires have proved to be unreliable, with their mechanical properties failing to match their improved aesthetic appearance.

One of the commonest complaints from patients wearing aesthetic brackets with conventional ligation is that the elastomeric modules or 'o' ring that holds the wire in the place have a good appearance initially (Fig. 20.7), but discolour with time, usually due to highly coloured food or drink. Self-ligating aesthetic brackets are available to overcome this problem, as they require no elastomeric modules (see Fig. 20.8).

20.6.2 Clear plastic orthodontic aligners

There has been a recent increase in the popularity of clear plastic orthodontic aligners (Fig. 20.9) as a result of improvements in digital technology and plastic materials, increased demand for more aesthetic

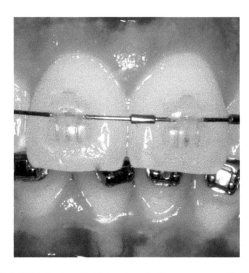

Fig. 20.8 Self-ligating aesthetic brackets in the upper arch. Both the bracket and the sliding clip mechanism are made from polycrystalline ceramic material. This removes the need for the wire to be held in place by elastomeric modules, which can discolour.

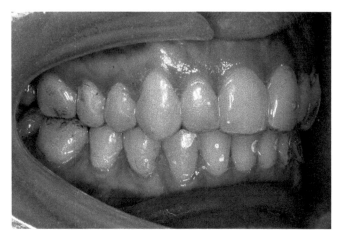

Fig. 20.9 Invisalign® clear orthodontic aligners.

orthodontic appliances and extensive marketing by the manufacturers to both clinicians and patients. Chapter 21 discusses orthodontic aligners in detail.

20.6.3 Lingual orthodontics

Lingual appliances (Fig. 20.10) in many ways offer the ultimate in aesthetic appliances, as the whole system is bonded to the lingual aspect of the teeth. They were first described in Japan in 1968. After much attention in the early 1980s, their popularity fell, partly due to the introduction of ceramic brackets, but also due to a number of problems with the appliance. However, the introduction of the Incognito® lingual appliance, using computer-assisted design/manufacture (CAD/CAM) technology to develop a fully customized appliance and robotically bent individual wires, in addition to an increased demand for 'invisible' appliances, has led to a recent increase in interest in lingual orthodontics.

Lingual orthodontics offers a number of advantages:

- Aesthetics.
- No risk to the labial enamel through decalcification.
- Position of the teeth can be seen more accurately as not obscured by the appliance.
- Some lingual brackets create a bite-plane effect on the upper incisors and canines, making these types of brackets useful for treating deep overbites.

Lingual orthodontics also has some potential disadvantages:

- Speech alteration.
- Discomfort to the patient's tongue (particularly for patients with a retrognathic mandible).
- Masticatory difficulties.
- More technically demanding for the operator, which increases the chair-time.
- Operator proficiency in indirect bonding is required for customized appliances and rebonding failed brackets can be difficult.
- More difficult to clean.
- Increased cost.

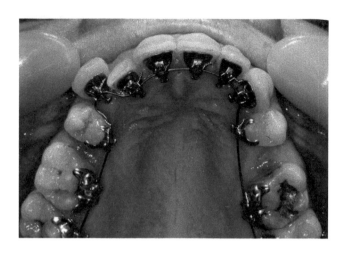

Fig. 20.10 Lingual orthodontics. Customized Incognito® lingual appliance. This patient has an Incognito® lingual appliance with customized brackets and wires. Courtesy of Dr Rob Slater.

The majority of tongue discomfort is related to the mandibular arch, so patients may choose to have a lingual appliance in the upper arch, where aesthetics is more crucial, and a labial appliance in the lower.

Lingual orthodontics can range from simple alignment of the upper labial segment (the so-called social six) using round wires, to comprehensive treatment using appliances made using state-of-the-art CAD/CAM technology (Fig. 20.10). CAD/CAM has allowed the production of fully customized appliances, with individualized production of brackets and wires. One of the challenges of aligning teeth from the lingual aspect is the unique morphology of the lingual aspect of teeth, and the range of buccolingual thickness of teeth. Customization of appliances overcomes these problems, improving the fit of the appliances, increasing the finishing control, as well as reducing speech problems and tongue irritation. Also, if the customized brackets debond during treatment they can be rebonded directly, as the bracket base-to-tooth fit is so good that incorrect positioning is unlikely.

At the present time, lingual appliances, particularly customized appliances, are more expensive, and they are more technically difficult than labial appliances for the clinician, so it remains to be seen if further developments in this field will lead to more widespread use of lingual orthodontics.

20.7 Obstructive sleep apnoea and mandibular advancement splints

20.7.1 Introduction to obstructive sleep apnoea (OSA)

Removable mandibular advancement splints can be successfully used in the treatment of adults suffering from OSA, a sleep-related breathing disorder. These splints are similar to orthodontic functional appliances that are used for the treatment of Class II problems in children, because they posture the mandible forwards.

OSA is characterized by repeated collapse of the upper airway during sleep, with cessation of breathing. The aetiology is complex, but involves anatomical and pathophysiological factors that produce obstruction of the airflow in the upper airway, often in the pharyngeal region. The compromised airflow often leads to snoring noise and occlusion of the airway. The collapse of the upper airway can lead to periodic cessation of breathing (apnoea) or reduced airflow (hypopnoea). This can lead to serious cardiovascular and respiratory complications, as well as affecting the quality of life of both the patient and their families. It is estimated that over 100 million people worldwide have the condition. The symptoms of OSA are summarized in Box 20.2. These symptoms can be worsened by certain aggravating factors:

- Alcohol consumption before bedtime
- Obesity
- Supine sleeping position
- Coexisting respiratory disease
- Medication that suppresses the central nervous system, which may lead to further relaxation of the pharyngeal musculature.

Box 20.2 Symptoms of OSA

Nocturnal symptoms

- Antisocial snoring
- Choking/gasping and witnessed apnoeas
- Restlessness
- Nocturia.

Daytime symptoms

- Excessive daytime sleepiness
- Depression
- Headaches.

20.7.2 Diagnosis of OSA

Accurate diagnosis of OSA requires a comprehensive history, examination, use of screening questionnaires, and specialist sleep tests.

The history should include a dental, medical, and sleep history, and if appropriate, a history from the partner can be useful to describe the sleep disturbances. Validated screening questionnaires, such as the STOP-BANG questionnaire and the Epworth Sleepiness Scale, may be used to determine whether formal sleep tests are indicated.

In addition to a normal extra-oral and intra-oral examination, a specialist ear, nose, and throat examination may be indicated to identify any clear physical obstructions that may be compromising the airway. The patient's body mass index (providing a measurement of possible obesity) and the neck circumference are both measured, as both are known to affect the patency of the upper airway.

If the history, examination, and screening questionnaires are suggestive of OSA, then the diagnosis can be confirmed using sleep tests. This can be done with an overnight sleep study, known as polysomnography, or more recently multichannel monitoring systems, which the patient can wear at home while they are asleep, and the data from these can help confirm the diagnosis of OSA.

20.7.3 Treatment of OSA including the use of mandibular advancement splints

Treatment of OSA may be surgical or non-surgical. Unless a clear anatomical problem can be identified, the surgical approaches to treatment are controversial and success can be unpredictable. As a result, non-surgical approaches are often the first choice of treatment.

Non-surgical approaches include the following:

1. Removal of aggravating factors
2. Continuous positive airway pressure (CPAP)
3. Mandibular advancement splints.

The first stage of treatment for all patients suffering from OSA is to identify, and if possible remove, the aggravating factors discussed earlier. This can often reduce the severity of OSA.

CPAP is a continuous stream of filtered air delivered via a nasal mask and is considered the gold standard for the treatment of OSA. To be effective, the CPAP needs to be worn at least 4–6 hours per night, 7 days a week. However, some patients find it difficult to wear the mask and long-term compliance can be a problem.

Mandibular advancement splints are used for the treatment of simple snoring, mild to moderate OSA, and for patients with severe OSA who cannot tolerate CPAP. By advancing the mandible, they increase the pharyngeal airway, pulling the tongue anteriorly and increasing the muscle tone of the palatal muscles and reducing airway collapsibility.

There are various designs of mandibular advancement appliances, but customized appliances constructed from accurate impressions have been shown to be more successful than semi-customized versions that the patient adapts to their dentition. Both types of appliances protrude the mandible. Fig. 20.11 shows a custom-made, one-piece mandibular advancement splint. The key to success is a comfortable, retentive appliance, which protrudes the mandible, with minimal vertical opening, and a motivated patient. Excessive vertical opening tends to rotate the mandible backwards and downwards, which may compromise the airway.

For patients with more severe OSA, titratable mandibular advancement splints are recommended, where the mandible can be advanced gradually to a level where the signs and symptoms are addressed (see Fig. 20.12).

Patients need to be made aware that the splints can reduce the symptoms of OSA, but they are not a cure, so long-term wear is usually required. They also need to be aware of the possible side effects (see Box 20.3). The sleep physician may suggest a repeat sleep test with the splint in place to ensure that it has addressed the OSA, particularly in more severe cases.

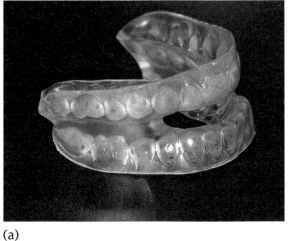

(a)

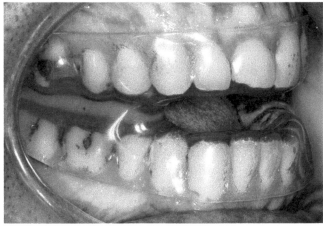

(b)

Fig. 20.11 (a, b). A custom-made, one-piece mandibular advancement splint, protruding the mandible forwards, with limited vertical opening.

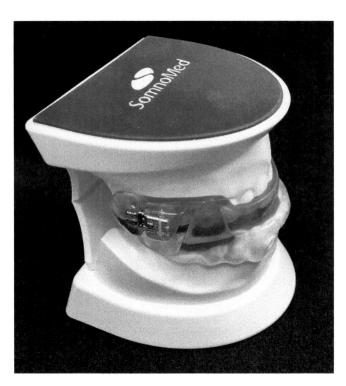

Fig. 20.12 SomnoMed® titratable two-piece mandibular advancement splint. There is a screw present on each side that can be turned to advance the mandible to a level where the signs and symptoms are addressed. © SomnoMed AG.

Box 20.3 Possible side effects of mandibular advancement splints

Short term

- Discomfort of teeth, muscles of mastication, temporomandibular joints
- Excess salivation
- Dry mouth
- Occlusion is incorrect on wakening, before gradually returning to normal.

Long term

- Possible minor dento-alveolar changes, with long-term changes in the occlusion.

20.7.4 Conclusion about mandibular advancement splints and OSA

Mandibular advancement splints can play a vital role in the treatment of OSA. Due to the multifactorial nature of OSA, these patients must be treated as part of a team, involving not only the dentist, but also sleep physicians and ear, nose, and throat surgeons. With a careful diagnosis and liaison with the other team members, mandibular advancement splints clearly have an important role in the treatment of some patients with OSA.

Key points

- The demand for adult orthodontics is increasing.
- Adult orthodontics may be comprehensive, adjunctive, or have limited objectives.
- Certain problems are particularly relevant in adult orthodontics: lack of growth, periodontal disease, missing or heavily restored teeth, different physiological response in tooth movement, motivation for treatment, previous orthodontic treatment, and request for more aesthetic appliances.
- Adult patients are more likely to present with periodontal disease. Orthodontic treatment is possible in patients with periodontal disease, provided this is treated, stabilized, and maintained throughout treatment. Treatment mechanics and retention must be adapted to allow for the reduced periodontal support.
- Adjunctive orthodontic treatment is tooth movement to facilitate other dental procedures and is more common in adults.
- There is an increased demand for aesthetic orthodontic appliances in adults. This can include aesthetic labial fixed appliances, clear aligners, and lingual appliances.
- Orthodontists may be involved in the treatment of the sleep disorder OSA using mandibular advancement splints.

Principal sources and further reading

Boyd, R. L., Leggot, P. J., Quinn, R. S., Eakle, W. S., and Chambers, D. (1989). Periodontal implications of orthodontic treatment in adults with reduced or normal periodontal tissues versus those of adolescents. *American Journal of Orthodontics and Dentofacial Orthopedics*, **96**, 191–9. [DOI: 10.1016/0889-5406(89)90455-1] [PubMed: 2773862]
The periodontal implications of orthodontic treatments in adults are discussed.

Johal, A. and Battagel, J. M. (2001). Current principles in the management of obstructive sleep apnoea with mandibular advancement appliances. *British Dental Journal*, **190**, 532–6. [DOI: 10.1038/sj.bdj.4801025] [PubMed: 11411887]
This paper provides a good overview of the use of mandibular advancement splints in the treatment of OSA, emphasizing a multidisciplinary approach to treatment.

Nattrass, C. and Sandy, J. R. (1995). Adult orthodontics – a review. *British Journal of Orthodontics*, **22**, 331–7. [DOI: 10.1179/bjo.22.4.331] [PubMed: 8580099].
This review covers a range of issues involved in adult orthodontics.

Ong, M. A., Wang, H. -L., and Smith, F. N. (1998). Interrelationship between periodontics and adult orthodontics. *Journal of Clinical Periodontology*, **25**, 271–7. [DOI: 10.1111/j.1600-051X.1998.tb02440.x] [PubMed: 9565276]

As the title suggests, this review describes the interface between periodontal and orthodontic treatment.

Shah, H. V., Boyd, S. A., Sandy, J. R., and Ireland, A. J. (2011). Aesthetic labial appliances – an update. *Orthodontic Update*, **4**, 70–7. [DOI: 10.12968/ortu.2011.4.3.70]

Shelton, A. T., Hodge, T. M., and Scott, P. (2018). Lingual orthodontics – clinical applications and patient information. *Dental Update*, **45**, 141–8. [DOI: 10.12968/denu.2018.45.2.141]
This paper provides a contemporary view of lingual orthodontics.

Wiechmann, D., Rummel, V., Thalheim, A., Simon, J. -S., and Wiechmann, L. (2003). Customized brackets and archwires for lingual orthodontic treatment. *American Journal of Orthodontics and Dentofacial Orthopedics*, **124**, 593–9. [DOI: 10.1016/j.ajodo.2003.08.008] [PubMed: 14614428]
This paper describes how computer-aided design and manufacturing technology was initially used to produce custom-made brackets to overcome some of the problems of lingual orthodontics.

References for this chapter can also be found at: **www.oup.com/uk/orthodontics5e**. Where possible, these are presented as active links which direct you to the electronic version of the work, to help facilitate onward study. If you are a subscriber to that work (either individually or through an institution), and depending on your level of access, you may be able to peruse an abstract or the full article if available.

21

Orthodontic aligners

S. K. Barber

Orthodontic aligners are growing in popularity. This chapter provides an overview of the key features of orthodontic aligners but those interested in more detailed information are guided to the 'Principal sources and further reading' section.

21.1 Definition of orthodontic aligners

The term 'orthodontic aligner' most commonly refers to clear, removable, plastic appliances that can produce small tooth movements (Fig. 21.1). The name aligner reflects the origin of the appliances in correction of mild irregularity, often in cases where post-orthodontic relapse had occurred. Contemporary aligner treatment usually refers to the process of providing a series of aligners to deliver comprehensive treatment for a range of malocclusions.

21.2 History of aligners

Removable appliances were first used in orthodontics in Europe in the nineteenth century as a method for straightening teeth. Later advances in enamel bonding technology and recognition of better results with fixed appliances resulted in greater use of fixed appliances with removable appliances becoming a largely adjunctive treatment. The discovery of vacuum-formable thermoplastic sheets in the 1980s led to a resurgence in the popularity of removable appliances as a stand-alone treatment in the form of aligners.

21.2.1 Thermoplastic aligners

Initially aligners were used in cases where one or two teeth required a small amount of movement. These aligners were referred to as 'positioners'.

The aligners were constructed by laboratory technicians, who sectioned and repositioned any teeth, usually with a maximum tooth movement of approximately 0.2 mm. The teeth were secured in the new position and the subsequent cast was used to construct the aligner using thermoplastic vacuum-formed sheets (Fig. 21.2).

The Hilliard thermoforming pliers were later developed to enable tooth-moving forces to be added to the aligner by the clinician at the chair-side. The pliers were used to create a projection in the appliance which then applied force to the tooth as the plastic returned to its original state. Various pliers were designed to apply different forces to the teeth and to modify the projections as the teeth moved.

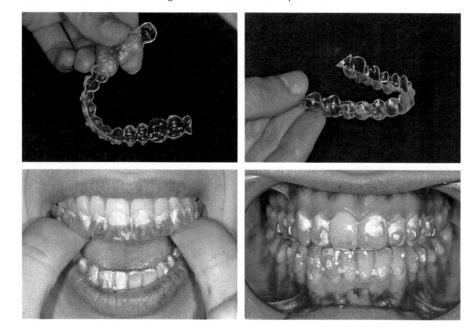

Fig. 21.1 The term orthodontic aligner most commonly refers to clear, removable, plastic appliances.

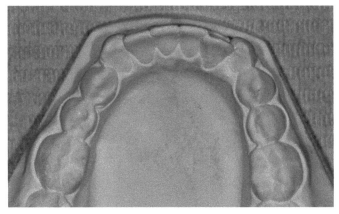

(a)

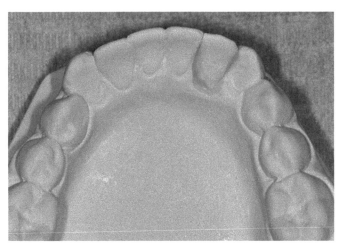

(b)

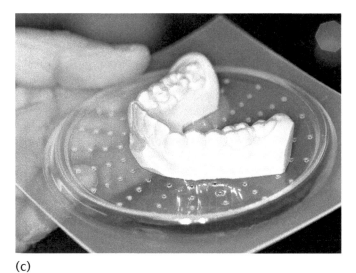

(c)

Fig. 21.2 The laboratory stages in construction of a simple orthodontic aligner to procline the mandibular right lateral incisor. (a) A dental cast is produced from the impression; (b) the tooth that requires movement is sectioned from the cast, repositioned, and secured; (c) a working cast is produced to make the aligner using vacuum-formed thermoplastic sheets.

Even with the introduction of pliers to create projections, individual thermoplastic aligners had limited ability to move teeth due to the stiffness of the material. To overcome this, sequential aligners were used to incrementally move the teeth and achieve greater overall tooth movement. Using the method previously described, laboratory technicians would perform multiple incremental tooth movements, producing an aligner at each stage. The considerable time requirements and technical difficulties associated with modifying multiple casts to produce a series of aligners by hand limited the scope of this method.

21.2.2 Spring aligners

The spring aligner was developed as an alternative method for aligning anterior teeth. These appliances employ two opposing nickel-titanium sprung bows, which straighten teeth by applying reciprocal force labially and palatally (Fig. 21.3). The appliances are designed

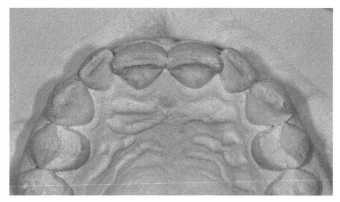

(a)

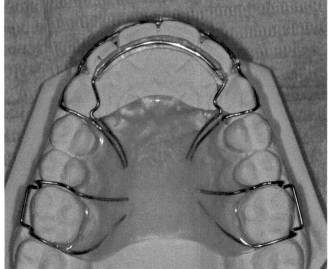

(b)

Fig. 21.3 Alignment with a spring aligner appliance. (a) The maxillary central incisors are retroclined and the lateral incisors are rotated. (b) The opposing palatal and labial bows simultaneously apply force to the palatal surface of the central incisors to procline the teeth and to the mesial corner of the lateral incisors to de-rotate the teeth.

to provide a short course of treatment (usually less than 4 months) and are limited to mild crowding of rotated or labiolingually displaced incisors. The most common commercially manufactured spring aligner is the Inman Aligner™, but most laboratory technicians can produce a spring aligner from a standard appliance prescription.

21.2.3 Contemporary aligners

Contemporary orthodontic aligner treatment has been driven by the research and development arising from the Invisalign® system, which was introduced by Align Technology (San Jose, California, USA) in 1998. Invisalign® is a proprietary orthodontic technique that uses sequential computer-generated plastic aligners to deliver a course of treatment. Other manufacturers have emerged to offer complete aligner treatment that follow similar principles, but Invisalign® remains the most popular system worldwide. The combined benefits of three-dimensional (3D) planning technology, improved materials, mechanics arising from understanding of aligner tooth movement, and computer-aided manufacture of multiple aligners have led to a much broader scope for orthodontic aligner treatment. This is discussed more in the following sections.

The popularity of contemporary aligner treatment may be attributed to a number of factors (Box 21.1). Although designed for adults with fully erupted permanent dentitions, there is a growing demand for aligner

> **Box 21.1 Factors that may have contributed to the popularity of contemporary orthodontic aligners**
>
> - Advances in technology providing greater tooth movement and versatility.
> - Advances in technology leading to improved treatment outcome.
> - Increased treatment demand by adults.
> - Increased demand for aesthetic orthodontic treatment.
> - Extensive marketing by manufacturers to clinicians and patients leading to increasing awareness.

treatment for teenage patients. This younger age group presents particular challenges for aligner treatment, such as changes to the dentition with continued tooth eruption, difficulties in gaining sufficient purchase on partially erupted teeth to fully control tooth movements and retain the aligners, and potential compliance issues. Manufacturers are rapidly developing solutions to address these potential difficulties and it is likely that through continued research and development, aligner treatment will evolve further and become established as an adjunct or alternative to other orthodontic treatment modalities in many countries.

21.3 Tooth movement with aligners

21.3.1 Understanding tooth movement with aligners

Application of force to achieve tooth movement with aligners is different to other orthodontic appliances. For aligners, the plastic enclosing the tooth has two functions: application of force for tooth movement and retention of the appliance. Tooth movement is achieved by elastic deformation of the aligner and the composition of the plastic is therefore important. The material needs to be stiff enough to deliver the correct level of force, but also highly elastic so it will return to its original shape when stretched, moving the tooth with it. Retention for the appliance is usually provided by the natural undercuts of the tooth, however, in some cases the functions of retention and elastic deformation can compete, for example, displacement of the aligner when trying to extrude teeth. This has been addressed to some extent by adding composite attachments to the teeth. Attachments provide a surface for the retainer to grip on to and prevent unwanted displacement of the aligner in addition to providing a point of force application to achieve more difficult tooth movements.

An understanding of the biomechanics of tooth movement with aligners will help clinicians to achieve more predictable results. For further information, readers are directed to the sources given in 'Principal sources and further reading'.

21.3.2 Scope of tooth movement with aligners

Much like other removable appliances, early aligners were largely restricted to tipping movements of the crown due to limitations in the force vectors that could be transmitted to the teeth. The ability to apply adequate forces to correct buccolingual tip and rotational movement of flat teeth, such as incisors, allowed aligners to manage rotated, proclined, or retroclined anterior teeth; however, there was little scope for mesiodistal or vertical tooth movement, or root torque.

Advances in understanding of tooth movement mechanics have enabled the development of a range of different shaped attachments that are placed on teeth to increase engagement between the aligner and tooth. These attachments have been carefully designed using biomechanical knowledge to allow the aligner to exert a range of force vectors. Attachments, in conjunction with advanced plastic aligner materials, enable more difficult tooth movements to be achieved, such as derotation of round teeth (canines and premolars), relative intrusion/extrusion of one or multiple teeth, and root torque. With appropriate understanding, planning, and use of modern aligner technologies it is possible to achieve a scope of tooth movement with aligners that is comparable to fixed appliances.

21.4 Clinical stages in aligner treatment

It is a common misconception that the brand of aligner is important to the eventual success of aligner treatment. The type and brand of aligner may determine the scope of potential tooth movements, however, as with all orthodontic treatment, success depends on accurate diagnosis of malocclusion, establishing patients' expectations from treatment, careful treatment planning, and understanding of mechanics.

21.4.1 Case selection

When deciding whether alignment treatment is a viable option, it is important to elicit the patient's key concerns and establish treatment goals. If significant tooth movement is required or there is an underlying skeletal discrepancy that requires correction, other forms of treatment may be preferable. It is essential that treatment objectives are measured against the scope of the appliance to deliver the necessary tooth movements and any biological limitations posed by the malocclusion. Advances in aligner technology have broadened the scope of treatment with aligners but this will not compensate for poor case selection by inexperienced clinicians.

21.4.2 Treatment planning

Regardless of the aligner system, full diagnostic records are required for treatment planning. This includes clinical information, photographs,

radiographs, and detailed impressions in a stable material. Bite registration is usually taken in maximum intercuspation and should be checked carefully, as errors in bite registration increase the risk of unattainable treatment plans.

A prescription is sent by the clinician with the records to the manufacturer to allow the technician to deliver a preliminary sequence of tooth movements. In the prescription, the clinician specifies the aims of treatment, including which aspects of malocclusion are to be corrected or accepted. The manufacturer will usually produce a virtual set-up that reflects the desired outcome described in the prescription. The virtual set-up can often be viewed in a software program, such as the Invisalign® ClinCheck (Fig. 21.4).

The virtual set-up is not the treatment plan but simply the technician's 3D interpretation of the prescription provided by the clinician. It should be noted that the technician is usually not orthodontically trained and is

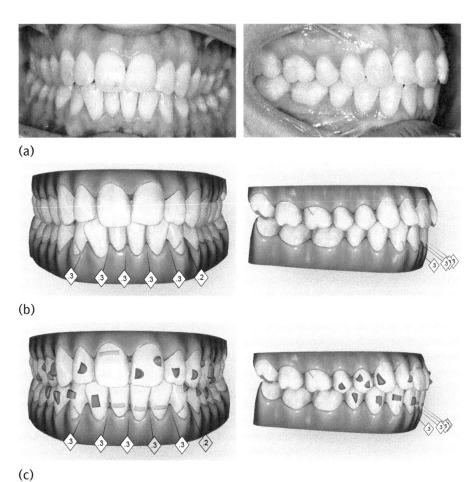

(a)

(b)

(c)

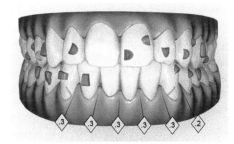

(d)

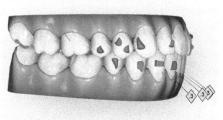

Fig. 21.4 Treatment planning check using the Invisalign® ClinCheck programme. Only select stages using front and right buccal views are included in this example, but the full programme provides a detailed 3D plan with an extensive range of views. (a) Pre-treatment intra-oral photographs; (b) pre-treatment digitization for treatment planning, created from impressions and wax bite; (c) mid-treatment stage with evidence of attachments and interproximal enamel reduction; (d) prediction for end of treatment.

not responsible for the treatment plan. The technician will follow the instructions on the prescription and ensure the tooth movements are within the software limits for that particular brand of aligner, but it is the clinician's responsibility to approve the virtual set-up. The preliminary set-up details the sequence of steps, the amount of movement per aligner, the use of adjunctive treatments such as attachments, elastics, and interproximal reduction. The clinician can view the virtual set-up and make adjustments to the treatment plan to ensure the treatment objectives are met.

21.4.3 Consent

Treatment planning and consent are covered in detail in Chapter 7; however, it is worthwhile highlighting the issues that are most pertinent to aligners. The effectiveness of aligners is not yet established and clinicians are wise to avoid overselling the alleged benefits of aligners compared to other types of treatment. Much like fixed appliance treatment, the outcome of treatment is influenced by the experience of the clinician and careful treatment planning and delivery.

Patients should be aware of any potential limitations posed by the biological constraints of the malocclusion and limited treatment objectives should be clearly stated. Aligners are not able to overcome the aspects of treatment that are biologically determined, such as any limitations in the final tooth position, the rate of tooth movement, and the need for long-term retention. Treatment time depends on the extent of tooth movement needed and compliance with aligner wear and conservative estimates are advised to allow time for detailing the occlusion with additional aligners if needed. Adjunctive treatments should be described and agreed during treatment planning and consent.

Aligners have similar potential side effects as other removable appliances, namely effects on speech, increased salivation, discomfort, and gagging, and these may be more marked in adults than children. The patient should be warned that in most cases aligners must be removed for eating and drinking, as this can impact eating habits and the number of hours of wear that are achievable. The benefit of being able to remove aligners for cleaning may be countered by the risk of non-compliance with wear and patients should be assessed on an individual basis.

21.4.4 Starting treatment

Following confirmation of the treatment plan and consent, aligners are manufactured and dispatched to the clinician to commence treatment. The first aligner is fitted, and instructions are provided including the hours of wear needed per day, usually a minimum of 22 hours, alongside dietary and oral hygiene advice. Advocates of aligner treatment claim patients report lower pain experience than with fixed appliances, however, there is no good evidence to support this claim. Pain depends on the individual and analgesia advice is recommended, as aligners often feel tight initially.

Where a series of aligners are to be used, patients should be instructed how and when to progress to the next aligner. Teeth should be 'tracking' with the series of aligners, meaning the teeth move as expected to fit

into the aligner, and teeth must be fully seated in the current aligner before moving to the next one.

21.4.5 Adjunctive treatments

Adjunctive treatments may be required to facilitate the required tooth movement. The most common adjunctive treatments are placement of attachments, interproximal reduction and use of inter-arch elastics.

Attachments are selected and located during the treatment planning stage to allow force application in the desired vector or to provide additional retention. The attachments are placed using a stent to allow composite to be bonded to the tooth in the correct shape and position (Fig. 21.5). There is anecdotal evidence that during treatment the attachments may be prone to some staining. Patients should be warned about this but reassured that at the end of treatment attachments will be removed without any permanent effect on the enamel if diet control and oral hygiene are satisfactory throughout treatment.

Interproximal reduction is often incorporated into treatment plans to provide space for alignment of teeth. The timing, location, and extent of interproximal reduction is specified in the prescription (Fig. 21.6). Usually a maximum of 0.3 mm and 0.5 mm of enamel removal is advised per interproximal surface for anterior and posterior teeth respectively, although the extent of reduction possible should be judged individually for each tooth based on enamel thickness and crown morphology. Current evidence suggests that interproximal enamel reduction used in appropriate cases and within recognized limits causes no long-term detriment to dental health.

Inter-arch elastics can be applied to notches or hooks incorporated during the aligner construction (Fig. 21.7) or by bonding metal or clear buttons directly to the tooth surface. Much like fixed orthodontics, inter-arch elastics allow correction of the anteroposterior relationship. If the application points for elastic traction are cut into the aligner, these need to be designed to prevent displacement of the aligner by the elastic force.

More advanced adaptations to aligners are also possible. Aligners have been designed to incorporate interlocking blocks to apply a Class II correction, working in the same way as other types of functional appliances. Aligners have reportedly been used in conjunction with other orthodontic auxiliaries, for example, temporary anchorage devices (mini-screws) to correct vertical discrepancies. This type of treatment is highly complex and should only be undertaken by experienced orthodontists who are competent in this approach

21.4.6 Monitoring progress

One potential benefit of aligner treatment is reduced chair-side time arising from patients being able to change their own aligners. The patient can be instructed how to monitor progress to determine when the next aligner can be started. However, it is still important that patients are seen regularly to allow the clinician to monitor progress and provide support. Progress is assessed by comparing actual tooth movement to expected tooth movement and this allows any problems to be

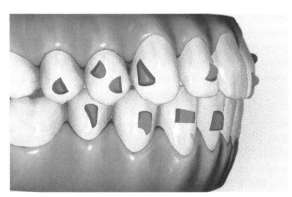

(a)

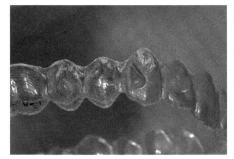 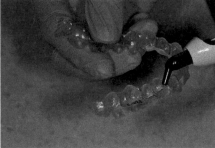 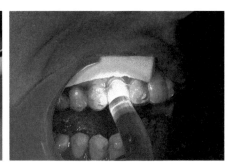

(b)

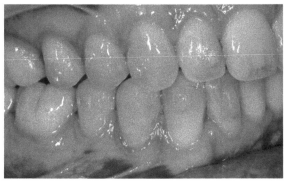

(c)

Fig. 21.5 Application of attachments. (a) Attachments are added to the teeth during the treatment planning stage. (b) A plastic flexible stent is produced from the treatment plan. The stent is used to place the composite attachments in the correct position and shape. (c) Composite attachments in place. Note there is some staining around the attachments and patients should be warned of this during the consent process.

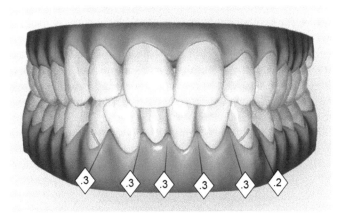

Fig. 21.6 A prescription for interproximal reduction is included in the treatment plan. In this case, 0.3 mm of enamel reduction is required between the mandibular incisors to allow alignment of the teeth.

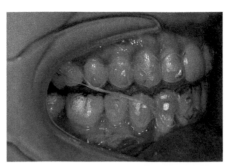 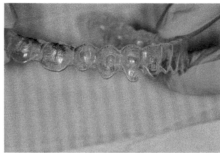

Fig. 21.7 Use of Class III inter-arch elastics with aligners. The elastic attaches to notches on the gingival margin of the aligner.

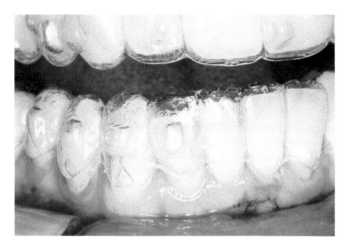

Fig. 21.8 The upper aligner is not seating fully on the lower right lateral incisor, indicating a problem with tracking.

identified and managed swiftly. The most common reasons for lack of progress are loss of tracking (Fig. 21.8) arising from insufficient wear, insufficient interproximal reduction, inadequate application of force on teeth, for example, from incorrect attachment placement, or as a result of an unfeasible plan where too much movement is planned from one aligner.

21.4.7 Retention

As with all forms of orthodontic treatment, retention is a key component of aligner treatment and the patient must be aware of the commitment to long-term retention from the outset of treatment. Removable, fixed, or combined retainers may be used depending on patient preference. Retention is discussed in detail in Chapter 16.

21.5 Digital aligner construction

Most manufacturers use their own proprietary software and processing equipment for computer-aided aligner construction, however, the systems tend to follow a common sequence. The key stages are summarized here but for further information about a specific system it is advisable to contact the manufacturer.

Firstly, a digital study model is creating using a direct scan of the impression or scan of a dental cast. The teeth are articulated using the bite registration and any obvious artefacts are removed at this stage. Some systems allow the teeth and bite to be scanned directly and transferred to the manufacturer without the need for an impression and this can reduce the time required for the digitization stage.

Tooth movements are executed by the technician using instructions from the prescribing dentist. The teeth are moved incrementally to ensure the forces applied are within physiologically acceptable limits, usually around 0.25 mm and 0.33 mm per aligner for anterior and posterior teeth respectively. Adjunctive treatments are added as required to achieve the range of desired tooth movements. Once the full sequence of movements has been executed, the final occlusion is provided and

this should correspond to the treatment objectives. At this stage, it is usual for the preliminary plan to be reviewed by the prescribing clinician. Ideally, software that enables 3D visualization of each aligner stage is used to allow real-time adjustments by the clinician to the tooth movements to finalize the treatment plan. Modifications can be made and rechecked until the clinician is satisfied that the treatment is feasible and will achieve the desired outcome. It is also possible to show the patient the proposed plan and expected tooth movements at this stage.

Following finalization of the treatment plan by the clinician, the digital study models are transferred to cast production. Previously a series of stereolithographic models were produced and each model was used to fabricate an aligner. However, developments in 3D printing technology now mean aligners can be produced directly from the computer software by the manufacturer. It is likely that with the reducing price of 3D printers and the increasing use of aligners, in the future, in-house 3D printers will enable the manufacturer to transfer the aligner details to the clinician for printing on site.

21.6 Uses for aligners

21.6.1 Types of cases

The type of case that can be successfully managed with orthodontic aligners depends on the tooth movements required to correct the malocclusion and the ability of the aligner system to achieve this movement. Different aligner systems are able to deliver different types of tooth movements and this, alongside clinician competence, will determine whether aligners are a suitable treatment method. More complex cases require a more sophisticated system that incorporates adjunctive treatments (Table 21.1). There is little evidence beyond the level of case reports to evaluate the efficacy of orthodontic aligners for correction of specific types of malocclusion and the rapid advances in technology combined with individual patient variation present challenges for generalization across cases.

Most aligner systems are suitable for simple cases where mostly tipping movements are required. Where there is moderate crowding, space for alignment is gained through interproximal reduction, expansion, or a combination of both. Alignment in the anterior region commonly results in proclination of the incisors and the effect of this should be considered in relation to the overjet and overbite. If proclination or expansion is not desirable, interproximal reduction will be necessary.

For more complex cases, where tooth movement beyond tipping is required, attachments are necessary to enable appropriate force application. Attempts to close spaces without attachments to drive root movement will result in tipped crowns. For intrusive or extrusive movement of one or two teeth, attachments enable differential force application on adjacent teeth. On round teeth, such as premolars and canines, attachments provide a point of force application. Inter-arch elastic traction may also be necessary to correct the buccal segment relationship.

Complex cases are those judged to require significant tooth movement, such as bodily movement of teeth over a distance after extraction (Fig. 21.9) or distalization of molars. For complex cases, the selection of an appropriately advanced aligner system and execution of treatment by an experienced clinician is essential for success.

21.6.2 Who should provide aligner treatment?

In the UK, the General Dental Council states dental treatment can be performed by any dentist who has the necessary skills and is appropriately trained, competent, and indemnified. Similar guidance exists in

Table 21.1 Uses for aligners

Simple	Alignment of anterior teeth by tipping
	Alignment of rotated incisors
	Mild–moderate anterior crowding (may require interproximal reduction or expansion)
	Posterior expansion
	Distal molar tip
Moderate	Closure of mild–moderate spacing
	Intrusion or extrusion of teeth
	Severe rotations on round teeth
Complex	Expansion to allow alignment of a totally blocked out tooth
	Severely ectopic teeth
	Molar uprighting or any teeth with significant undercuts
	Closure of extraction spaces
	Bodily distalization of molars
	Management of anterior open bite

other countries. Therefore, specialists and general dentists who have sought the appropriate training and are competent to perform the treatment to a satisfactory standard are generally allowed to offer orthodontic treatment. Competency will depend on the aligner system used, the complexity of the case, and clinician experience, so clinicians must decide on a case-by-case basis whether they feel able to offer treatment.

One area of concern has arisen around manufacturer training courses which only include information about the one specific system. In these cases, clinicians may not have sufficiently broad knowledge to be able to provide all treatment options in a balanced way to allow informed decision-making. It is important that patients are informed of the qualifications and experience of clinicians offering treatment, including any limitations in what they are able to offer, and if the patient requests additional information or a second opinion, a referral should be offered.

Evidence shows treatment outcomes are improved by accurate diagnosis, careful treatment planning, and operator experience. Those at the start of their aligner journey are encouraged to select cases carefully and seek mentoring from more experienced colleagues where possible to ensure patient care is optimized.

21.7 Advantages and limitations of orthodontic aligners

Many claims have been made by supporters and manufacturers of orthodontic aligners and while the body of evidence to support these claims is growing, there are few high-quality trials to determine the effectiveness of aligners compared to other treatment methods. The most commonly proposed advantages of aligners include more aesthetic appliance, improved dental health in terms of periodontal health and reduced risk of decalcification, and a reduction in chair-side time, overall treatment time, pain experience, and root resorption. The current body of evidence for orthodontic aligners is insufficient to conclusively support or refute these claims although future high-quality randomized trials are planned.

It is generally acknowledged that aligners are more aesthetic than metal buccal fixed appliances but not as inconspicuous as lingual fixed appliances. The appearance of aligners compared to ceramic fixed appliances is more difficult to judge and depends on the particular systems in use and personal preference. The ability to remove aligners for cleaning and eating might be expected to reduce the risk of periodontal problems and decalcification; however, this has not yet been substantiated and it is likely that the risk of treatment is related more to individual motivation than the appliance.

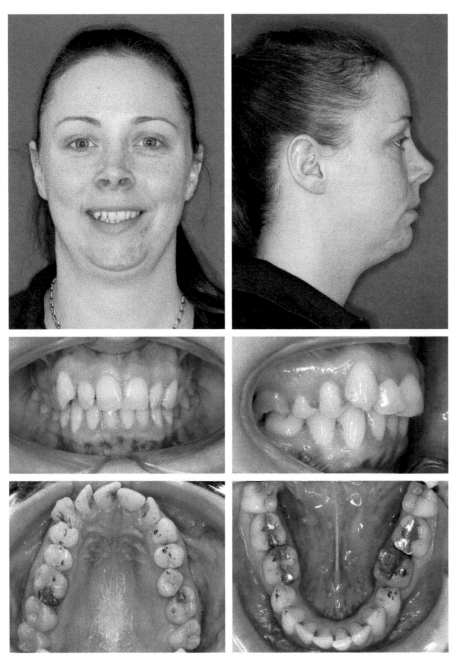

Fig. 21.9 A female adult patient who underwent comprehensive treatment with orthodontic aligners (treatment was provided by Catherine McCanny). The patient presented with a Class II division 1 incisor on a Class I skeletal base with moderate upper and mild lower arch crowding. The malocclusion was complicated by a Class II buccal segment relationship on the right side and a 2 mm centreline discrepancy. Treatment involved extraction of the maxillary right first premolar and treatment with the Invisalign® system. The malocclusion was successfully corrected in 30 months and bonded retainers were provided.

Key points

- Aligners have gained popularity over the last decade due to advances in the understanding of tooth movement with aligners and increased demand for aesthetic orthodontic appliances, particularly for adults.

- Aligners may provide an alternative to fixed appliances for amenable malocclusions in the hands of trained and competent clinicians.

- Diagnosis, treatment planning, and use of appropriate biomechanics is the responsibility of the treating clinician, not the aligner manufacturer.

- More complex cases may require aligners to be used in combination with fixed appliances or other adjunctive treatments.

- It is essential a full orthodontic assessment is undertaken and the full range of treatment options are discussed with the patient.

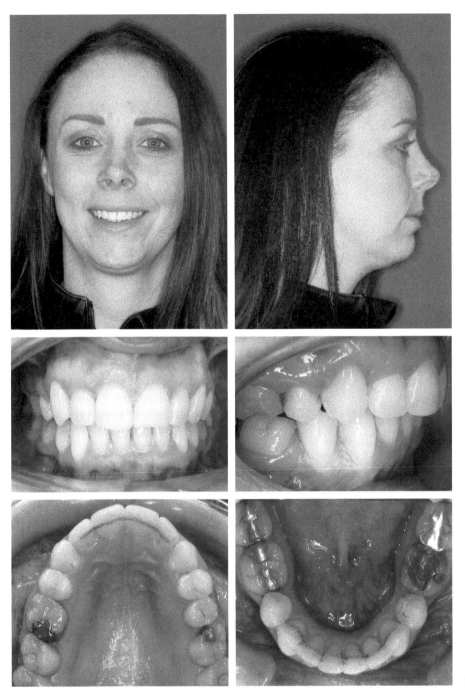

Fig. 21.9 (*Continued*)

Relevant Cochrane review

Yu, Y., Sun, J., Lai, W., Wu, T., Koshy, S., and Shi, Z. (2013). Interventions for managing relapse of the lower front teeth after orthodontic treatment. *Cochrane Database of Systematic Reviews*, Issue 9, Art. No.: CD008734. DOI: 10.1002/14651858.CD008734.pub2
This review included aligner treatment but no studies that fulfilled the inclusion criteria were identified.

Principal sources and further reading

Azaripour, A., Weusmann, J., Mahmoodi, B., Peppas, D., Gerhold-Ay, A., Van Noorden, C. J., et al. (2015). Braces versus Invisalign®: gingival parameters and patients' satisfaction during treatment: a cross-sectional study. *BMC Oral Health*, **15**, 69. [DOI: 10.1186/s12903-015-0060-4] [PubMed: 26104387]
Evidence that Invisalign® treatment is associated with better gingival health and patient satisfaction, but caution is advised due to limitations in the methodology.

Best, A. D., Shroff, B., Carrico, C. K., and Lindauer, S. J. (2017). Treatment management between orthodontists and general practitioners performing clear aligner therapy. *Angle Orthodontist*, **87**, 432–9. [DOI: 10.2319/062616-500.1] [PubMed: 27874282]
An interesting comparison of treatment perspectives between different types of clinicians from the USA.

Bowman, S. J. (2017). Improving the predictability of clear aligners. *Seminars in Orthodontics*, **23**, 65–75. [DOI: 10.1053/j.sodo.2016.10.005]
Discussion of some of the common aligner problems and possible solutions.

Gay, G., Ravera, S., Castrflorio, T., Garino, F., Rossini, G., Parrini, S., *et al.* (2017). Root resorption during orthodontic treatment with Invisalign®: a radiometric study. *Progress in Orthodontics*. **18**, 12. [DOI: 10.1186/s40510-017-0166-0] [PubMed: 28503724]
A prospective cohort study that suggests root resorption with aligners is similar to other systems using light forces.

Qureshi, A. (2008). The Inman Aligner for anterior tooth alignment. *Dental Update*, **35**, 569–71, 574–6. [DOI: 10.12968/denu.2008.35.8.569] [PubMed: 19055094]
A summary of the design and uses of the most commonly used commercial spring aligner appliance.

Noah, J. H., Sharma, S., Roberts-Harry, D., and Qureshi, T. (2015). A discerning approach to simple aesthetic orthodontics. *British Dental Journal*, **218**, 157–66. [DOI: 10.1038/sj.bdj.2015.55] [PubMed: 25686433]

An interesting discussion of the purpose and ethics of adult orthodontics, including the scope and limitations of aligner treatment.

Paquette, D. E., Colville, C., and Wheeler, T. (2016). Clear aligner treatment. In: Graber, L. W. and Vanarsdall, R. L. (eds) *Orthodontics: Current Principles and Techniques* (6th edn), pp. 778–811. St. Louis, MO: Elsevier.
This chapter provides a detailed overview of the history and current approach to the use of clear aligners, focusing principally on Invisalign®.

Tuncay, O. C. (2006). *The Invisalign® System*. New Malden: Quintessence Books.
The original Invisalign® textbook, which although slightly outdated now, does provide a historical perspective to the system.

Weihong, L., Wang, S., and Zhang, Y. (2015). The effectiveness of the Invisalign appliance in extraction cases using the ABO model grading system: a multicenter randomized controlled clinical trial. *International Journal of Clinical and Experimental Medicine*, **8**, 8276–82. [PubMed: 26221410]
A trial to compare fixed appliances and aligners for extraction treatment in adults. Limitations were noted in the methodology.

Wheeler, T. T. (2017). Orthodontic clear aligner treatment. *Seminars in Orthodontics*, **23**, 83–6. [DOI: 10.1053/j.sodo.2016.10.009]
A paper describing the types of malocclusion that can be treatment with aligners.

White, D. W., Julien, K. C., Jacob, H., Campbell, P. M., and Buschang, P. H. (2017). Discomfort associated with Invisalign and traditional brackets: a randomized prospective trial. *Angle Orthodontist*, **87**, 801–8. [DOI: 10.2319/091416-687.1] [PubMed: 28753032]
This trial suggests aligner treatment may slightly reduce pain experience and analgesic use.

Zheng, M., Lui, R., Ni, Z., and Yu, Z. (2017). Efficiency, effectiveness and treatment stability of clear aligners: a systematic review and meta-analysis. *Orthodontics and Craniofacial Research*, **20**, 127–33. [DOI: **10.1111/ocr.12177**] [PubMed: 28547915]
This review found a lack of evidence to support claims about the effectiveness of orthodontic aligners.

References for this chapter can also be found at: **www.oup.com/uk/orthodontics5e**. Where possible, these are presented as active links which direct you to the electronic version of the work, to help facilitate onward study. If you are a subscriber to that work (either individually or through an institution), and depending on your level of access, you may be able to peruse an abstract or the full article if available.

22

Orthodontics and orthognathic surgery

S. J. Littlewood

Chapter contents

22.1 Introduction

Orthognathic surgery is surgery aimed at correcting dentofacial deformity. A dentofacial deformity is a deviation from normal facial proportions and dental relationships that is severe enough to be handicapping to a patient. A malocclusion can be handicapping in two ways: problems with jaw function or aesthetics. It is estimated that 2–3% of the population has a dentofacial deformity.

Jaw function problems may include eating difficulties or speech problems. A malocclusion is rarely so extreme that eating is not possible at all, but it may be difficult and embarrassing for the patient to try and eat certain types of food, particularly in public (Fig. 22.1). Speech difficulties may also be related to an underlying dentofacial deformity. However, the most common reason for patients seeking combined orthodontic and surgical treatment is dental and/or facial aesthetic problems, which can lead to psychological and social problems. An index specifically designed to assess the need of orthognathic patients called the Index of Orthognathic Functional Treatment Need (IOFTN) has been developed to identify patients who would most benefit from combined orthodontics and orthognathic surgical treatment (see Chapter 2, Section 2.3.6).

For correction of a dentofacial deformity, a combined orthodontic and surgical approach is required. Successful treatment requires close interdisciplinary work involving a number of specialists. Joint planning sessions and combined clinics are helpful to ensure that the whole team provides a coordinated approach to treatment. The patient should also be provided with appropriate information leaflets and referred to appropriate online resources to help them fully understand the implications of treatment as part of the overall consent process (Fig. 22.2).

22.2 Indications for treatment

Combined orthodontics and orthognathic surgery is indicated for patients who have a severe skeletal or very severe dento-alveolar problem that is too extreme to correct with orthodontics alone. The presence of a skeletal discrepancy does not automatically mean that a patient requires surgical intervention. When faced with a skeletal discrepancy, the clinician has three choices:

- Growth modification
- Orthodontic camouflage
- Combined orthodontics and orthognathic surgery.

Growth modification is only possible in growing patients and usually means treatment with headgear or functional appliances (see Chapter 19). On average, growth modification can only alter skeletal relationships by a limited amount and is often unpredictable. There is inevitably some correction by displacement of the teeth, so when using growth modification at least part of the correction is due to dental compensation for the skeletal discrepancy.

Once growth is complete, the only non-surgical option is orthodontic camouflage. This means moving the teeth into the correct dental relationships, but accepting the skeletal discrepancy. Major tooth movements may help to produce a good dental occlusion, but there is a danger of compromising facial aesthetics (Fig. 22.3). In these cases, a combined surgical approach may be required.

Clinical examples of cases when orthognathic surgery is commonly used include:

- severe Class II skeletal malocclusions
- severe Class III skeletal malocclusions
- severe vertical disproportions leading to anterior open bite or a severely increased overbite
- skeletal asymmetries.

Combined orthodontic and surgical treatment is only started once growth has slowed to adult levels. This is important, because if the patient experiences significant facial growth after treatment has finished, this could compromise the result.

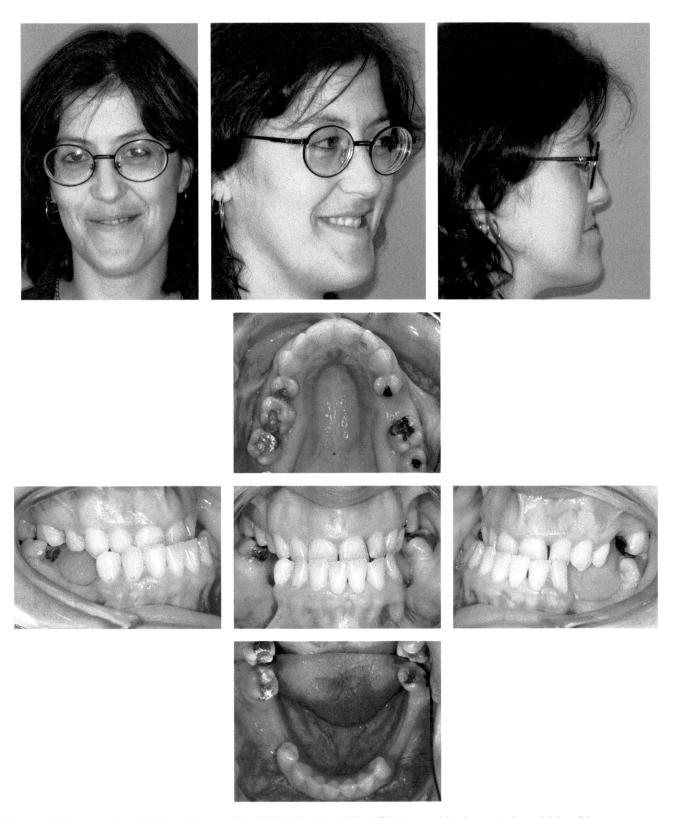

Fig. 22.1 Initial presentation of patient with severe Class III skeletal pattern. Patient IE is 35 years old and presented complaining of the poor appearance of her bite, her prominent chin, and difficulty eating in public. She had a marked Class III skeletal relationship with a reverse overjet. This patient's computer planning is shown in Fig. 22.9, her pre-surgical photographs in Fig. 22.12, and her end of treatment photographs in Fig. 22.15.

22.3 Objectives of combined orthodontics and orthognathic surgery

The objectives of treatment are the same as for orthodontic treatment:

- Acceptable dental and facial aesthetics
- Good function
- Optimal oral health
- Stability.

22.4 The importance of the soft tissues

For many years, diagnosis and treatment planning was focused on the hard tissues of the face (the dentition and the bony skeleton), with treatment aiming to achieve a perfect occlusion and ideal skeletal proportions. However, we are now aware that the soft tissues are key for two reasons:

- It is the soft tissues we see, so the soft tissue proportions are more important than the skeletal proportions for achieving an aesthetic result. The soft tissue proportions are related to, but not necessarily identical, to the underlying skeletal pattern.
- The soft tissues determine the limit of orthodontic and orthognathic treatment. It is not possible to create the same ideal dental and skeletal result in every case, as the outcome is strongly influenced by the

surrounding soft tissues and how well a patient can adapt to the new position of the teeth and jaws. This includes the pressures exerted by the lips, cheeks, tongue, and facial musculature, as well as soft tissues around the teeth—the periodontal ligament.

As a result, diagnosis should start with an analysis of the soft tissues, followed by an assessment of the underlying bones and teeth. In terms of planning, a process called 'reverse engineering' is used. This means the clinician decides what facial soft tissue and smile aesthetics outcomes are desirable, and then works backwards to determine what has to be done to the hard tissues (dentition and facial skeleton) to achieve these outcomes.

22.5 Diagnosis and treatment plan

For combined orthodontic and orthognathic surgical patients, the same logical sequence used for routine orthodontic treatment planning (see Chapter 7) should be followed. By taking an appropriate history, clinical examination, and diagnostic records, the necessary database of information can be collected. This database can then be used to make a problem list (see Chapter 7, Fig. 7.1). This chapter will focus on the areas of direct relevance to orthognathic surgical patients.

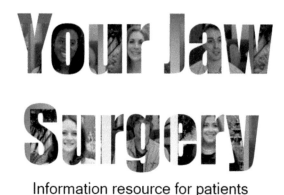

Your Jaw Surgery

Information resource for patients

Helping patients understand Jaw Surgery

Fig. 22.2 Screenshot of 'Your Jaw Surgery' website produced by the British Orthodontic Society. Reproduced with the kind permission of the British Orthodontic Society.

22.5.1 History

The purpose of the history is to determine the patient's concerns, motivation for treatment, expectations of treatment, psychological status, and medical and dental history.

Patient's concerns

The patient should be allowed to describe whether their concerns are aesthetic, functional, or both. Functional problems could be masticatory and/or speech problems. While masticatory problems can often be markedly improved, care should be taken when promising resolution of speech problems, which are often firmly established by adulthood. Full correction of the speech problems may not be possible with the orthodontics and orthognathic surgery, and it is wise to seek the expert advice of a speech therapist.

In addition to aesthetic and functional problems, the patient may present complaining of pain. This could be due to a traumatic overbite or temporomandibular joint dysfunction. Traumatic overbites can be successfully addressed during combined treatment, but there is no guarantee that surgery to correct a dentofacial deformity will correct temporomandibular joint dysfunction.

Patient's motivation, expectations, and psychological status

It is important to assess why the patient is seeking treatment at this time and what they expect the effect of the treatment will be. A small number of patients may have unrealistic expectations that combined treatment will not only improve their facial and dental appearance, but also have remarkable

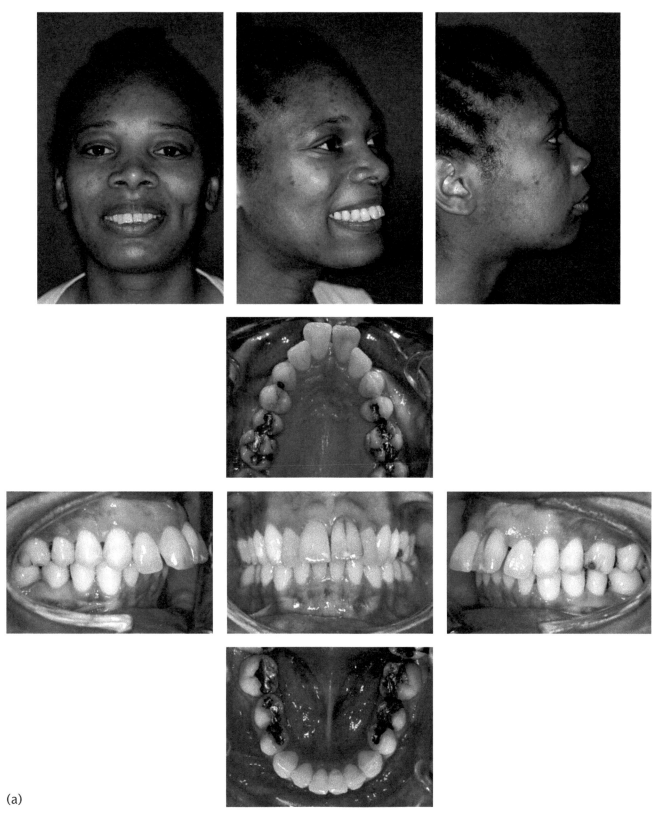

(a)

Fig. 22.3 Patient with Class II skeletal discrepancy. (a) Before treatment. This patient complained of her prominent upper teeth. She had a 14 mm overjet and a retrognathic mandible. It may have been possible to correct her dental malocclusion with orthodontics alone, but excessive retraction of the upper labial segment would have resulted in an unfavourable facial profile.

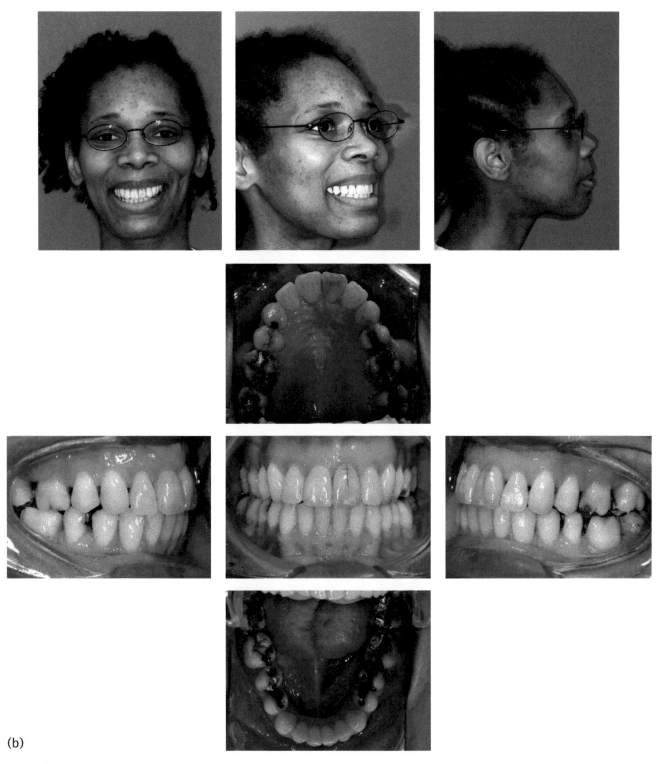

(b)

Fig. 22.3 (b) After treatment. The patient was treated with a combination of extractions, fixed appliances, and mandibular advancement surgery.

effects on their relationships and career prospects. A clinical psychologist should ideally be part of the interdisciplinary team as their involvement during the assessment and treatment planning of these cases is often helpful.

The psychologist can help to assess a patient's expectations and determine their ability to cope with the treatment. They can also identify patients who may have underlying psychological or psychiatric problems that need to be addressed before beginning any treatment. There is one particular group of patients to be aware of who suffer from a condition known as body dysmorphic disorder. These patients present with a non-existent or very minor facial deformity and have an obsession with this imagined or greatly exaggerated defect in their appearance. This excessive concern can cause significant psychological distress. A close liaison with a clinical psychologist or psychiatrist is required in the management of this group of patients.

Patients with dentofacial deformities may present expressing concerns about their facial appearance, but may have no concerns about their teeth. These patients may be surprised that prolonged fixed appliances are required as part of the treatment. In very rare circumstances it is possible to achieve a reasonable result with surgery alone. However, in most cases surgery without orthodontic involvement produces a compromised result.

Medical and dental history

Patients who will be undergoing combined treatment must be fully dentally fit. They must also have a medical history that is compatible with a general anaesthetic. Conditions such as diabetes, hypothyroidism, adrenal insufficiency, bleeding disorders, cardiac and respiratory disorders, and many other medical conditions may complicate or prevent treatment. If there is any doubt about this, then an early consultation with an anaesthetist and their general medical practitioner is advised, before embarking on treatment.

22.5.2 Clinical examination

A systematic approach to the clinical examination is required to assess the facial and dental aesthetics and the malocclusion and to identify any pathology.

When assessing the facial appearance, it is the proportions of the face that are important. The aim of combined orthodontic and orthognathic treatment is not necessarily to try and make the patient beautiful—it is about moving them towards more normal facial proportions (see section on 'Principal sources and further reading' for more details on this). When assessing facial proportions, it is important to take into account the patient's racial background, gender, and age. This will help the clinician to decide whether the clinical features are within normal limits.

The extra-oral assessment is really an assessment of the facial soft tissues and smile aesthetics. The information from the extra-oral examination can then be combined with the information obtained from the radiographs. The radiographs will explain the hard tissue (dental and skeletal) contribution to the facial appearance.

Full face assessment

The symmetry and vertical proportions of the face are assessed from the frontal view. No face is completely symmetrical, but marked deviations should be noted (Fig. 22.4).

The 'ideal' face can be vertically divided by horizontal lines at the hairline, nasal base, and the chin. The lower third can be further divided so that the meeting point of the lips is one-third of the way from the base of the nose to the chin (Fig. 22.5).

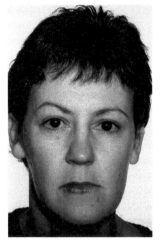
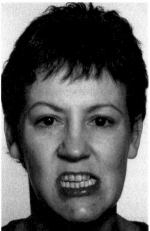
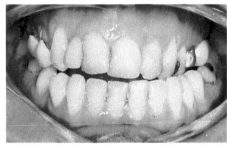

Fig. 22.4 Facial asymmetry. This patient shows a mandibular asymmetry to the left. Note the large centreline discrepancy between the arches. This is partly because the upper centreline is to the right by 2 mm (for dental reasons), but mostly because the lower centreline is to the left by 5 mm due to the underlying mandibular skeletal asymmetry.

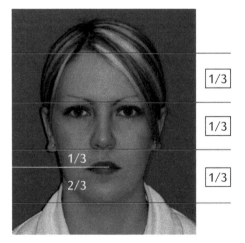

Fig. 22.5 Vertical proportions. In normal proportions, the face can be divided into three equal thirds, with the lower third further divided so that the commissures of the lips are one-third of the way from the base of the nose to the chin.

Profile assessment

For assessment of the patient's profile, the patient should be assessed in the natural head position: the position the head is held in when the patient is relaxed and looking into the distance. The middle and lower thirds are assessed in relation to the forehead area. In normal profile, the base of the nose lies approximately vertically below the most anterior portion of the forehead. The shape and size of the nose and paranasal areas should also be assessed. In general, the bigger the nose, the more lip and chin prominence is needed to achieve facial balance. The nasolabial angle should also be noted, as it can be affected by excessive retraction or proclination of the upper incisors.

It is worth noting at this point that a full assessment of the patient's nose should form part of the assessment. It is possible the patient may benefit from a rhinoplasty as part of the overall treatment plan. It is also important to recognize that surgery to the maxilla may affect the shape of the nose, and this needs to be assessed and discussed with the patient as part of the consent process.

The chin projection is affected by the position of the mandible, the prominence of the bony chin point, and the amount of soft tissue coverage. When a patient has a retrognathic mandible, it is possible to get an idea of the effect of surgery by asking the patient to posture their mandible forwards the desired amount. The likely effects of other surgical movements are more difficult to assess clinically, and usually involve manipulation of the patient's photographic and radiographic records. Surgical planning and predictions are discussed in more detail in Section 22.6.

Smile aesthetics

One of the most important features to assess is the position of the dentition in relation to the lips and face, anteroposteriorly, transversely, and vertically. See the section on 'Principal sources and further reading' at the end of the chapter for information about how best to assess the anteroposterior position of the incisors in the face. Transversely, it is important to check whether the centrelines of the upper and lower dentitions are coincident with each other, and whether they are coincident with the centre of the face. It should be noted whether any centreline problem is of dental or skeletal origin.

Vertically, the amount of upper incisor show should be assessed. At rest this should be 1 mm for males and 3 mm for females. On full smiling, the full height of the upper incisors should be visible. Any occlusal cant of the dentition should also be noted.

If there is excess gingival show, the patient may refer to this as a 'gummy smile'. When a 'gummy' smile is noted, it is important that the aetiology is understood, as this will dictate the type of treatment required. 'Gummy' smiles do not always require surgical treatment. Possible aetiological causes of a 'gummy' smile include true vertical maxillary excess (Fig. 22.6), a short upper lip, a localized dento-alveolar problem, short crowns (due to incisal wear), gingival overgrowth, or hyperactive lip musculature.

Temporomandibular joints

The presence of any signs or symptoms of temporomandibular joint dysfunction should be noted. Ideally any symptoms should be treated conservatively prior to treatment. Often placing fixed appliances will at

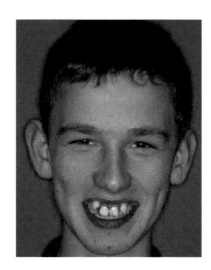

Fig. 22.6 'Gummy smile'. This 'gummy smile' is due to vertical maxillary excess.

least temporarily relieve some of the symptoms. This may be due to the tenderness of the teeth reducing parafunctional habits such as clenching and grinding. However, it is unwise to promise any marked long-term improvement in the temporomandibular dysfunction, as a direct result of the combined orthodontics and orthognathic surgery (see also Chapter 1, Section 1.4.6).

Intra-oral assessment

A full assessment of the dentition and occlusion needs to be undertaken. Any dental disease needs to be identified, treated, and stabilized before combined orthodontics and orthognathic surgery can begin.

The relationship of one arch to the other is less important in orthognathic cases, as this part of the problem is often addressed by the surgery. However, each arch should be individually assessed for alignment and symmetry. The amount of crowding in each arch should be evaluated, as well as the inclination of the teeth. The latter is important, because in most patients with a skeletal discrepancy the teeth have been tilted. This is due to the action of the lips and tongue attempting to achieve an anterior oral seal. This process is called 'dento-alveolar compensation' for the underlying skeletal pattern. In a Class II skeletal problem, the lower incisors are often proclined by the tongue. Conversely, in a Class III skeletal pattern the lower incisors are often retroclined by the lower lip, with the upper incisors proclined by the tongue (Fig. 22.7). It is important to recognize any dento-alveolar compensation, as one of the aims of pre-surgical orthodontic treatment is to undo this compensation—a process known as 'decompensation'—to allow appropriate positioning of the jaws to create the best facial and smile aesthetics (see Chapter 11, Fig. 11.6).

22.5.3 Radiographic examination

This usually includes those radiographs taken as part of the routine orthodontic assessment of a patient with a skeletal discrepancy: a dental panoramic tomogram (DPT), a lateral cephalometric radiograph, and if indicated a view of the upper incisors. Additional views may be needed, depending on the case. For example, a posteroanterior skull radiograph may be taken to assess asymmetry.

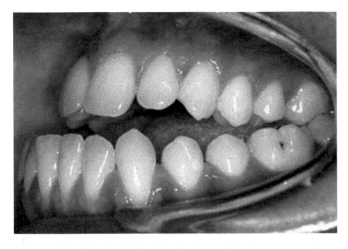

Fig. 22.7 Class III malocclusion showing dento-alveolar compensation. In this case, the lower lip has retroclined the lower incisors and the upper incisors have been proclined by the tongue.

22.5.4 Cephalometric assessment

In addition to a routine cephalometric analysis (see Chapter 6), many surgeons and orthodontists will carry out more specialized analyses to determine the underlying aetiology of the particular problem. Many such analyses exist, and for further details the reader is referred to the section on 'Principal sources and further reading' at the end of the chapter. The purpose of the analysis is to provide detailed information about the relationships between the different parts of the dentofacial complex:

- Cranium and cranial base
- Nasomaxillary complex
- Mandible
- Maxillary dentition
- Mandibular dentition.

The detection of any imbalances and disproportions in these dentofacial relationships is based on comparing the values for the individual with so-called normal data. As with the assessment of soft tissue proportions, the normal data for the hard tissues must be relevant to the patient being treated, in terms of age, gender, and racial background.

There is an increasing move towards three-dimensional (3D) assessment using cone beam computed tomography (CBCT), which is discussed in Section 22.10.

22.6 Planning

Using the information gathered from the history, examination, and diagnostic records, it should be possible to create a problem list, followed by the aims of treatment. This is discussed in greater detail in Chapter 7, Sections 7.3 and 7.4. Once the aims of the treatment are identified, the various specialists involved in the case should consider, as a team, the advantages and disadvantages of different approaches to treatment.

One of the orthodontist's responsibilities in the planning process is to consider reversing any dento-alveolar decompensation. It may not always be possible, or desirable, to fully decompensate incisors. For example, a narrow mandibular symphysis and/or thin labial periodontal tissues may make full decompensation impossible without compromising the periodontal support around the teeth. Fig. 22.8 shows lower incisors that were decompensated to their ideal angulations, but this resulted in perforation of the labial plate, producing gingival recession. This is an example of a treatment aimed at producing an ideal occlusal result that has produced a compromised result, because it was beyond the limitations of the soft tissues (see Section 22.4).

One of the principal aims of combined orthodontics and orthognathic surgery is to obtain ideal facial aesthetics. This means appropriate soft tissue positioning in 3D. The treatment actually moves the hard tissues: the orthodontist positions the teeth and the surgeon positions the facial skeleton. The challenge is to move the hard tissues to produce the best possible position of the soft tissues. Accurately predicting the soft tissue changes in response to hard tissue treatment changes is not an exact art, as the hard and soft tissues do not move in a one-to-one ratio.

Planning can be undertaken with a combination of cephalometric tracings, digital photographs, and dental casts. Computer prediction software can predict the likely responses of the soft tissues, so when the proposed orthodontic and surgical movements are undertaken virtually on the computer, the likely soft tissue profile can be produced. Specialist planning software can be used to link the patient's digital photograph with their cephalometric tracing, so that the patient's image can be automatically 'morphed' in response to the planned surgical and orthodontic movements (Fig. 22.9). These predictions provide the clinicians with an idea of the feasibility and likely success of different treatment plans. The computerized prediction can be shown to the patient to give them a better understanding of the likely possible outcome, but it must be made clear that this is simply a prediction and not a guarantee of the final outcome.

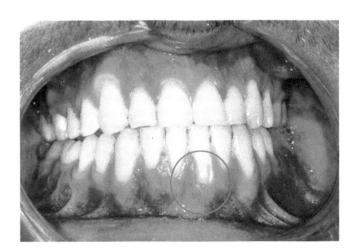

Fig. 22.8 Periodontal problems associated with proclination of the lower incisors during decompensation in a Class III skeletal case.
© The Cleft Lip and Palate Association, 2012.

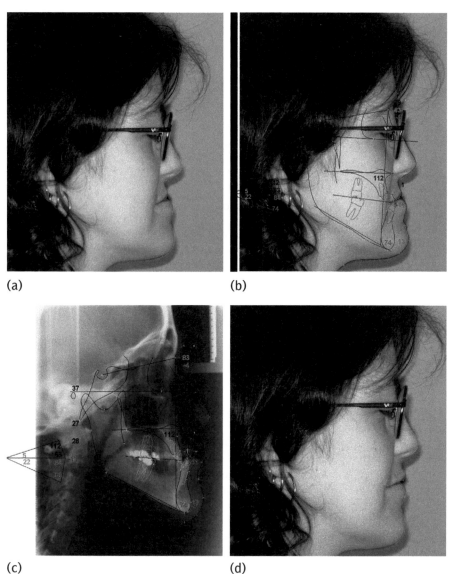

(a)

(b)

(c)

(d)

Fig. 22.9 Computer predictions. This figure demonstrates the use of Dolphin Imaging® software to predict the facial appearance of the proposed plan for the patient shown in Fig. 22.1. The proposed plan is a Le Fort I maxillary advancement of 5 mm and mandibular sagittal split setback of 3 mm. The actual result of surgery is shown in Fig. 22.15. (a) Lateral facial photograph before treatment. (b) Analysis superimposed on lateral facial photograph. (c) Analysis superimposed on lateral cephalometric radiograph. (d) Computer prediction of proposed plan.

22.7 Common surgical procedures

Only a brief overview of some of the more popular surgical techniques is included here. Additional information is available in the literature cited in the section on 'Principal sources and further reading'.

As aesthetics are of major importance, where possible an intra-oral approach should be used to avoid unsightly scars. Segmental procedures have an increased morbidity, as damage to the teeth or disruption of the blood supply to a segment is more likely.

22.7.1 Maxillary procedures

Le Fort I

This is the most widely used maxillary technique (Fig. 22.10). The standard approach is a horseshoe incision of the buccal mucosa and underlying bone, which results in the maxilla being pedicled on the palatal soft tissues and blood supply. The maxilla can then be moved upwards (after removal of the intervening bone), downwards (with interpositional bone graft), or forwards. Movement of the maxilla backwards is not feasible in practice.

Le Fort II

This is employed to achieve mid-face advancement. The surgery is more extensive than for a Le Fort I and therefore carries more risks.

Le Fort III

This usually necessitates the raising of a bicoronal flap for access and is commonly used in the management of craniofacial anomalies.

Surgically assisted rapid palatal expansion (SARPE)

Stable correction of the transverse dimension is notoriously difficult. SARPE is an attempt to address the transverse problem, without

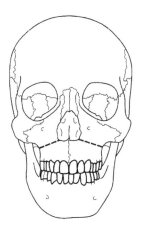

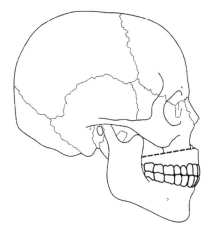

Fig. 22.10 Diagram showing the position of the surgical incisions (broken lines) for a Le Fort I procedure.

resorting to segmental surgery of the maxilla and its inherent risks. It involves the use of corticotomies, and the use of a rapid palatal expander that is used to rapidly widen the upper arch. The advantage of the technique is that it enlarges the maxilla transversely, expanding the upper arch considerably more than can be achieved with orthodontic appliances alone. The disadvantage is that an additional surgical intervention is required.

22.7.2 Mandibular procedures

Ramus procedures

The most commonly used ramus techniques are the following:

- Sagittal split osteotomy (Fig. 22.11). This procedure can be used to advance or push back the mandible or to correct mild asymmetry. The bony cut extends obliquely from above the lingula, across the retromolar region, and vertically down the buccal plate to the lower border. The main complication is damage to the inferior alveolar nerve.
- Vertical subsigmoid osteotomy. This is used for mandibular prognathism and involves a bone cut from the sigmoid notch to the lower border. This can be performed intra-orally using special instruments or extra-orally using standard instruments at the expense of a scar.

- Body osteotomy. This operation is useful if there is a natural gap in the lower arch anterior to the mental foramen in a patient with mandibular prognathism. It is rarely used.

Genioplasty

The tip of the chin can be moved in almost any direction, limited by sliding bony contact and the muscle pedicle. This technique may be used to supplement mandibular ramus surgery where there is a localized abnormality of the chin area in addition to the general mandibular position. It can also be usefully employed as an isolated operation, where it is used as a masking procedure, thus avoiding more complex treatment (e.g. mild mandibular asymmetry).

22.7.3 Bimaxillary surgery

Many patients require surgery to both jaws to correct the underlying skeletal discrepancy (see clinical case illustrated in Figs 22.1, 22.9, 22.12, and 22.15).

22.7.4 Distraction osteogenesis

This is a technique that involves osteotomy cuts followed by a slow mechanical separation of the bone fragments with an expandable device.

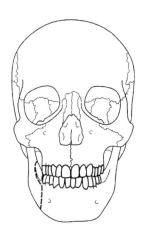

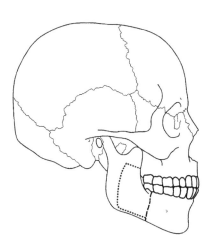

Fig. 22.11 Diagram to show the position of the surgical incisions (broken and dotted lines) for a sagittal split osteotomy.

It is a technique that was originally developed for lengthening limbs. It offers exciting potential for larger movements than can be achieved with traditional orthognathic surgery, and has been found to be useful in the treatment of patients with severe jaw deficiencies, particularly those associated with craniofacial syndromes.

After the bone cuts, there is a latent period of 4–5 days allowing a soft bony callus to form, before the bones are separated gradually by the mechanical device. The mechanism is turned each day and the tension leads to the production of new bone, while allowing time for the soft tissues to adapt. The technique avoids the problems of harvesting and maintaining a viable bone graft, and in addition the adaptation of the soft tissues allows larger movements than with traditional approaches.

Initially external fixators were used, but there are now an increasing number of intra-oral devices available, which reduce the risk of extra-oral scarring. The potential problems of the devices—discomfort, difficulty achieving the correct vector of force, and the need for good patient compliance—have meant that this technique has not been seen as a replacement for conventional osteotomies in routine cases. However, cases that were previously thought to be beyond the scope of orthognathic treatment (principally due to soft tissue restrictions) can now be treated.

22.8 Sequence of treatment

22.8.1 Extractions

Extractions may be required to relieve crowding, level arches, and allow correction of the inclination of the incisors (decompensation). In addition, the surgeon may wish to extract unerupted third molars before the start of treatment, in case they interfere with the future osteotomy site. This is particularly true for mandibular ramus surgery.

22.8.2 Pre-surgical orthodontics

There are four aims of pre-surgical orthodontics:

- Alignment and levelling
- Coordination (ensuring arches will be compatible with each other after surgery)
- Decompensation
- Creation of space for osteotomy cuts if segmental surgery is required.

The pre-surgical orthodontics is undertaken with fixed appliances to allow the correct anteroposterior and vertical positioning of the incisors. The fixed appliances also act as a method of intraoperative intermaxillary fixation and a means of attaching the intermaxillary elastics used postoperatively.

Although levelling of the arches is typically undertaken before surgery, there are two exceptions to this:

- In cases of anterior open bite, attempts to level the arch before surgery will lead to extrusion of the upper incisors, which is unstable. In cases where there is a 'step' in the occlusion, the anterior and posterior segments are aligned in separate segments. Space is made between these segments and the arch is levelled by aligning the segments surgically.
- In Class II cases presenting with deep overbite and a reduced face height, the lower arch is not levelled before surgery. When the mandible is advanced, the lower incisor position ensures the lower face height is increased. This approach is called a 'three-point landing' because immediately after surgery the only tooth contact is between the incisors and the posterior molars. The arch is levelled after surgery by extruding the premolar teeth.

Decompensation is undertaken to correct the angulations of the incisors. There is a tendency for the decompensation during pre-surgical orthodontics to make the patient look worse, as the full extent of the skeletal discrepancy becomes clear (Fig. 22.12). The patient should be warned about this before treatment begins and reassured that this is just temporary until the surgery is completed.

Traditionally, the majority of orthodontic treatment is undertaken before surgery, producing aligned, levelled, coordinated, and decompensated arches. The advantage of this approach is that it offers a more predictable surgical phase and more accurate planning immediately prior to surgery. An alternative view, sometimes referred to as 'Surgery First', is that minimal orthodontics should be undertaken before surgery, as the soft tissue environment may be more conducive to some orthodontic movements once the skeletal pattern is corrected and also total treatment time may be reduced.

22.8.3 Preparing for surgery

Pre-surgical orthodontics takes about 12–18 months, depending on the complexity of the case. At the end of this stage, a new set of records are taken to check the pre-surgical movements have been achieved and to modify or confirm the surgical plan. Rigid stainless steel archwires are placed. Intermaxillary fixation is required during surgery, so hooks are usually added to the archwire (Fig. 22.13) or brackets. Alternatively, the orthodontist can use brackets that incorporate a hook on every tooth from the start.

Study models are produced which can be used for model surgery to mimic the surgical plan. Model surgery is undertaken to verify that the planned surgical moves are appropriate, and to allow construction of intermaxillary wafers. These acrylic wafers are used during surgery to help the surgeon position the jaws correctly. A face-bow recording is required to mount the models on a semi-adjustable articulator, for single jaw maxillary procedures and bimaxillary procedures (Fig. 22.14). If the condyles are to be separated from the dentition by mandibular surgery alone, then the semi-adjustable articulator (and therefore face-bow recording) is not required.

22.8.4 Surgery

This is an in-patient procedure usually involving a stay of 1–3 days in hospital, depending on the complexity of the surgery. In the past, patients were placed in intermaxillary wires to fix the bony segments in place during healing. This meant the patient's upper and lower arches were tied together for 6 weeks. This is now rarely required due to the introduction of small bone plates that are used to fix the bony segments semi-rigidly in

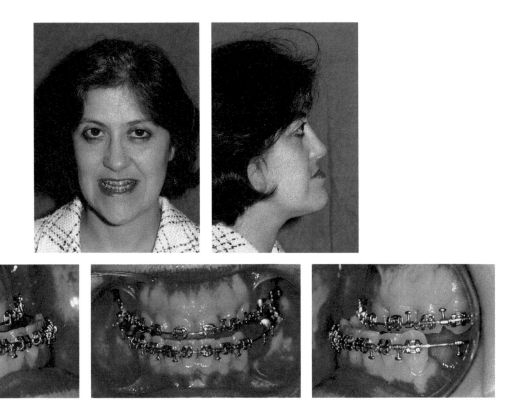

Fig. 22.12 End of pre-surgical orthodontics. Patient IE (from Fig. 22.1) has now been decompensated for surgery. Note the upright lower incisors and the associated worsening of the facial aesthetics due to the protruding lower lip. The patient was warned about this temporary worsening of the profile before surgery.

the maxilla and the use of plates and/or screws in the mandible. This has significantly reduced the morbidity postoperatively, with a reduced risk to the airway, early mobilization of the jaws, earlier return to a good palatable diet, and easier oral hygiene. As a result, the procedure is much better tolerated by patients and also has resulted in better final bone stability.

The surgery carries a number of risks, the exact nature of these risks depend on the procedure undertaken. These risks should be explained by the surgeon before any treatment is started as part of the consent process (see Box 22.1).

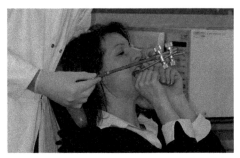

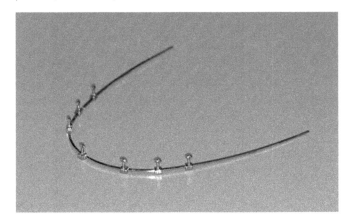

Fig. 22.13 Crimpable hooks added to the archwire. These can be used for intermaxillary fixation during surgery and for attachment of intermaxillary elastics postoperatively.

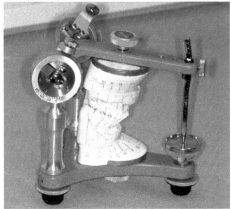

Fig. 22.14 Model surgery. A face-bow recording is taken and the models mounted on a semi-adjustable articulator.

Box 22.1 Possible risks of orthognathic surgery

These depend on the type and extent of the surgery. The patient needs to be made aware of these surgical risks before treatment begins as part of the consent process.

Expected surgical risk

- Swelling
- Bleeding
- Limited mouth opening
- Dietary changes and associated weight loss in the short term
- Time off work and recovery
- Changes in facial appearance
- Changes in nerve sensation.

Possible surgical risks

- Permanent nerve damage to inferior dental nerve

- Need for reoperation
- Infection
- Need to remove plates
- Temporomandibular joint problems
- Relapse
- Problems swallowing
- Bleeding requiring further intervention
- Tooth avulsion or other damage to periodontal support
- Ophthalmic complications
- Reduction in auditory capacity.

Risks of anaesthetic

- The risks associated with a general anaesthetic need to be discussed.

Adapted from *Journal of Orthodontics*, 38, 2, Ryan F., Shute J., Cedro M. et al., A new style of orthognathic clinic, pp.234–33. Copyright (2011) with permission from Taylor & Francis.

22.8.5 Post-surgical orthodontics

Immediately after surgery, intermaxillary traction is usually employed to guide the arches into the desired position. The aims of post-surgical orthodontics are:

- to complete any movements not undertaken prior to surgery (e.g. correction of posterior crossbite and levelling by extrusion of premolars)

- root paralleling at any segmental osteotomy sites
- detailing and settling.

Within a few weeks, lighter, round stainless steel wires are often used in conjunction with the intermaxillary elastics to aid settling. Final detailing can then be undertaken to produce a well-interdigitated occlusion (Fig. 22.15). Post-surgical orthodontics typically takes 3–9 months.

22.9 Retention and relapse

Orthodontic retainers are used to retain the teeth in the correct position at the end of treatment, along similar lines as for conventional fixed appliance therapy (see Chapter 16). However, in addition to the usual relapse factors, there are additional aetiological factors of relapse in combined orthodontic and orthognathic surgery.

22.9.1 Surgical factors

- Poor planning.
- The size of the movement required. Movement of the maxilla by more than 5–6 mm in any direction is more susceptible to relapse, as is movement of the mandible by more than 8 mm.
- Direction of movement required (see Box 22.2).
- Distraction or 'torqueing' of the condylar heads in the glenoid fossa during surgery.
- Inadequate fixation.

22.9.2 Orthodontic factors

- Poor planning.

- Movement of the teeth into zones of soft tissue pressure will lead to relapse when appliances are removed. Treatment should therefore be planned to ensure that the teeth will be in a zone of soft tissue balance postoperatively and that the lips will be competent.
- Extrusion of the teeth during alignment tends to relapse post treatment, particularly in cases of anterior open bite.

22.9.3 Patient factors

- The nature of the problem; for example, anterior open bites associated with abnormal soft tissue behaviour, are notoriously difficult to treat successfully, and have a marked potential to relapse. Patients should be warned of this prior to treatment.
- In patients with cleft lip and palate, advancement of the maxilla is difficult and prone to relapse because of the scar tissue of the primary repair.
- Failure to comply with treatment; for example, patient does not wear intermaxillary elastic traction as instructed.

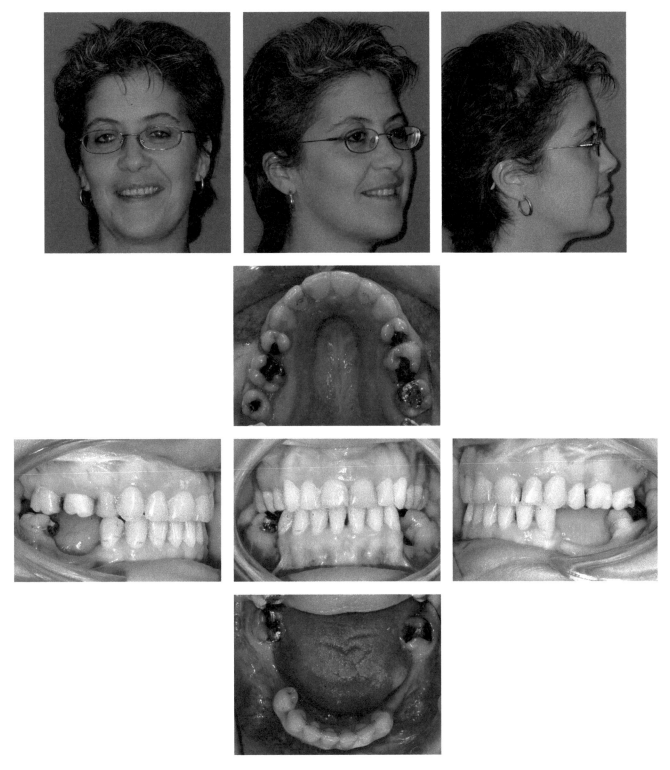

Fig. 22.15 End of treatment following orthodontics and bimaxillary osteotomy. This shows the end-of-treatment photographs for patient IE shown in Figs 22.1, 22.9, and 22.12.

Box 22.2 Stability of orthognathic surgery

(Most stable at the top, gradually moving down to the least stable at the bottom of the list.)

Very stable

- Maxillary impaction
- Mandibular advancement
- Genioplasty (any direction).

Stable

- Maxillary advancement
- Correction of maxillary asymmetry.

Stable (with rigid fixation)

- Maxillary impaction with mandibular advancement
- Maxillary advancement with mandibular setback
- Correction of mandibular asymmetry.

Problems with stability

- Mandibular setback
- Movement of maxilla downwards
- Surgical expansion of maxilla.

Source data from *Head & Face Medicine*, 3, 21, 2007, Proffit W. R., Turvey T. A., and Phillips C., The hierarchy of stability and predictability in orthognathic surgery with rigid fixation: an update and extension.

22.10 3D developments in orthognathic surgery: planning, simulation, and guided surgery

The conventional methods used to plan orthognathic surgery described in this chapter rely on lateral radiographic images (often combined with lateral facial views), and occasionally posteroanterior radiographs in cases of asymmetry. These radiographs only provide a two-dimensional (2D) presentation of the dentition and facial skeleton. Model surgery allows some appreciation of the dentition and occlusion in 3D, but not the maxilla and mandible.

The traditional approach provides only a limited understanding of the complex 3D structures of the dentofacial skeleton. It is only at the time of surgery that the surgeon has a better understanding of the contours, thickness, and quality of bone, and is able to gain a more detailed appreciation of the position of key anatomical structures, such as the inferior dental nerve. Osteotomy cuts, alignment of the segments, and fixation are effectively undertaken in a freehand manner, and are reliant on the skill and experience of the surgeon. The anatomy of the region is complex and slightly different in every patient, and the surgeon is often working in a field with restricted visibility.

22.10.1 Use of cone beam computed tomography technology and implications for orthognathic surgery

CBCT now allows the acquisition of detailed 3D images of the face in high resolution. Using this 'virtual' 3D information, software is being used which has the potential to revolutionize the way that orthognathic planning and surgery is undertaken. In dentistry we are familiar with the use of CAD/CAM (computer-aided design/computer-aided manufacture) for the manufacture of complex 3D restorations. Computer-aided surgery (CAS) is now being introduced that will allow surgical planning

and simulation using the information captured from CBCT, as well as intraoperative guidance.

This technology offers a number of potential exciting possibilities:

- A more detailed appreciation of the anatomy of the patient in 3D (Fig. 22.16a).

- The data from CBCT can be combined with the data captured from 3D facial camera systems. This allows the clinicians to see the relationship of the soft tissues with the underlying hard tissues. Virtual surgery can then be undertaken on this 3D model and the effect on the overlying soft tissues assessed. The accuracy of these 3D predictions will improve as we gather more data on the 3D effects on soft tissues of combined orthodontics and orthognathic surgical treatment.

- Fig. 22.16b, c shows virtual surgery that allows the surgeon to calculate the most appropriate and safest osteotomy lines in advance of the operation (Fig. 22.16d, e).

- Once the team is happy with the final virtual surgery, this virtual setup can be used to manufacture positioning splints (Fig. 22.16f, g). It can also be used to construct customized fixation plates, as well as customized cutting guides to ensure the surgeon makes the cuts in the same position as the virtual plan.

- The developments described so far have been based on the surgery being planned and executed virtually. However, the surgeon, not the computer, will perform the actual surgery, so the next challenge is to ensure the surgeon follows the virtual plan. While current surgical splints are successful in positioning the maxilla and mandible correctly in relation to each other, there is potential for more inaccuracies when positioning the jaws in relation to the rest of the face,

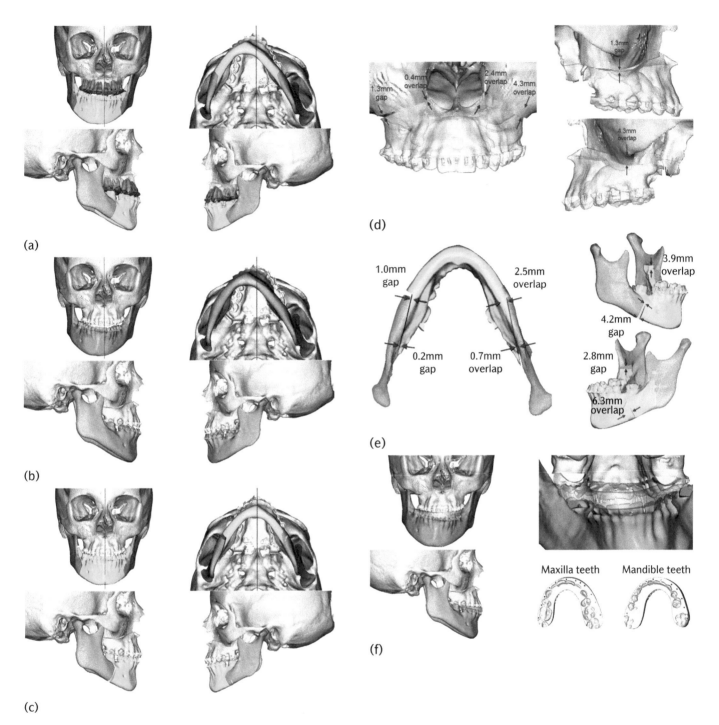

Fig. 22.16 3D planning of an asymmetry case, treated using a combination of orthodontics and orthognathic surgery. The case was treated by Nicholas Lee (maxillofacial surgeon) and Friedy Luther (orthodontist), Sheffield Teaching Hospitals, UK). (a) Preoperative scan of a patient showing asymmetry. Note the mandible is asymmetric to the right and there is a cant of the maxilla (the left side of the maxilla is more inferior than the right side). The patient is planned for bimaxillary surgery (maxillary Le Fort I osteotomy and mandibular bilateral sagittal split osteotomy). (b) Surgical plan (intermediate position) after correction of the maxilla. (c) Surgical plan showing final position (after second stage of mandibular surgery). (d) Overview of surgical movements of maxilla. This shows the amount of bone that needs to be removed on the left side to allow more impaction of the left side of the maxilla, and the slight inferior movement of the right side of the maxilla. (e) Overview of surgical movements of mandible. This shows the amount of bone that needs to be removed on the left side to allow distal movement on the left side of the proximal mandibular segment, and the slight advancement needed on the right side. This helps the surgeon to virtually visualize the movements that are required to correct the asymmetry in 3D, in advance of the surgery. Customized fixation plates (not shown here) could also be produced using these scans. (f) Virtual intermediate splint is produced to correctly position the maxilla after the Le Fort I osteotomy. The holes in the splint are used to wire the splint to the fixed appliance during the operation. A 3D printer is used to produce the splints from these virtual scans.

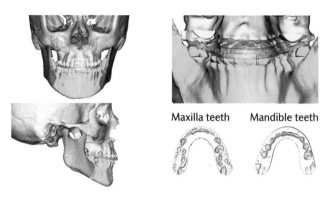

Maxilla teeth   Mandible teeth

(g)

Fig. 22.16 (g) Virtual final splint. This is used to position the mandible, after the maxilla has been fixed in its final position.

particularly in the vertical plane. Surgical navigation systems are being developed to help transfer the information from the virtual plan into the operating room. They use tracking devices to follow surgical instruments and the mobilized fragment of bone. Use of a navigation screen will help to guide the surgeon in making the appropriate cuts and ensure correct positioning and fixation of the bone segments.

Developments in 3D technology are beginning to change our approach to combined orthodontic and orthognathic treatment in terms of diagnosis, treatment planning, and execution of the surgery, and in the future will improve our assessments of outcomes and stability.

Key points

- Orthognathic surgery is aimed at correcting dentofacial deformity.

- It is indicated for patients that have a severe skeletal or very severe dento-alveolar problem that is beyond the scope of orthodontics alone.

- Planning and treatment should be undertaken by an interdisciplinary team.

- The typical sequence of treatment is extractions, a phase of pre-surgical orthodontics, the surgery, and then a shorter phase of post-surgical orthodontics.

- The aims of pre-surgical orthodontics are alignment and levelling, coordination of the arches, decompensation, and creation of space for osteotomy cuts if segmental surgery is used.

- Fixed appliances are used to fulfil the pre-surgical aims, provide a method of intermaxillary fixation during surgery, and offer a means of attaching intermaxillary elastics postoperatively.

- Post-surgical orthodontics aims to correct any movements not undertaken at surgery, root paralleling at any segmental osteotomy sites, and detailing and settling.

- Developments in 3D technology are changing our approach to combined orthodontic and orthognathic treatment in terms of diagnosis, treatment plan, execution of the surgery, as well as assessment of the outcomes.

Principal sources and further reading

Arnett, G. W. and McLaughlin R. P. (2004). *Facial and Dental Planning for Orthodontists and Oral Surgeons*. Edinburgh: Mosby.
This practical textbook provides information on how to position the jaws and dentition to optimize the facial aesthetics.

Cevidanes, L. H. S., Boen, B., Paniagua, P., Styner, M., and Nguyen, T. (2017). Orthodontic and orthognathic surgery planning using CBCT. In: Naini, F. B. and Gill, D. S. (eds) *Orthognathic Surgery: Principles, Planning and Practice*, pp. 221–34. Chichester: John Wiley & Sons, Ltd.
This chapter provides an overview of the use of CBCT for orthognathic surgery planning and virtual simulation.

Cunningham, S. J. and Feinmann, C. (1998). Psychological assessment of patients requiring orthognathic surgery and the relevance of body dysmorphic disorder. *British Journal of Orthodontics*, **25**, 293–8. [DOI: 10.1093/ortho/25.4.293] [PubMed: 9884781]
An article alerting the clinician to the condition body dysmorphic disorder.

Hunt, N. P. and Rudge, S. J. (1984). Facial profile and orthognathic surgery. *British Journal of Orthodontics*, **11**, 126–36. [DOI: 10.1179/bjo.11.3.126] [PubMed: 6591951]
A detailed account of assessment of a patient for orthognathic surgery.

Naini, F. B. (2011). *Facial Aesthetics: Concepts and Clinical Diagnosis*. Oxford: Wiley-Blackwell.
This textbook provides a beautifully illustrated overview of facial aesthetics.

Proffit, W. R., Turvey, T. A., and Phillips, C. (2007). The hierarchy of stability and predictability in orthognathic surgery with rigid fixation: an update and extension. *Head & Face Medicine*, **3**, 21. [DOI: 10.1186/1746-160X-3-21] [PubMed: 17470277]
  The stability of various types of orthognath\ic procedures is described.

Proffit, W. R., White, R. P., and Sarver, D. M. (2003). *Contemporary Treatment of Dentofacial Deformity*. St. Louis, MO: Mosby.

This textbook is highly recommended for readers wanting more information on this subject. It is a comprehensive and well-written account of the treatment of dentofacial deformity.

Ryan, F., Shute, J., Cedro, M., Singh, J., Lee, E., Lee, S., et al. (2011). A new style of orthognathic clinic. *Journal of Orthodontics*, **38**, 124–33. [DOI: 10.1179/14653121141353] [PubMed: 21677104]
An innovative approach to the orthognathic clinic, aiming to provide key information to patients deciding on whether or not to proceed with treatment.

 References for this chapter can also be found at: **www.oup.com/uk/orthodontics5e**. Where possible, these are presented as active links which direct you to the electronic version of the work, to help facilitate onward study. If you are a subscriber to that work (either individually or through an institution), and depending on your level of access, you may be able to peruse an abstract or the full article if available.

23.1 Definition

Hypodontia is the developmental absence or one or more primary or secondary teeth, excluding the third molars. Hypodontia is classified based on severity:

- **Mild hypodontia:** one or two missing teeth (Fig. 23.1).
- **Moderate hypodontia:** three to six missing teeth (Fig. 23.2).

- **Severe hypodontia/oligodontia:** more than six missing teeth (Fig. 23.3).
- **Anodontia:** complete absence of teeth in one or both dentitions.

More than 80% of people affected have mild hypodontia, 10% or less have moderate hypodontia, and less than 1% have severe hypodontia.

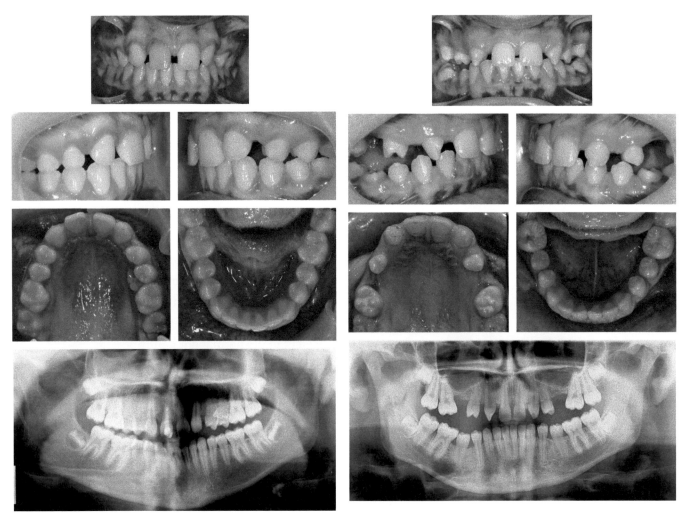

Fig. 23.1 Mild hypodontia: a 13-year-old female with developmentally absent maxillary lateral incisors. The malocclusion was complicated by previous trauma to the maxillary right central incisor requiring endodontic treatment.

Fig. 23.2 Moderate hypodontia: a 13-year-old female with hypodontia affecting the maxillary lateral incisors and second premolars.

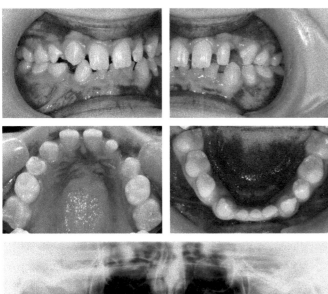

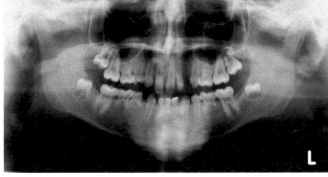

Fig. 23.3 Severe hypodontia: a 12-year-old female with developmental absence of UL4,5; UR 2,5; LL1,2,5; and LR1,2,4,5.

23.1.1 Prevalence

The prevalence of hypodontia in the primary dentition is estimated to be 0.1–0.9% with the primary lateral incisors being the most commonly missing teeth. The absence of a primary tooth increases the likelihood of hypodontia in the permanent dentition.

In the permanent dentition, the prevalence of hypodontia is approximately 3.5–6.5%. Excluding third molars, the most commonly missing teeth in Caucasians are mandibular second premolars and maxillary lateral incisors (Table 23.1). Hypodontia has a female predilection of approximately 3:2 and racial variation. The cause for unequal distribution between the sexes is still unknown.

Table 23.1 Frequency of missing teeth in Caucasians

Third molars (not considered to be hypodontia)	25–35%
Mandibular second premolars	3%
Maxillary lateral incisors	2%
Maxillary second premolars	1.5%
Mandibular incisors	0.5%
Maxillary canines, first premolars, mandibular second molars	0.1%
Maxillary central incisors, mandibular canines, first permanent molars	<0.1%

23.2 Aetiology

Hypodontia may be an isolated trait, known as non-syndromic or familial hypodontia. Non-syndromic hypodontia is thought to have a multifactorial aetiology arising from a complex interaction between genetic and environmental factors. Syndromic hypodontia is the term given to hypodontia that occurs with accompanying genetic disorders.

Hypodontia is more common in people with a cleft lip and/or palate, with prevalence estimated by some studies to be as high as 75%. Commonly hypodontia affects the cleft site as a result of absent or damaged tooth germs in the bony defect (Fig. 23.4). Interestingly, hypodontia is also higher in those born with cleft lip and/or palate than in the general population in sites unrelated to the cleft.

23.2.1 Non-syndromic hypodontia

Environmental factors

Environmental factors associated with hypodontia include systemic disturbances, local factors such as pathology, physical, and chemical trauma, irradiation, infection, and medical treatment. It is thought that environmental factors cause the threshold for an anomaly to be reached in those with a genetic predisposition.

Genetic factors

Twin and family studies have demonstrated that non-syndromic hypodontia may arise from a sporadic mutation or be inherited through dominant, recessive, or X-linked patterns with variable expressivity and dominance. Hypodontia is genetically and phenotypically heterogeneous and it is hypothesized that different genes and expression of these genes causes certain presentations of agenesis. Three key genes have been identified in non-syndromic hypodontia; muscle segment homeobox 1 (*MSX1*), paired box gene 9 (*PAX9*), and axis inhibition protein 2 (*AXIN2*). These are regulatory genes in the morphogenesis stages of tooth development and mutations have been linked to different phenotypes. Mutations in the *MSX1* gene are predominantly linked to familial oligodontia and premolar agenesis, those in the *PAX9* gene to molar agenesis, while mutations in *AXIN2* involve a wide range of teeth. It has been suggested that the combined, overlapping expression domains of genes within the tooth-forming regions is key for normal development of the dentition and this explains the vulnerability of teeth in certain regions (lateral incisor, second premolar, and third molar) to hypodontia.

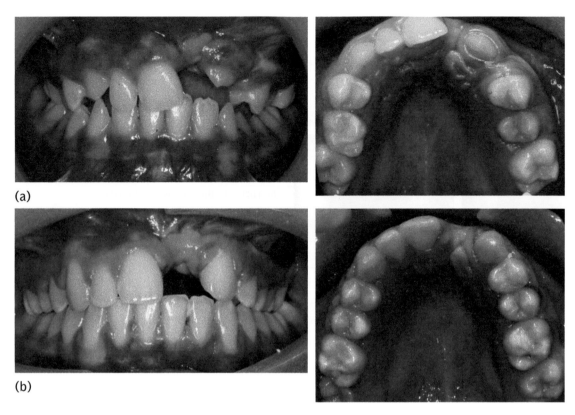

Fig. 23.4 Hypodontia associated with a unilateral left-sided cleft lip and palate in a 13-year-old female. (a) Pre-treatment: the maxillary left central and lateral incisors were absent and the canine was partially erupted. (b) Treatment aimed to align the teeth, correct the centreline, and reduce the agenesis site to a single tooth size. The left canine was moved into the lateral incisor position and the patient is awaiting canine camouflage and placement of a resin-bonded bridge.

23.2.2 Syndromic hypodontia

According to the Online Mendelian Inheritance in Man (OMIM) compendium of human genes and genetic disorders, hypodontia and oligodontia are associated with over 100 and 70 syndromes respectively. Some of the most common syndromes that feature hypodontia are listed in Box 23.1. Syndromes occur as a result of a number of different gene mutations. As well as non-syndromic hypodontia, *MSX1* mutations have been associated with some cleft lip and palate syndromes and Wiktop syndrome.

The associated features of syndromes can be highly variable and this can influence the approach to the management of hypodontia. Complex medical conditions may affect the suitability of patients for certain treatments and medical treatment for other problems may reduce the amount of dental care people are able or willing to accept.

Box 23.1 Syndromes associated with hypodontia—the OMIM catalogue number is given for further reference

- Cleft lip and palate syndromes, e.g. ectrodactyly, ectodermal dysplasia, and cleft lip/palate syndrome 1
- Ectodermal dysplasias
- Oral–facial–digital syndromes
- Incontinentia pigmenti (OMIM 308300)
- Down syndrome (OMIM 190685)
- Wiktop syndrome (OMIM 189500)
- Van de Woude syndrome (OMIM 119300)
- Ehlers–Danlos syndrome (OMIM 225410).

23.3 Features of hypodontia

23.3.1 Clinical presentation

Absence of teeth usually causes spacing in the dental arches unless the hypodontia is mild and there is notable tooth-arch size discrepancy (crowding) or primary teeth are retained. Retained primary teeth may appear smaller than the surrounding permanent teeth due to their naturally smaller size or as a consequence of tooth surface loss.

Hypodontia can be associated with a number of other dental anomalies, suggesting a common genetic origin (Box 23.2). The combination

Box 23.2 Dental anomalies commonly associated with hypodontia

- Hypoplastic enamel
- Ectopic maxillary canine tooth position
- Microdontia—localized or generalized, may affect crown or root
- Molar taurodontism
- Conical crown shape, such as peg-shaped lateral incisors

- Transposition, particularly between the maxillary canine and first premolar
- Supernumerary teeth
- Infra-occlusion of retained primary teeth
- Delayed eruption of teeth.

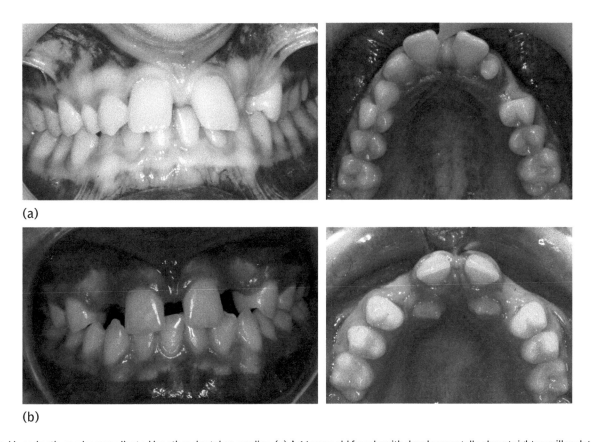

(a)

(b)

Fig. 23.5 Hypodontia can be complicated by other dental anomalies. (a) A 14-year-old female with developmentally absent right maxillary lateral incisor. The left lateral incisor is microdont, the left maxillary canine is ectopic, and the right primary canine is retained. (b) A 13-year-old female with bilateral maxillary incisor agenesis associated with bilateral ectopic canines, which have been surgically exposed prior to commencing orthodontic treatment.

of other dental anomalies with hypodontia can accentuate occlusal problems, such as spacing, malpositioned teeth, centreline shift, over-eruption of opposing teeth, and uneven gingival margins (Fig. 23.5). People with hypodontia may have atrophic alveolar ridges or local bone deficit due to underdevelopment of the alveolus in the absence of teeth (Fig. 23.6). Hypodontia is also commonly associated with reduced lower face height and deep overbite (Fig. 23.7).

23.3.2 Diagnosis

The most common indication of hypodontia is abnormalities in the eruption of teeth. Prolonged retention of primary teeth, inconsistencies in eruption timing between contralateral teeth of more than 6 months,

or deviation from the normal eruption sequence should prompt further investigation. Hypodontia may be associated with a generalized delay in dental development, although the extent of delay is variable.

Radiographic examination provides a definitive diagnosis of hypodontia and dental panoramic radiographs should be used to confirm the presence or absence of teeth where indicated by specific clinical signs or symptoms. Screening radiographs are not advised for young patients, as diagnosis of absent teeth radiographically before 10 years old may be erroneous due to late development of the second premolars. The approximate age of tooth development will determine the age at which the absence of a particular tooth can be accurately diagnosed (see Chapter 3, Table 3.1).

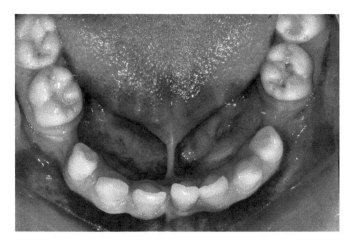

Fig. 23.6 Bone deficit may be associated with hypodontia. In this case, the mandible is narrow buccolingually in the second premolar region where the teeth are developmentally absent.

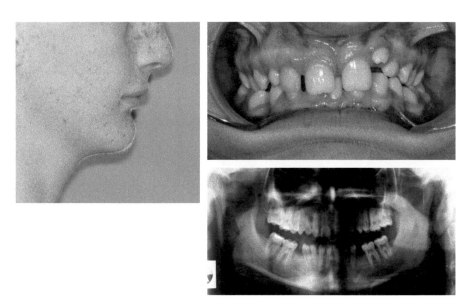

Fig. 23.7 Decreased lower face height and deep overbite are commonly associated with hypodontia.

23.4 Impact of hypodontia

23.4.1 Impact of untreated hypodontia

Hypodontia has been shown to reduce quality of life for those affected due to detrimental effects on appearance, function, and psychosocial well-being. Concerns regarding dental appearance are a key motivator for seeking treatment, with 'gaps' being reported as a source of bullying and anxiety for young people. Hypodontia can cause functional difficulties with eating and speech, such as avoidance of certain foods, difficulty biting hard food, and lisping. Oral health-related quality of life (OHRQoL) scales indicate that hypodontia can affect everyday activities such as brushing, speech, eating, and playing musical instruments.

23.4.2 Impact of hypodontia treatment

The impact of undergoing treatment for hypodontia depends on the type of treatment, service delivery factors, and individual patient factors. Active treatment most commonly starts in early adolescence, around 11–12 years old when the permanent dentition is established, and can continue throughout late childhood and into early adulthood depending on the treatment plan. The length and complexity of dental treatment influences patient experience and research has found that waiting for treatment and/or delays in treatment can be a source of frustration for patients. Burdensome appointments schedules can have an impact in terms of travel time and cost, time off work and school, and childcare for siblings, and treatment may also have temporary effects on appearance, talking, and eating. The potential impact of treatment should be considered during treatment planning and discussed with the patient and family to ensure the most appropriate care is provided.

23.5 Treatment in the primary dentition

Hypodontia in the primary dentition is relatively uncommon and for milder hypodontia often no active intervention is required. Developmental absence of primary teeth increases the index of suspicion for other developmental anomalies and as such, dental development should be carefully monitored. Any concerns about the possibility of an associated syndrome should prompt referral to an appropriate medical practitioner for further investigation. In addition, the dental team has an important role in providing support and advice to the young child and family. Parents may require counselling about the diagnosis of hypodontia and the likelihood of hypodontia in the permanent dentition or in siblings. The long-term management of hypodontia can be burdensome to the patient and family so providing advice about future treatment can allow time for preparation.

In cases of severe hypodontia or anodontia, tooth replacement in the form of removable dentures may be desirable to improve aesthetics and function. Dentures may be difficult to retain in those with poorly developed alveolar ridges and often require regular adjustments. Dentures can cause initial problems with speech, eating, and increased saliva but adaptation is usually good and may help speech development.

23.6 Treatment in the mixed dentition

Hypodontia affecting the permanent dentition may only become apparent during the transition from the primary to permanent dentition. Preventative advice to maintain primary teeth in the optimum condition is a priority to maximize future treatment options. This includes diet analysis, oral hygiene regimens tailored to the patient's needs, fluoride use, and fissure sealants. The risk of other dental anomalies should prompt careful and thorough monitoring of dental development.

Concerns about aesthetics and function may become evident during the mixed dentition, particularly around the time of progression to secondary school when peer influence increases. Any interim treatment provided in the mixed dentition should be minimally invasive and provided with consideration to the long-term treatment plan. The benefits of interim treatment must be judged against any potential risks, such as an ability to maintain oral health and increased treatment burden for the patient and family.

Adhesive, non-invasive restorative dentistry techniques can be used to reduce spacing by enlarging or reshaping small teeth with placement of composite restorations. Missing teeth can be replaced temporarily with an adhesive fixed prosthesis, such as a resin-bonded bridge placed without any prior preparation of the tooth surface. Where there are multiple missing teeth or no suitable abutment teeth, a removable prosthesis may be preferable. Dentures often require regular adaptation during the mixed dentition phase and compliance may be low in patients who are not significantly affected by their missing teeth.

Interceptive orthodontic treatment can aid space redistribution in the mixed dentition phase and improve aesthetics. Consideration must be given to how any orthodontic correction will be maintained until definitive treatment can be provided, as the risk of relapse is often high. In addition, orthodontic movement of primary teeth can cause accelerated root resorption and reduce long-term prognosis, and care must be taken if moving teeth in areas where there are unerupted teeth.

Judicious extraction of primary teeth may promote spontaneous space closure in agenesis sites if undertaken at the ideal time. However, it can be difficult to predict future tooth eruption and likelihood of crowding so it is strongly recommended that advice is sought from an orthodontic specialist prior to undertaking extractions in children with hypodontia. Extraction of the maxillary primary lateral incisors and canines may encourage mesial eruption of the permanent canines into a favourable position to replace developmentally absent lateral incisors. Similarly, a definite diagnosis of missing second premolars in those with some degree of crowding may indicate early extraction of the primary molars to relieve the crowding and promote spontaneous space closure, ideally before second permanent molar eruption around 11 years old.

23.7 Treatment in the permanent dentition

23.7.1 Treatment planning considerations

In most cases, treatment planning for hypodontia should be undertaken within an interdisciplinary team that usually includes paediatric dentists, restorative dentists, and orthodontists. Less commonly, oral surgeons, clinical psychologists, and genetic scientists may also be involved. General dentists often assist with monitoring dental development and provision of routine care and the patient's own dentist should therefore be included in correspondence to ensure continuity of care.

A number of treatment strategies are available for managing hypodontia in the permanent dentition, which may be undertaken alone or in combination:

1. No active treatment.

Table 23.2 Considerations during treatment planning for hypodontia

Patient factors	Concerns—aesthetic, functional Desired outcome in short, medium, and long term Motivation and cooperation with dental treatment Willingness to commit to long-term maintenance Use of fluoride and diet control Other medical considerations Social factors such as home circumstances, ability to attend appointments
Intra-oral features	Severity of hypodontia and position of teeth Dental health status: oral hygiene, dental disease Occlusal factors, e.g. crowding, inter-arch relationship Dental aesthetics Bone quality for implant placement
Extra-oral features	Skeletal pattern in three planes: anteroposterior, vertical, transverse Soft tissues: lip support, smile line Smile aesthetics
Availability of dental care	Access to services Cost of treatment

2. Management of retained primary teeth—maintenance or extraction.

3. Restorative camouflage to alter the shape, size, or colour of existing primary or permanent teeth.

4. Orthodontic treatment to change the position of teeth.

5. Tooth replacement.

A successful treatment outcome will depend on whether the patient's concerns and expectations have been addressed. Alongside patient factors, the extra-oral and intra-oral features and availability of dental care will influence the choice of treatment (Table 23.2). Treatment decisions should be made jointly between clinicians and the patient and family.

23.7.2 No active treatment

People with hypodontia may decide for a number of reasons that they do not wish to undergo any dental treatment, usually because they feel their dental appearance and function are acceptable and there is little to gain from treatment. Provided the patient and family have been given sufficient information to make this choice and are doing so freely, the choice to decline active treatment should be supported. For people with poor dental health or medical contraindications to dental treatment, the dental team may feel the risks of treatment outweigh any potential benefits and no treatment may be advisable. Where no active dental treatment is planned, the patient should be seen for routine care by his or her own general dentist. This provides an opportunity to reassess patient and family wishes and to monitor dental health status. Understanding around hypodontia and expectations around dental health can change over time and patients may later request a referral to the interdisciplinary team for further discussion of possible treatment options.

23.7.3 Management of primary teeth

Primary teeth may be retained in the mouth for longer than usual in sites where the permanent teeth are missing. Management of the retained primary tooth is a choice between maintaining the tooth or extraction of the tooth to enable spontaneous or active closure of the space. Alternatively, the primary tooth may be removed with no space closure. In this case a decision is made whether to accept the space or consider tooth replacement. The decision for management of primary teeth is influenced by a number of clinical factors, such as the number and location of missing teeth, the health of the primary tooth, the position of the primary tooth relative to other teeth, and other aspects of malocclusion such as spacing, crowding, and the inter-arch relationship (Fig. 23.8).

Infra-occlusion is the process where a tooth fails to maintain its occlusal relationship with adjacent teeth (see Chapter 3, Section 3.3.3).

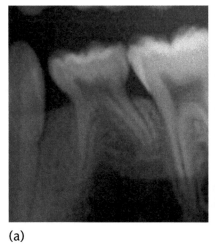
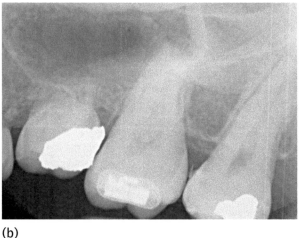

(a)   (b)

Fig. 23.8 The prognosis of the primary teeth is influenced by the coronal health and root length. (a) Mandibular primary second molar with a non-carious crown, minimal tooth surface loss, and good root length. Prognosis of the tooth is favourable. (b) A maxillary primary second molar with a large restoration and extensive root resorption. The prognosis of the tooth is poor.

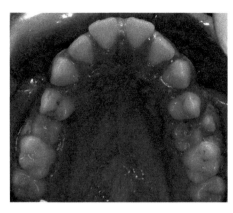
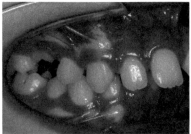

Fig. 23.9 Infra-occlusion of mandibular primary second molars where the right maxillary second premolar is developmentally absent. The severity of the infra-occlusion indicated extraction was necessary to prevent submergence of the tooth below the gingiva.

Infra-occlusion is most commonly seen in hypodontia in relation to primary second molars (Fig. 23.9) and in severe cases, extraction of the infra-occluding tooth may be necessary to prevent a localized vertical bony defect forming.

Primary teeth with good coronal health and adequate root length may be maintained for as long as possible. The teeth act as natural space maintainers and keeping the tooth is advantageous for reducing alveolar bone resorption, preserving soft tissue architecture, and improving appearance and function. Retained primary teeth can significantly reduce the impact of missing teeth and improve oral health-related quality of life. Primary teeth often appear small compared to adjacent permanent teeth so primary teeth may be modified with direct or indirect restorations to improve aesthetics and protect the primary tooth (Fig. 23.10). Onlays can be placed on primary molars to restore occlusal height in cases of tooth surface loss or mild–moderate infra-occlusion to improve function and prevent tipping of adjacent teeth (Fig. 23.11).

Generally primary teeth do not have the expected lifespan of a permanent tooth and long-term survival of primary teeth depends on the extent and rate of root resorption, dental pathology such as caries, non-carious tooth surface loss and periodontal disease, and infra-occlusion secondary to ankylosis. Primary second molars have been shown to have a good long-term prognosis if they are present at 20 years old, while primary canines usually have a shorter lifespan. Restoring primary teeth may reduce the long-term survival due to a less favourable crown–root ratio and increased occlusal loading.

Where primary teeth are to be retained for as long as possible, a long-term plan should be agreed to manage the eventual tooth loss. This usually involves a treatment plan that positions adjacent teeth in a favourable position to facilitate tooth replacement when the primary tooth is lost. Primary canine teeth are considerably smaller than the successor and space may need to be created around the primary tooth to facilitate implant placement or a better-proportioned prosthetic replacement in the future. On the other hand, primary second molar crowns are larger than the ideal size of a subsequent premolar tooth replacement and it may be desirable to reduce the mesiodistal width of the primary molar to allow orthodontic space closure to premolar size. The scope for crown reduction depends

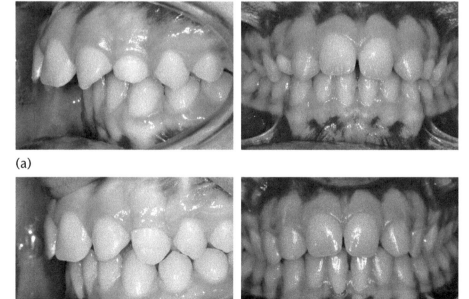

(a)

(b)

Fig. 23.10 A 14-year-old female, who presented with missing maxillary lateral incisors. (a) The patient was unhappy with the shape of her primary and permanent maxillary canines. (b) During the functional appliance phase, the permanent canine cusps were incrementally reduced and temporary restorations were placed on the primary canines.

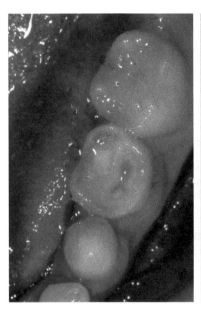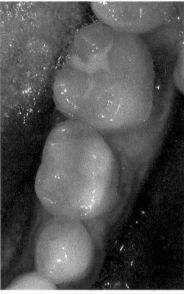

Fig. 23.11 Restoration of primary second molar where the permanent successor is absent. A direct composite onlay was used to restore occlusal height following non-carious tooth surface loss and mild infra-occlusion.

on the divergence of the primary molar roots and the thickness of interproximal enamel (Fig. 23.12).

23.7.4 Orthodontic treatment

Orthodontic treatment for hypodontia aims to adjust tooth position to either eliminate the spaces where teeth are missing or optimize the spaces for tooth replacement. Treatment planning of the final tooth position depends on the severity and presentation of hypodontia, extraoral features, dental health and suitability for orthodontic treatment, and other aspects of the malocclusion.

Maxillary lateral incisor agenesis

In cases with maxillary lateral incisor agenesis, a decision is made whether to open the space for tooth replacement (Fig. 23.13) or close

the space and accept the canine in the lateral incisor position and the first premolar as a substitute for the canine (Fig. 23.14). A number of clinical factors should be considered (Table 23.3). Space closure may be preferable for those wishing to minimize the long-term commitment to dental treatment and there is some evidence that periodontal health is better in cases where tooth replacement is avoided. In cases where both space opening or space closure are possible, a mock-up of the treatment options, known as a Kesling's set-up, can be used to aid visualization for the patient (see Fig. 23.15).

Canine teeth can be challenging to camouflage as lateral incisors due to the increased buccolingual, mesiodistal, and gingival–apical proportions, the higher gingival contour, prominent canine eminence, and darker coronal colour. These issues can be managed to some extent with adjustment of the canine position and enamel recontouring during orthodontic treatment and/or single tooth whitening and restorative camouflage following orthodontic treatment.

Mandibular second premolar agenesis

In mild hypodontia where premolars are absent, similar decisions are required regarding orthodontic space closure or space optimization for tooth replacement. Space closure may be challenging, particularly for larger spaces resulting from late loss of a primary second molar. Successful space closure of posterior spaces of 8–11 mm has been

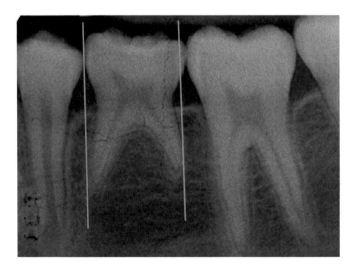

Fig. 23.12 Interproximal reduction of retained primary second molars enables some orthodontic space closure to optimize the space for premolar-sized tooth replacement in the future. However, divergent roots may limit the scope for space closure.

Table 23.3 Management of missing maxillary lateral incisors

Space opening	Space closure
Class III skeletal pattern	Class II skeletal pattern
No crowding or spacing in arch	Crowding
Class I buccal segment	Class II buccal segment
Unfavourable canine colour and morphology	Favourable canine colour and morphology
Hypodontia or teeth of poor prognosis in the same quadrant	Patient does not want prosthesis

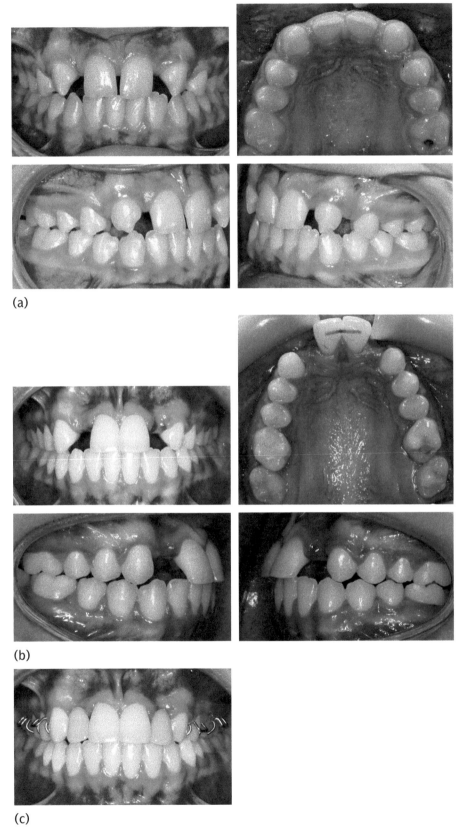

(a)

(b)

(c)

Fig. 23.13 Orthodontic space opening in bilateral maxillary incisor agenesis. (a) A 14-year-old female with bilateral maxillary lateral incisor agenesis. (b) The maxillary canine teeth were retracted into the correct position using fixed appliances, creating space for tooth replacement in the lateral incisor position. (c) A Hawley retainer with artificial teeth in the lateral incisor spaces. Treatment was provided by Gavin Bell.

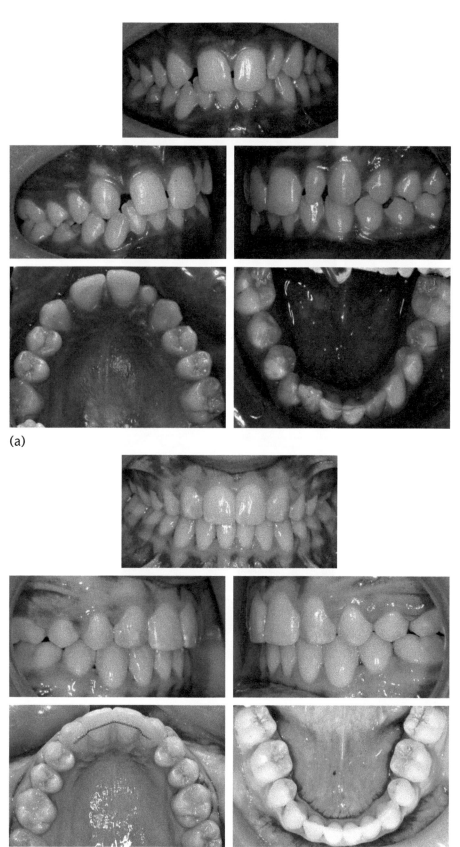

(a)

(b)

Fig. 23.14 Orthodontic space closure. (a) A 14-year-old female with a developmentally absent right maxillary incisor and a microdont left maxillary incisor. (b) Treatment involved extraction of the microdont incisor and orthodontic space closure with canine substitution into the lateral incisor spaces. The canines were reshaped throughout orthodontic treatment. Lower arch extractions were indicated to relieve crowding and maintain the incisor relationship. Treatment was provided by Zynab Jawad.

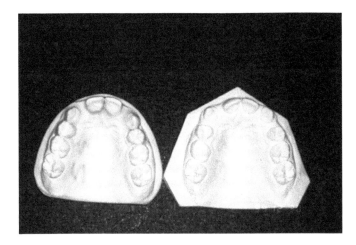

Fig. 23.15 Trial (Kesling's) set-up can be used to help the patient visualize the treatment options where more than one treatment option is feasible.

demonstrated without detrimental effects to the occlusion but often additional anchorage is required to encourage molar protraction and reduce the risk of over-retraction of the anterior teeth. The aesthetic impact of missing posterior teeth is lower than anterior teeth and patients may opt to accept a posterior space rather than undergo tooth replacement or extensive orthodontic treatment to close the space.

Mandibular incisor agenesis

The management of mandibular incisor agenesis will be guided by the incisor relationship and the number of missing teeth (Fig. 23.16). In cases where the overbite and overjet are reduced and there is a Class III incisor tendency, space closure may improve the incisor relationship. On the other hand, where the overbite and overjet are increased, space closure in the lower labial segment is likely to worsen the incisor relationship and should generally be avoided. If two incisor spaces are to be created for tooth replacement, it is generally preferable to locate the spaces in the lateral incisor position, as the adjacent lower canine teeth are ideal abutment teeth to support pontics.

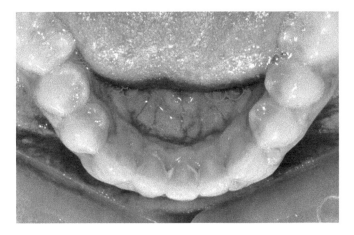

Fig. 23.16 Orthodontic space closure for a single missing lower incisor.

Unilateral hypodontia

Unilateral tooth agenesis poses specific challenges for orthodontic treatment, particularly maintaining symmetry between the teeth and ensuring centrelines are coincident to the face. Management of unilateral maxillary lateral incisor agenesis depends on the factors previously listed but in addition, the ability to gain a symmetrical result from either space closure with canine camouflage or space opening with replacement of a single lateral incisor needs to be assessed. Unilateral agenesis often presents in conjunction with peg-shaped lateral incisors and it can be difficult to achieve symmetry between a small lateral incisor and a contralateral canine if space closure is undertaken. In these cases, the orthodontist may elect to extract the peg-shaped lateral incisor (Fig. 23.14). Alternatively, if the space is to be opened, the peg tooth may require restoration to match the contralateral prosthesis.

Moderate–severe hypodontia

In moderate–severe hypodontia, for example, cases with more than one missing tooth per quadrant, interdisciplinary input is required to allow a holistic treatment plan to be developed. Tooth position is likely to be guided by the proposed method of tooth replacement and the scope for tooth movement (Fig. 23.17). Ideally, spaces are located to optimize aesthetics and reduce the occlusal load on artificial replacement teeth. In severe hypodontia, with multiple missing teeth per quadrant, orthodontic treatment can be challenging as there may be insufficient teeth to gain anchorage for significant tooth movement using fixed appliances. In these cases, it may be necessary to accept the tooth position or plan only minimal tooth movements. Tooth replacement is often reliant on implant-retained prostheses and it may also be helpful to delay orthodontic treatment until nearer the age of growth cessation (see Section 23.7.6).

Orthodontic appliances

Fixed appliances are generally the treatment of choice for repositioning teeth but treatment mechanics may be complicated by a lack of teeth for anchorage, long spans of wire in edentulous sites that are prone to deformation and breakage, and challenges posed by a reduced face height and deep overbite. Where spaces have been created, acrylic pontic teeth can be ligated to the archwire via a bracket attached to the artificial tooth to improve aesthetics (Fig. 23.18). Anchorage support can be gained from removable appliances or adjuncts such as transpalatal or lingual arches, headgear, or skeletal anchorage from temporary anchorage devices.

Upper removable appliances with a flat anterior bite plane can be used to aid overbite reduction (see Chapter 10, Section 10.3.2) or to move teeth where there are insufficient teeth for fixed appliances. In growing patients with an underlying skeletal discrepancy, growth modification may be indicated. In Class II malocclusion with reduced face height, functional appliances might be useful to encourage anteroposterior and vertical correction and in Class III cases protraction headgear may be used (see Chapter 11, Section 11.4). In non-growing patients with a significant underlying skeletal discrepancy, orthognathic treatment may be required (see Chapter 20).

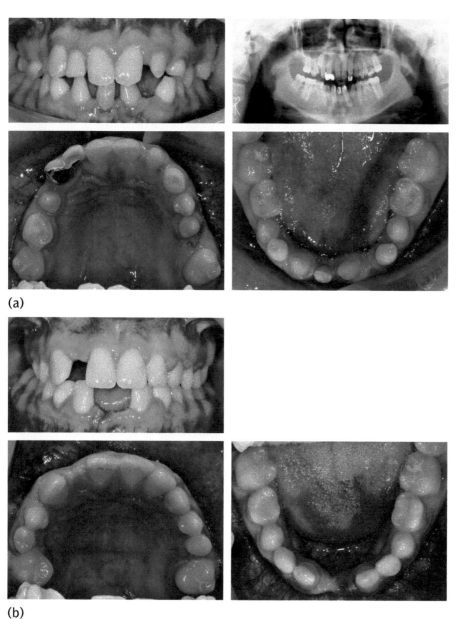

(a)

(b)

Fig. 23.17 Orthodontic treatment for severe hypodontia.(a) A 14-year-old male missing 13 permanent teeth with retained primary teeth and a number of microdont and conical-shaped permanent teeth. The right second premolar was impacted. A temporary bridge had been provided to replace the right maxillary lateral incisor. (b) Treatment involved extraction of the maxillary right primary second molar (URE) to encourage eruption of the premolar. Fixed appliances were used to redistribute space and temporary restorations were placed on the central incisors, conical permanent canine teeth, and primary teeth to improve the appearance of the teeth. The patient is awaiting tooth whitening followed by permanent restorations and provision of tooth replacement (RBBs) in the lower incisor and upper right maxillary incisor position.

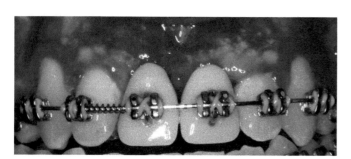

Fig. 23.18 Acrylic teeth (in this case, upper central incisors) can be ligated to the archwire using brackets glued to the teeth to provide an aesthetic solution to edentulous spaces during orthodontic treatment.

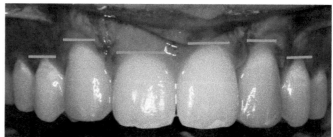

Fig. 23.19 Despite favourable canine morphology and reshaping throughout orthodontic treatment, the aesthetics of the canine substitution into the lateral incisor position is reduced by the darker colour of the canine crowns and discrepancies in the gingival height of the anterior teeth.

Retention

As with other malocclusions, retention is a key component of treatment (see Chapter 16). Spaces that have been closed orthodontically are prone to reopening and fixed retention is often indicated. In sites where space has been opened for tooth replacement, it is essential appropriate retention is planned to prevent relapse in tooth crown or root position that would complicate future restorative work. Artificial teeth can be added to a Hawley retainer as a temporary method of tooth replacement (Fig. 23.13). It is advisable that metal stops are included on the mesial and distal aspects of the edentulous space to prevent space loss if the artificial tooth/teeth are fractured. Artificial teeth can also be added to vacuum-formed retainers to improve aesthetics, but the patient must be instructed to remove the retainer for eating and drinking.

23.7.5 Restorative camouflage

Minimally invasive, adhesive restorative dentistry techniques can be used to alter the morphology of primary and permanent teeth (Fig. 23.17). This may be a stand-alone treatment if the tooth position and occlusion are acceptable, or undertaken in conjunction with orthodontic treatment.

In cases where permanent teeth have erupted or been orthodontically moved into the position of other teeth, restorative techniques can be used to camouflage the crown morphology to improve aesthetics. This is most commonly undertaken for canines acting as lateral incisors, where composite is added to the mesial and distal incisal corners to make the canines more square, and premolars in the canine position where the crown may require some enlargement. Recontouring of the gingival margins may also be desirable to optimize the aesthetics, particularly for people with a high smile line. Single-tooth whitening can improve the colour harmony between darker canines and adjacent teeth in space closure cases (Fig. 23.19).

23.7.6 Tooth replacement

A number of methods are available for replacing missing teeth depending on the number and position of missing teeth and adjacent structures. Tooth replacement includes:

- removable prostheses
- tooth-supported fixed prostheses
- implant-supported fixed prostheses
- tooth autotransplantation.

The method of tooth replacement should be agreed during initial treatment planning to ensure orthodontic treatment achieves the ideal tooth position to facilitate restoration. It is advisable to seek a restorative opinion before completion of fixed appliances to enable any final adjustments to the occlusion or spaces to be made to optimize the prognosis of the tooth replacement.

Removable prostheses

Removable prostheses (dentures) may be used to replace a single tooth or multiple teeth as a short-term or long-term solution. For patients with severe hypodontia and significant bony deficits, such as those with ectodermal dysplasia, dentures may be the preferred method for replacing a large number of teeth. Dentures may be constructed from acrylic or cobalt-chrome and can gain support and retention from the soft tissues as well as the dentition. Dentures have a number of advantages that are often overlooked; they are relatively quick and simple to make, versatile in design, and can provide good aesthetics and replace soft tissues. The main disadvantages of dentures are that some patients may find them hard to adapt to, both physically and psychologically, and bony remodelling during growth means the prosthesis will require adjustment or replacement over time.

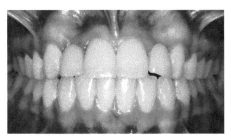
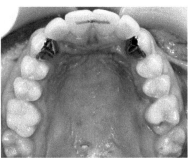
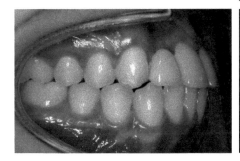
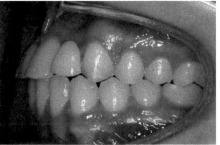

Fig. 23.20 Orthodontic space opening and tooth replacement with RBBs in a 13-year-old female with bilateral maxillary incisor agenesis. The restorations were provided by the patient's general dentist.

high, around 85%, but success depends on the design of the bridge, selection of the abutment tooth, occlusal factors, and patient factors. Conventional bridges with more extensive coronal coverage of abutment teeth are rarely used in younger patients, as the coronal preparation is often excessively destructive and there is an increased risk of pulpal damage in immature teeth. The exception is patients with conical or worn abutment teeth where existing inter-occlusal space means little preparation is required to enable placement of a full coverage crown, or older patients with previously restored abutment teeth.

Implant-supported fixed prostheses

Fixed tooth replacement can also be achieved by attaching crowns or bridges to dental implants. Implants require osseointegration for stability and as a result, it is necessary to wait for facial growth to have slowed to adult level to prevent infra-occlusion of the implant and restoration. The success rate of single-tooth implant-supported restorations in adults with hypodontia has been estimated to be greater than 95% over 3 years. Implant placement requires adequate alveolar bone height and width in the edentulous site to support the preferred implant size. Bone augmentation is possible where bone is deficient, most commonly using autogenous grafts from donor sites in the patient, although synthetic alloplastic materials are gaining popularity. As well as adequate alveolar bone, it is also necessary to have sufficient space between the roots of adjacent teeth for the implant, and between the crowns of adjacent and opposing teeth for the restoration (Fig. 23.21). Root parallelism achieved by orthodontic treatment in preparation for implant placement is prone to relapse so careful retention and minimal delay between orthodontic treatment and implant placement are advised. In cases where implants are planned, it may be prudent to delay the start of orthodontic treatment where possible, so that growth has slowed to adult levels and the implant can be safely placed once orthodontics is complete.

Tooth autotransplantation

Tooth autotransplantation is a procedure in which a tooth is carefully extracted under controlled conditions and implanted into another site in the same patient. In hypodontia, this treatment may be considered where there is crowding in one segment and a missing tooth in another. Transplantation most commonly involves premolars, although other teeth can be transplanted depending on the size of the agenesis space and the availability of donor tooth. Maxillary lateral incisors may be challenging to replace with premolars due to the relative size difference between premolar and lateral incisor crowns. Case reports have highlighted the potential for transplanting mandibular incisors into the maxillary lateral incisor position but this will depend on the scope for extracting a mandibular incisor without compromising the occlusal result.

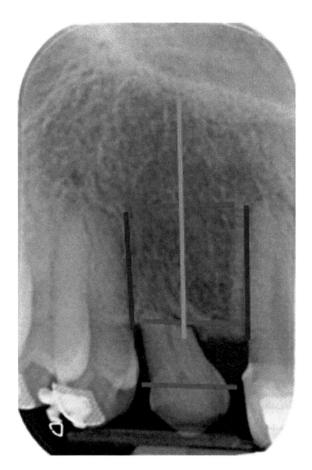

Fig. 23.21 Consideration for placement of an implant: root parallelism of adjacent teeth (red), mesiodistal width at the height of the crown, marginal bone and apical bone (blue), and the vertical height of the alveolar bone (green).

Tooth-supported fixed prostheses

Tooth-supported fixed prostheses include various designs of bridges that are retained through attachment to abutment teeth. Bridges can be used for short edentulous spans but the quality of abutment teeth and the occlusion must be assessed carefully to determine suitability. Microdont teeth or teeth with immature gingival margins may have inadequate enamel surface for bonding, while teeth with short roots or previous periodontal bone loss may not be able to support an increased occlusal load.

The most commonly used bridges are resin-bonded bridges (RBBs), which require minimal or no preparation to the abutment tooth (Fig. 23.20). Retention is achieved through enamel bonding with a resin-based adhesive. Survival of RBBs over 5 years have been shown to be

Key points

- Hypodontia is a relatively common dental anomaly, affecting permanent teeth in 3.5–6.5% of the population.
- Hypodontia is often associated with other dental anomalies and the impact of hypodontia and its treatment can be significant for those affected.
- Treatment may require an interdisciplinary approach involving the management of retained primary teeth, orthodontic treatment, and restorative treatment.

Principal sources and further reading

Akram, A. J., Jerreat, A. S., Woodford, J., Sandy, J. R., and Ireland, A. J. (2011). Development of a condition-specific measure to assess quality of life in patients with hypodontia. *Orthodontics and Craniofacial Research*, **14**, 160–7. [DOI: **10.1111/j.1601-6343.2011.01517.x**] [PubMed: 21771271]
This paper highlights the potential issues for people with hypodontia.

Allen, P. F., Anweigi, L., and Ziada, H. (2016). A prospective study of the performance of resin-bonded bridgework in patients with hypodontia. *Journal of Dentistry*, **50**, 69–73. [DOI: 10.1016/j.jdent.2016.05.003] [PubMed: 27178339]

Bacetti, T. (1998). A controlled study of associated dental anomalies. *Angle Orthodontist*, **68**, 267–74. [DOI: 10.1043/0003-3219(1998)068<0267:ACSOAD>2.3.CO;2] [PubMed: 9622764]

Bjerklin, K., Al-Najjar, M., Karestedt, H., and Andren, A. (2008). Agenesis of mandibular second premolars with retained primary molars. A longitudinal radiographic study of 99 subjects from 12 years of age to adulthood. *European Journal of Orthodontics*, **20**, 254–61. [DOI: 10.1093/ejo/cjn027] [PubMed: 18540014]
A key paper providing evidence about the longevity of primary teeth.

Cobourne, M. T. (2007). Familial human hypodontia – is it all in the genes? *British Dental Journal*, **203**, 203–8. [DOI: 10.1038/bdj.2007.732] [PubMed: 17721480]
An accessible introduction to the role of genes in hypodontia.

Durey, K. A., Nixon, P. J., Robinson, S., and Chan, M. F. W. Y. (2011). Resin bonded bridges: techniques for success. *British Dental Journal*, **211**, 113–8. [DOI: 10.1038/sj.bdj.2011.619] [PubMed: 21836574]
A useful overview of considerations when planning resin-bonded bridges.

Garnett, M. J., Wassell, R. W., Jepson, N. J., and Nohl, F. S. (2006). Survival of resin-bonded bridgework provided for post-orthodontic hypodontia patients with missing maxillary lateral incisors. *British Dental Journal*, **201**, 527–34. [DOI: 10.1038/sj.bdj.4814160] [PubMed: 17057683]

Gill, D. S. and Barker, C. S. (2015). The multidisciplinary management of hypodontia: a team approach. *British Dental Journal*, **218**, 143–9. [DOI: 10.1038/sj.bdj.2015.52] [PubMed: 25686431]
A summary of treatment approaches for hypodontia throughout dental development.

Hosseini, M., Worsaae, N., Schiodt, M., and Gotfredsen, K. (2013). A 3-year prospective study of implant-supported, single-tooth restorations of all-ceramic and metal-ceramic materials in patients with tooth agenesis. *Clinical Oral Implant Research*, **24**, 1078–87. [DOI: **10.1111/j.1600-0501.2012.02514.x**] [PubMed: 22708959]

Jonsson, T. and Sigurdsson, T. J. (2004). Autotransplantation of premolars to premolar sites. A long-term follow-up study of 40 consecutive patients. *American Journal of Orthodontics Dentofacial Orthopedics*, **125**, 668–75. [DOI: 10.1016/S088954060301031X] [PubMed: 15179391]
This study demonstrates the success of tooth transplantation in hypodontia.

Khalaf, K., Miskelly, J., Voge, E., and Macfarlane, T. V. (2014). Prevalence of hypodontia and associated factors: a systematic review and meta-analysis. *Journal of Orthodontics*, **41**, 299–316. [DOI: 10.1179/1465313314Y.0000000116] [PubMed: 25404667]

King, P., Maiorana, C., Luthardt, R. G., Sondell, K., Oland, J., Galindo-Moreno, P., et al. (2016). Clinical and radiographic evaluation of a small diameter dental implant used for the restoration of patients with permanent tooth agenesis in the maxillary and mandibular incisor regions: a 36-month follow-up. *International Journal of Prosthodontics*, **29**, 147–53. [DOI: 10.11607/ijp.4444] [PubMed: 26929953]

Kotecha S., Turner P. J., Dietrich T., and Dhopatkar A. (2013). The impact of tooth agenesis on oral health-related quality of life in children. *Journal of Orthodontics*, **20**, 122–9. [DOI: 10.1179/1465313312Y.0000000035] [PubMed: 23794692]

Lindqvist, B. (1980). Extraction of deciduous second molar in hypodontia. *European Journal of Orthodontics*. **2**, 173–81. [DOI: 10.1093/ejo/2.3.173] [PubMed: 6935067]
An early study promoting the early extraction of primary molars to encourage spontaneous space closure.

Locker, D., Jokovic, A., Prakash, P., and Tompson, B. (2010). Oral health-related quality of life in children with oligodontia. *International Journal of Paediatric Dentistry*, **20**, 8–14. [DOI: **10.1111/j.1365-263X.2009.01001.x**] [PubMed: 20059588]
This study found children with hypodontia have worse OHRQoL than children with caries or other malocclusions.

Meaney, S., Anweigi, L., Ziada, H., and Allen, F. (2012). The impact of hypodontia: a qualitative study on the experiences of patients. *European Journal of Orthodontics*, **34**, 547–52. [DOI: 10.1093/ejo/cjr061] [PubMed: 21693681]
An interesting paper outlining the impact of the hypodontia treatment journey.

Nordquist, G. G. and McNeil, R. W. (1975). Orthodontic vs. restorative treatment of congenitally absent lateral incisor – long term occlusal and periodontal evaluation. *Journal of Periodontology*, **46**, 139–43. [DOI: 10.1902/jop.1975.46.3.139] [PubMed: 1054757]
A classic paper—findings indicate space closure has periodontal health benefits and no detriment to the occlusion.

Olsen, T. M. and Kokich, V. G. (2010). Postorthodontic root approximation after opening space for maxillary lateral incisor implants. *American Journal of Orthodontics Dentofacial Orthopedics*, **137**, e1–158. [DOI: 10.1016/j.ajodo.2009.08.024] [PubMed: 20152659]
This study emphasizes the risk of post-treatment relapse of root position.

Polder, B. J., Van't Hof, M. A., Van der Linder, F. P. G. M., and Kuijpers-Jagtman, A. M. (2004). A meta-analysis of the prevalence of dental agenesis of permanent teeth. *Community Dental Oral Epidemiology*, **32**, 217–26. [DOI: 10.1111/j.1600-0528.2004.00158.x] [PubMed: 15151692]

Robertsson, S. and Mohlin, B. (2000). The congenitally missing upper lateral incisor. A retrospective study of orthodontic space closure versus restorative treatment. *European Journal of Orthodontics*, **22**, 697–710. [DOI: 10.1093/ejo/22.6.697] [PubMed: 11212605]
A more recent study of space opening compared to space closure with similar findings.

Savarrio, L. and McIntyre, G. T. (2005). To open or close the space – that is the missing lateral incisor question. *Dental Update*, **32**, 16–25. [DOI: 10.12968/denu.2005.32.1.16] [PubMed: 15739660]
A discussion around decision-making for maxillary lateral incisor agenesis including useful summaries of the decision pathway and factors to consider.

Zimmer, B., Schelper, I., and Seifi-Shirvandeh, N. (2007). Localized orthodontic space closure for unilateral aplasia of lower second premolars. *European Journal of Orthodontics*, **29**, 210–16. [DOI: 10.1093/ejo/cjm009] [PubMed: 17489002]
This study demonstrated the scope for closing premolar agenesis sites without detriment to the occlusion.

References for this chapter can also be found at: **www.oup.com/uk/orthodontics5e**. Where possible, these are presented as active links which direct you to the electronic version of the work, to help facilitate onward study. If you are a subscriber to that work (either individually or through an institution), and depending on your level of access, you may be able to peruse an abstract or the full article if available.

24

Cleft lip and palate and other craniofacial anomalies

L. Mitchell

Chapter contents

Relevant sections in other chapters

4.2 Early cranofacial development

Learning objectives for this chapter

- Gain an appreciation of the different presentations of cleft lip and/or palate and the problems they present for the patient and the clinician.
- Gain an understanding of the basic principles of management of patients with a cleft.

24.1 Prevalence

Cleft lip and palate is the most common craniofacial malformation, comprising 65% of all anomalies affecting the head and neck. There are two distinct types of cleft anomaly: cleft lip with or without cleft palate, and isolated cleft palate, which result from failure of fusion at two different stages of dentofacial development (see Chapter 4, Section 4.2).

24.1.1 Cleft lip and palate

The prevalence of cleft lip and palate varies geographically and between different racial groups. Among Caucasians, this anomaly occurs in approximately 1 in every 700 live births and the prevalence is increasing. A family history can be found in around 40% of cases of cleft lip with or without cleft palate, and the risk of unaffected parents having another child with this anomaly is 1 in 25 (Box 24.1). Males are affected more frequently than females, and the left side is involved more commonly than the right. Interestingly, the severity of the cleft is usually more marked when it arises in the less common variant.

Box 24.1 Genetic risks of cleft lip and palate

- Parents with no cleft but with one affected child: risk for next child = 1 in 25 (4%).
- One parent with cleft lip and palate: risk for first child = 1 in 50 (2%).
- One parent with cleft lip and palate and first child with cleft lip and palate: risk for next child = 1 in 10 (10%).
- Both parents affected: risk for first child = 3 in 5 (60%).

24.1.2 Isolated cleft of the secondary palate

Isolated cleft occurs in around 1 in 2000 live births and affects females more often than males. Clefts of the secondary palate have a lesser genetic component, with a family history in around 20% and a reduced risk of further affected offspring to normal parents (1 in 80).

Isolated cleft palate is also found as a feature in a number of syndromes including Down, Treacher–Collins, Pierre–Robin, and Klippel–Fiel syndromes.

24.2 Aetiology

In normal development, fusion of the embryological processes that comprise the upper lip occurs around the sixth week of intrauterine life. 'Flip-up' of the palatal shelves from a vertical to a horizontal position followed by fusion to form the secondary palate occurs around the eighth week. Before fusion can take place, the embryological processes must grow until they come into contact. Then breakdown of the overlying epithelium is followed by invasion of mesenchyme. If this process is to take place successfully, a number of different factors need to interact at the right time. Evidence from population studies and experimental data suggests that both genetic and environmental factors play a part in the aetiology of clefts. Specific gene mutations have been shown to be linked to cleft lip and/or cleft palate. Environmental factors that have been implicated include anticonvulsant drugs, folic acid deficiency, and maternal smoking.

It is postulated that isolated cleft palate is more common in females than males because transposition of the palatal shelves occurs later in the female fetus. Thus, greater opportunity exists for an environmental insult to affect successful elevation, which is further hampered by widening of the face as a result of growth in the intervening period (see Chapter 4, Section 4.2.4).

24.3 Classification

A number of classifications exist but, given the wide variation in clinical presentation, in practice it is often preferable to describe the presenting deformity in words (Fig. 24.1).

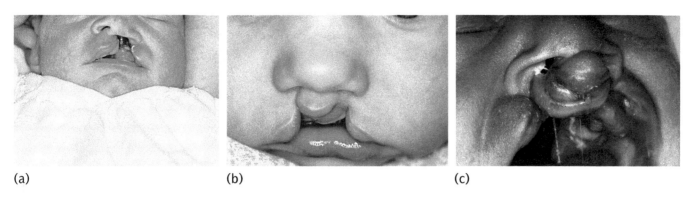

(a)   (b)   (c)

Fig. 24.1 (a) Baby with a complete unilateral cleft lip and palate on the left side; (b) baby with a bilateral incomplete cleft lip; (c) baby with a complete bilateral cleft lip and palate.

24.4 Problems in management

24.4.1 Congenital anomalies

The disturbances in dental and skeletal development caused by the clefting process itself depend upon the site and severity of the cleft.

Lip only

There is little effect in this type, although notching of the alveolus adjacent to the cleft lip may sometimes be seen.

Lip and alveolus

A unilateral cleft of the lip and alveolus is not usually associated with segmental displacement. However, in bilateral cases the premaxilla may be rotated forwards. The lateral incisor on the side of the cleft may exhibit some of the following dental anomalies:

- Congenital absence
- An abnormality of tooth size and/or shape
- Defects of the enamel
- Or present as two conical teeth, one on each side of the cleft.

Lip and palate

In unilateral clefts, rotation and collapse of both segments inwards anteriorly is usually seen, although this is usually more marked on the side of the cleft (the lesser segment). In bilateral clefts, both lateral segments are often collapsed behind a prominent premaxilla (Fig. 24.2).

Palate only

A widening of the arch posteriorly is usually seen.

It has been shown that individuals with a cleft have a more concave profile, and while a degree of this is due to a restriction of growth (see later), research indicates that cleft patients have a tendency towards a more retrognathic maxilla and mandible and also a reduced upper face height compared with the normal population.

24.4.2 Post-surgical distortions

Studies of individuals with unoperated clefts (usually in Third World countries) show that they do not experience a significant restriction of facial growth, although there is a lack of development in the region of the cleft itself, possibly because of tissue hypoplasia. In contrast, individuals who have undergone surgical repair of a cleft lip and palate exhibit marked restriction of mid-face growth anteroposteriorly and transversely (Fig. 24.3). This is attributed to the restraining effect of the scar tissue, which results from surgical intervention. It has been estimated that approximately 40% of cleft patients exhibit marked maxillary retrusion. Limitation of vertical growth of the maxilla coupled with a tendency for an increased lower facial height results in an excessive freeway space, and frequently overclosure (Fig. 24.4).

24.4.3 Hearing and speech

Speech development is adversely affected by the presence of fistulae in the palate and by velopharyngeal insufficiency, where the soft palate is not able to make an adequate contact with the back of the pharynx to close off the nasal airway (Fig. 24.5). This can result in hypernasal speech.

A cleft involving the posterior part of the hard and soft palate will also involve the tensor palati muscles, which act on the Eustachian tube. This predisposes the patient to problems with middle-ear effusion (known colloquially as 'glue ear'). Obviously, hearing difficulties will also retard a child's speech development. Therefore, management of the child with a cleft involving the posterior palate must include audiological assessments and myringotomy with or without grommets as indicated.

24.4.4 Other congenital abnormalities

Cleft lip with or without cleft palate, and isolated cleft palate are associated with other congenital abnormalities (Box 24.2). The actual figures vary between populations, but the prevalence is greater in babies with isolated cleft palate. The most common anomalies affect the heart and extremities.

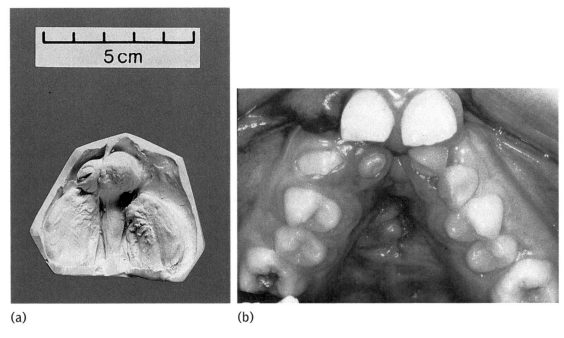

Fig. 24.2 (a) Upper model of a bilateral complete cleft lip and palate showing the inward collapse of the lateral segments behind the pre-maxillary segment; (b) upper arch of a patient in the late mixed dentition with a bilateral complete cleft lip and palate.

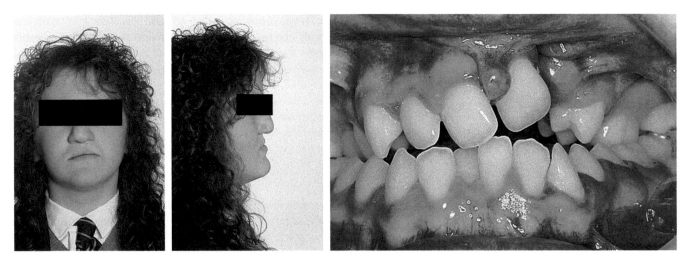

Fig. 24.3 Patient with a repaired unilateral cleft lip and palate of the left side showing mid-face retrusion.

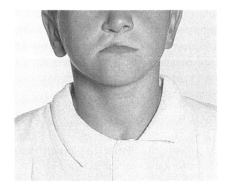

Fig. 24.4 Patient with a repaired cleft lip and palate of the right side who had a degree of overclosure, believed to be due to the restricting effect of the primary repair on vertical growth.

24.4.5 Dental anomalies

In addition to the effects on the teeth in the region of the cleft discussed above, the following anomalies are more prevalent in the remainder of the dentition:

- Delayed eruption (delay increases with severity of cleft)
- Hypodontia
- Supernumerary teeth
- General reduction in tooth size
- Abnormalities of tooth size and shape (Fig. 24.6)
- Enamel defects.

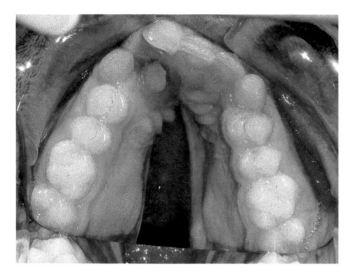

Fig. 24.5 Patient with unrepaired cleft palate. As a result, their speech was unintelligible.

Box 24.2 In a study of nearly 4000 patients with isolated cleft palate

- 55% had cleft palate only.
- 27% had a recognized syndrome.
- 18% had other anomalies.

Source data from *Cleft Palate – Craniofacial Journal*, 41, Calzolari, E. Bianchi et al, EUROCAT working group. Epidemiology of cleft palate in Europe: implications for genetic research 2004.

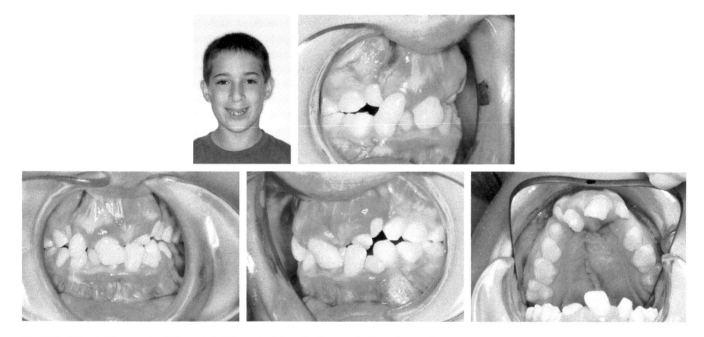

Fig. 24.6 Patient with a repaired bilateral cleft lip and palate with abnormally shaped upper incisors.

24.5 Coordination of care

In order to minimize the number of hospital visits and to ensure integrated interdisciplinary management, it is essential to employ a team approach with joint clinics. In order to build up expertise within the team and for meaningful audit, care should be centralized within a region. The core members usually include the following:

- Cleft surgeon
- Orthodontist
- Psychologist
- Speech and language therapist
- Health visitor/specialized nurse
- Ear, nose, and throat (ENT) surgeon.

24.6 Management

It is now accepted practice that patients with a cleft lip and/or palate should be managed to a standardized protocol. The rationale for this is twofold. Firstly, a standard regimen reduces the temptation for additional 'touch-up' surgical procedures, the benefits of which are limited. A standardized protocol also permits useful audit of the outcome of all aspects of cleft care and thereby leads to the refinement and improvement of the management of subsequent generations of cleft children (see Section 24.7).

24.6.1 At birth

With improved fetal ultrasound screening, an increasing proportion of clefts are detected prenatally. This has the advantage that the parents can be counselled and prepared for the arrival of a child with a cleft. Otherwise, the birth of a child with a cleft anomaly will come as a shock and a disappointment for the parents. It is common for them to experience feelings of guilt and they will need time to grieve for the emotional loss of the 'normal' child that they anticipated. It is important to provide support for the mother at this time to ensure that bonding develops normally and that help with feeding is available straightaway for those infants with a cleft. This is now usually provided by a trained cleft health visitor. Because an affected child will have difficulty in sucking, a bottle and teat which help direct the flow of milk into the mouth is helpful, for example a soft bottle which can be squeezed (Fig. 24.7). An early explanation from a member(s) of the cleft team of probable future management and the possibilities of modern treatment is appreciated by parents. Further support

can be obtained from CLAPA (the Cleft Lip and Palate Association: http://www.clapa.com), which is a voluntary group largely comprising parents of, and individuals with a cleft (Fig. 24.8).

Some centres advocate the use of acrylic plates designed to help with feeding or to move the displaced cleft segments actively towards a more normal relationship to aid subsequent surgical apposition. This is known as pre-surgical orthopaedics and has recently come back into fashion especially in America with the introduction of an extension from the acrylic plate into the cleft nostril(s) to help mould the cleft nose. This modified technique is called naso-alveolar moulding (or NAM). There is currently no robust long-term data to support the routine use of this approach, which does impose an additional burden on the parents in the time before initial lip repair.

24.6.2 Lip repair

There is a wide variation in the timing of primary lip repair, depending upon the preference and protocol of the surgeon and cleft team involved. Neonatal repair is still being evaluated. In the UK, primary lip repair is, on average, carried out around 3 months of age. A number of different surgical techniques have been described (e.g. Millard, Delaire, and straight line) but the main aim is to dissect out and reoppose the muscles of the lip and alar base in their correct anatomical position.

Most centres repair bilateral cleft lips at the same procedure, but some still carry out two separate operations. Primary bone grafting of the alveolus at the time of lip repair has fallen into disrepute due to the adverse effects upon subsequent growth.

24.6.3 Palate repair

The goal of hard palate closure is to separate the oral and nasal cavities, with minimal effects upon normal growth and development. In order to achieve the latter, surgery should avoid wide undermining of the palatal soft tissues. Two-layered closure is currently often employed with vomer flaps used to close the nasal layer and mucoperiosteal flaps with minimal bone exposure used for the oral layer.

The aim of soft palate surgery is to facilitate normal velopharyngeal function and closure for intelligible speech.

In some European centres, closure of the hard palate is delayed until 5 years of age or older in an effort to reduce the unwanted effects of early surgery upon growth. There is some evidence to suggest that transverse growth of the maxilla is improved. However, the adverse effect upon speech development has been well documented. In the UK, hard and soft palate repair is undertaken, on average, between 6 and 9 months of

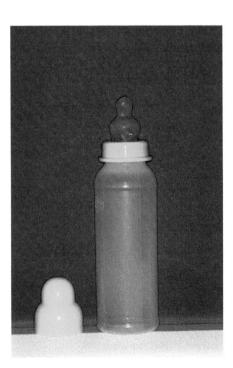

Fig. 24.7 A soft squeezable bottle and special teat for feeding cleft babies.

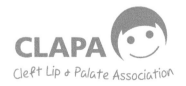

Fig. 24.8 The Cleft Lip and Palate Association logo.

age with the philosophy that any unwanted effects upon growth caused by repair at this stage (which can be compensated for to a degree by orthodontics and surgery) are preferable to fostering the development of poor articulatory speech habits, which can be extremely difficult to eradicate after the age of 5 years.

24.6.4 Primary dentition

The first formal speech assessment is usually carried out around 18 months of age, however, monitoring of a patient's speech should continue throughout childhood. This is usually done at certain pre-defined ages, but will depend upon the needs and circumstances of the child.

If the cleft involves the palate, an assessment with an ENT surgeon should also be arranged, if this specialty has not been involved at the time of primary repair.

It is important to minimize surgical interference with the cleft child's life and 'minor' touch-ups should be avoided. Lip revision, prior to the start of schooling, should be performed only if clearly indicated. Closure of any residual palatal fistulae may be considered to help speech development. In a proportion of cases, the repaired cleft palate does not completely seal off the nasopharynx during speech and nasal escape of air may occur, resulting in a nasal intonation to the child's speech. This is called velopharyngeal incompetence (VPI). If from evidence from investigations such as speech assessment, videofluoroscopy, and nasoendoscopy, VPI is diagnosed, a pharyngoplasty may help. This operation involves moving mucosal or musculomucosal pharyngeal flaps to augment the shape and function of the soft palate. If indicated, this should be carried out around 4–5 years of age.

Orthodontic treatment in the primary dentition is not warranted. However, during this stage it is important to develop good dental care habits, instituting fluoride supplements in non-fluoridated areas.

24.6.5 Mixed dentition

During this stage, the restraining effect of surgery upon growth becomes more apparent, initially transversely in the upper arch and then anteroposteriorly as growth in the latter dimension predominates. With the eruption of the permanent incisors, defects in tooth number, formation, and position can be assessed. Often the upper incisors erupt into lingual occlusion and commonly are also displaced or rotated (Fig. 24.9).

In order to avoid straining patient cooperation, it is better if orthodontic intervention is concentrated into two phases. The first stage is usually carried out during the mixed dentition with the specific aim of preparing the patient for alveolar or secondary bone grafting. Subsequent management is discussed in Section 24.6.6.

Alveolar (secondary) bone grafting

This technique has significantly improved the orthodontic care of patients with an alveolar cleft involving the alveolus as it involves repairing the defect with cancellous bone (Box 24.3).

For optimal results, this procedure should be timed before the eruption of the permanent canines, at around 9–10 years, particularly as eruption of a tooth through the graft helps to stabilize it. However, in some patients, earlier bone grafting is indicated to provide bone for an unerupted viable lateral incisor to erupt.

Before bone grafting is carried out, any transverse collapse of the segments should be corrected to allow complete exposure of the alveolar defect and to improve access for the surgeon. This is most commonly carried out by using a fixed expansion appliance called the quadhelix (see Chapter 13, Section 13.4.4). This appliance has the advantage that the arms can be extended anteriorly, if indicated, to procline the upper incisors, but in cases with more severe displacement and/or rotation of the incisors, a simple fixed appliance can be used concurrently (Fig. 24.11). However, care is required to ensure that the roots of the teeth adjacent to the cleft are not moved out of their bony support, and it may be necessary to defer their complete alignment to the post-grafting stage. A palatal arch may be fitted to retain the expansion achieved while bone grafting is carried out (Fig. 24.12).

In patients with a bilateral complete cleft lip and palate the premaxillary segment is often mobile. In these cases, in order to ensure that the graft takes and bony healing occurs, it is necessary to stabilize the premaxilla during the healing period after bone grafting. This can be accomplished by placement of a relatively rigid buccal archwire prior to bone grafting, which is left *in situ* for around 3 months after the operation.

If space closure on the side of the cleft is planned, consideration should be given to the need to extract the deciduous molars on that side prior to grafting in order to facilitate forward movement of the first permanent molar. However, any extractions should be carried out at

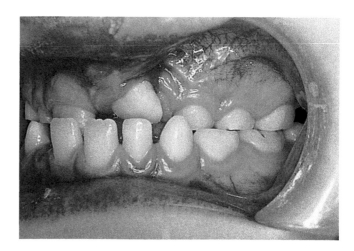

Fig. 24.9 A repaired unilateral cleft lip and palate in the mixed dentition.

Box 24.3 Benefits of alveolar bone grafting

- Provision of bone through which the permanent canine (or lateral incisor) can erupt into the arch (Fig. 24.10).
- The possibility of providing the patient with an intact arch.
- Improved alar base support.
- Aids closure of residual oronasal fistulae.
- Stabilization of a mobile premaxilla in a bilateral cleft.

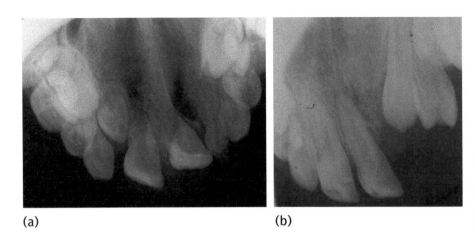

Fig. 24.10 Radiographs of the patient shown in Fig. 24.13, who had an alveolar bone graft: (a) prior to bone grafting showing cleft of left alveolus; (b) 1 month after bone grafting. The supernumerary tooth lying in the cleft was removed at the time of surgery.

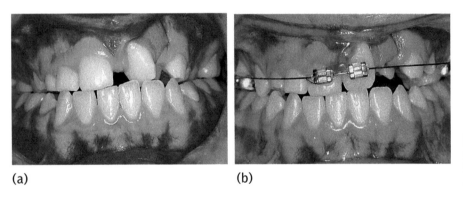

Fig. 24.11 Patient with a repaired unilateral cleft of the lip and palate of the left side: (a) pre-treatment; (b) following expansion and alignment of the rotated upper left central incisor.

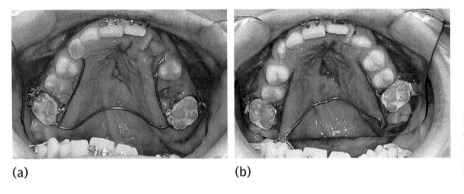

Fig. 24.12 The same patient as in Fig. 24.11: (a) palatal arch and sectional archwire to retain position of the upper central incisors, prior to bone grafting; (b) after bone grafting, showing the upper left canine erupting.

least 3 weeks prior to bone grafting in order to allow healing of the keratinized mucosa for the surgeon to raise flaps.

Cancellous bone is currently used for bone grafting because it assumes the characteristics of the adjacent bone; however, this may change in the future as bone morphogenesis proteins become cheaper and more readily available. Cancellous bone can be harvested from a number of sites, but the iliac crest is currently the most popular site. Keratinized flaps should be raised and utilized for closure, as mucosal flaps may interfere with subsequent tooth eruption. Unerupted supernumerary teeth are commonly found in the cleft itself, and these can be removed at the time of operation. There is no substantive evidence to support the contention that simultaneous bone grafting of bilateral alveolar clefts jeopardizes the integrity of the premaxilla.

The complications of this technique include:

- granuloma formation in the region of the graft—this often resolves with increased oral hygiene, but surgical removal may be required
- failure of the graft to take—this usually only occurs to a partial degree
- root resorption—relatively rare
- around 10–15% of canines on the grafted side subsequently require exposure.

24.6.6 Permanent dentition

Once the permanent dentition has been established, but before further orthodontic treatment is planned, the patient should be assessed as to the likely need for orthognathic surgery to correct mid-face retrusion (see Chapter 22). The degree of maxillary retrognathia, the magnitude and effect of any future growth, and the patient's wishes should all be taken into consideration; however, it has been shown that around 25% of cleft lip and palate patients treated to a standardized protocol require orthognathic surgery. This is because scar tissue from the original primary repair restricts growth of the maxilla. If surgical correction is indicated, this should be deferred until the growth rate has slowed to adult levels (and be preceded by pre-surgical orthodontic alignment) (Box 24.4).

If orthodontics alone is indicated, this can be commenced once the permanent dentition is established. Usually fixed appliances are necessary (Fig. 24.13). If space closure in the region of the cleft is not feasible, treatment planning should be carried out in collaboration with a restorative opinion regarding how the resultant space will be restored in the longer term (e.g. implant, bridgework).

At the end of orthodontic treatment, retention will be required. If the maxillary arch has been expanded, this will be particularly prone to

---

Box 24.4 Orthognathic surgery in cleft patients

- Surgical advancement of the maxilla may affect velopharyngeal function therefore a speech assessment should be carried out before planning surgery.
- Scar tissue may restrict the amount of forward movement of the maxilla that is possible.
- Reduced blood supply to the maxilla due to scarring.
- Maxillary distraction may overcome these problems (see Chapter 22, Section 22.7.4).

---

relapse therefore long-term retention is advisable. For further details on retention and the different types of retainer, see Chapter 16 and Section 16.6 in particular.

24.6.7 Completion of growth

A final surgical revision of the nose (rhinoplasty) may be carried out at this stage. However, if orthognathic surgery is planned this should be carried out first, as movement of the underlying facial bones will affect the contour of the nose.

24.7 Audit of cleft palate care

Audit of cleft palate management is difficult because of the different disciplines involved in providing care and the range of clinical presentations. As in all branches of medicine, concentration of expertise and experience at a centre of excellence produces superior results to those obtained by a lone practitioner carrying out small numbers of a particular procedure each year. Therefore, it has been suggested that each team should 'treat' a minimum of 50 cleft patients per year to provide sufficient numbers for meaningful audit and to develop adequate expertise. In order to try to evaluate the effects of treatment, careful records taken before and after any intervention (surgical or orthodontic) must be a priority. If the results of one surgical team carrying out a particular treatment protocol are to be compared with another treatment regimen carried out at a different centre, some standardization of these records is required. These should include study models and photographs of the cleft prior to primary closure, so that the size and morphology of the original cleft can be taken into consideration.

24.8 Other craniofacial anomalies

24.8.1 Craniofacial microsomia

This is the second most common craniofacial anomaly, with a prevalence of between 1 in 3500 to 1 in 5000 live births. It is a congenital defect characterized by a lack of both hard and soft tissue on one or both sides of the face, usually in the area of the mandibular ramus and external ear (i.e. in the region of the first and second branchial arches). This anomaly usually affects one side of the face (Fig. 24.14), but does present bilaterally in around 30% of cases. A wide spectrum of ear and cranial nerve deformities are found. In the milder forms it is known as oculoauriculovertebral dysplasia, while Goldenhar syndrome is commonly used to refer to the more severe presentation.

Management usually involves a combination of surgery and orthodontic treatment. However, milder cases can sometimes be managed with orthodontic appliances alone. Orthodontic treatment usually involves the use of a specialized type of functional appliance known as a hybrid appliance, so called because components are selected according to the needs of the individual malocclusion, for example, encouraging eruption of the buccal segment teeth on the affected side.

The degree and type of surgery depends upon the severity of the defect:

- Early reconstruction (5–8 years of age)—is usually reserved for severe cases with no functioning temporomandibular joint (TMJ).
- In the growing child—distraction osteogenesis (see Chapter 22, Section 22.7.4) where a functioning TMJ exists.
- Late teens—to enhance the contour of the skeleton and soft tissues—conventional orthognathic and reconstructive techniques.

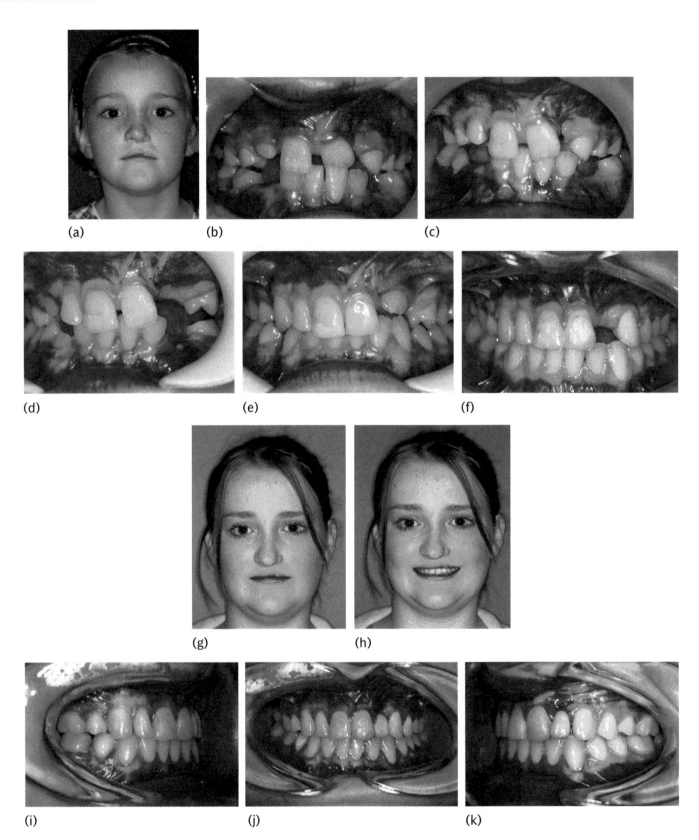

Fig. 24.13 Patient with a repaired unilateral left cleft lip and palate (see also Fig. 24.10 which shows radiographs of same patient before and after bone graft). (a, b) Aged 9 years, pre-treatment; (c) following correction of anterior crossbite and prior to alveolar bone graft of left alveolus; (d) post-alveolar bone graft; (e) at age 12 years after eruption of upper left canine; (f) following comprehensive fixed appliance treatment to localize space for prosthetic replacement of absent upper left lateral incisor; (g–k) following bridgework to replace absent upper left lateral incisor.

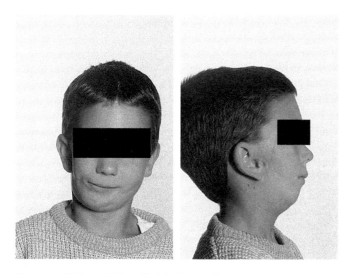

Fig. 24.14 Patient with hemifacial microsomia.

24.8.2 Mandibulofacial dystosis

This syndrome is also known as Treacher–Collins syndrome. It is inherited in an autosomal dominant manner and consists of the following features, which present bilaterally:

- Downward sloping (anti-mongoloid slant) palpebral fissures and colobomas (notched iris with a displaced pupil).
- Hypoplastic malar bones.
- Mandibular retrognathia.
- Deformed ears, including middle and inner ear which can result in deafness.
- Hypoplastic air sinuses.
- Cleft palate in one-third of cases.
- Most have completely normal intellectual function.

The specifics of management depend upon the features of the case, but usually staged craniofacial surgery is required.

24.8.3 Pierre–Robin sequence

This anomaly consists of retrognathia of the mandible, cleft palate, and glossoptosis (the tongue position restricts the pharynx), which together cause airway problems in the infant. The exact cause is unknown but it is likely to involve a genetic component as it occurs in other genetically associated anomalies (e.g. Stickler syndrome). The first priority at birth is to maintain the airway; in a proportion of cases it is necessary to use a nasopharyngeal airway for the first few days, but once the child is older, or in less severe cases, prone nursing will suffice. Rarely, tracheostomy for medium-term airway protection is required. Subsequent management is as for cleft palate (see earlier in chapter). For affected patients with a compromised airway or poor aesthetics, early distraction osteogenesis can be considered, or alternatively, orthognathic surgery towards the end of growth (see Chapter 22). In milder cases, conventional orthodontic mechanotherapy for Class II skeletal patterns can be planned.

24.8.4 Craniosynostoses

In craniosynostosis and craniofacial synostoses, premature fusion of one or more of the sutures of the bones of the cranial base or vault occurs. The effects depend upon the site and extent of the premature fusion, but all have a marked effect upon growth. In some cases, restriction of skull vault growth can lead to an increase in intracranial pressure which, if untreated, can lead to brain damage. If raised intracranial pressure is detected, release of the affected suture(s) before 6 months of age is indicated. This may be the only intervention needed in isolated craniosynostoses. Combined craniofacial synostoses (e.g. Crouzon syndrome; Apert syndrome) require subsequent staged orthodontic and surgical intervention. This may become the prime indication for telemetric distraction osteogenesis.

Key points

- Cleft care is complex and requires a coordinated multidisciplinary team approach.
- Each team should manage sufficient cases to build up expertise and provide numbers for meaningful audit.
- Management should be to a predetermined protocol.
- To facilitate audit and inter-centre comparisons, records should be collected to a standardized national protocol.
- Interventions should be restricted to the minimum to reduce the burden on the cleft patient and their family.

Relevant Cochrane reviews

Bessell, A., Hooper, L., Shaw, W. C., Reilly, S., Reid, J., and Glenny, A. M. (2011). Feeding interventions for growth and development in infants with cleft lip, cleft palate or cleft lip and palate. *Cochrane Database of Systematic Reviews*, Issue 2, Art. No.: CD003315. DOI: 10.1002/14651858.CD003315.pub3 https://www.cochranelibrary.com/cdsr/doi/10.1002/14651858.CD003315.pub3/full

Guo, J., Li, C., Zhang, Q., Wu, G., Deacon, S. A., Chen, J., et al. (2011). Secondary bone grafting for alveolar cleft in children with cleft lip or cleft lip and palate. *Cochrane Database of Systematic Reviews*, Issue 6, Art. No.: CD008050. DOI: 10.1002/14651858.CD008050.pub2 https://www.cochranelibrary.com/cdsr/doi/10.1002/14651858.CD008050.pub2/full

Principal sources and further reading

Bergland, O., Semb, G., and Abyholm, F. E. (1986). Elimination of the residual alveolar cleft by secondary bone grafting and subsequent orthodontic treatment. *Cleft Lip and Palate Journal*, **23**, 175–205. [PubMed: 3524905]
This paper is now a classic. It describes the pioneering work by the Oslo cleft team on alveolar bone grafting.

Calzolari, E., Bianchi, F., Rubini, M., Ritvanen, A., and Neville, A. J. (2004). EUROCAT working group. Epidemiology of cleft palate in Europe: implications for genetic research. *Cleft Palate – Craniofacial Journal*, **41**, 244–9. [DOI: 10.1597/02-074.1] [PubMed: 15151454]
The source of the figures for the study of nearly 4000 patients with isolated cleft palate referred to in Box 24.2.

Clinical Standards Advisory Group (1998). *Cleft Lip and/or Palate*. London: Stationery Office.
The results of a national audit of cleft care in the UK that led to a transformation in the way cleft care is delivered.

Eppley, B. L. and Sadove, A. M. (2000). Management of alveolar cleft bone grafting – state of the art. *Cleft Palate – Craniofacial Journal*, **37**, 229–33. [DOI: 10.1597/1545-1569(2000)037] [PubMed: 10830800]
An interesting read for those clinicians involved in alveolar bone grafting.

Mossey, P., Little, J., Munger, R. G., Dixon, M. J., and Shaw, W. C. (2009). Cleft lip and palate. *The Lancet*, **374**, 1773–85. [DOI: 10.1016/S0140-6736(09)60695-4] [PubMed: 19747722]
An excellent review article which focuses on the aetiology of clefts.

Ranta, R. (1986). A review of tooth formation in children in cleft lip/palate. *American Journal of Orthodontics and Dentofacial Orthopedics*, **90**, 11–18. [DOI: 10.1016/0889-5406(86)90022-3] [PubMed: 3524249]
Details of the dental anomalies found in patients with a cleft.

Uzel A. and Alparslan, N. (2010). Long-term effects of presurgical infant orthopedics in patients with cleft lip and palate: a systematic review. *Cleft Palate – Craniofacial Journal*, **48**, 587–95. [DOI: 10.1597/10-008] [PubMed: 20858135]
This review found no long-term benefits from the use of pre-surgical orthopaedic plates prior to primary surgery.

Wyatt, R., Sell, D., Russell, J, Harding, A., Harland, K., and Albery, E. (1996). Cleft palate speech dissected: a review of current knowledge and analysis. *British Journal of Plastic Surgery*, **49**, 143–9.[DOI: 10.1016/S0007-1226(96)90216-7] [PubMed: 8785593]
An excellent article—recommended reading for any professional treating cleft children.

 References for this chapter can also be found at **www.oup.com/uk/orthodontics5e**. Where possible, these are presented as active links which direct you to the electronic version of the work, to help facilitate onward study. If you are a subscriber to that work (either individually or through an institution), and depending on your level of access, you may be able to peruse an abstract or the full article if available.

25

Orthodontic first aid

L. Mitchell

Whenever a patient presents with an orthodontic problem, the following points are important:

- Take a medical history.
- Take a full history of the 'problem'.

- If the patient is the patient of another operator, then a history of the treatment should also be taken.
- Do a thorough examination.
- When in doubt, seek expert advice.

25.1 Fixed appliance

See Table 25.1 for further information about fixed appliances.

Table 25.1 Fixed appliance

Patient's presenting complaint	Possible causes	Management	Learning points
Wire sticking out distally from molar tube/band	Ends of wire not trimmed	(1) NT round wires: cut leaving 1–2 mm, remove wire, flame ends, and turn-in (2) SS round wires: cut leaving 1–2 mm to turn-in (3) Rectangular wires: cut flush with distal aspect of tube (Fig. 25.1)	Always check with patient that ends are not sticking out before they leave chair
	Archwire has moved round	(1) Round wires: reposition archwire and turn ends in (2) Rectangular wires: reposition archwire and crimp hook or piece of tubing; or bond composite blob onto wire in convenient position	This is a particular problem with reduced friction bracket systems. Use a 'stop' (see 'Management' column) to prevent wire sliding round when using these systems
	In initial stages as teeth align, excess wire has moved distally through tubes	NT round wires: cut leaving 1–2 mm, remove wire, flame ends, and turn-in	
Wire sticking out mesial to molar	Ligature wire end turned out	Turn end in	
	Ligature wire has broken	Replace	
Bracket has detached from tooth	Bracket is in traumatic occlusion with opposing tooth	Consider these options: (1) Use a band instead of a bonded attachment (2) Place GI cement blob to either occlusal surface of molar teeth or palatally to upper incisors (depending upon overbite) (3) Fit a removable bite-plane appliance (4) Place an intrusion bend in wire in opposing arch (5) Leave off bond until further overbite reduction has been achieved	
	Archwire over-activated to engage bracket	Replace bracket and then place more flexible archwire to align tooth	
	Patient has knocked bracket off	Replace bracket in 'ideal position' on tooth. May need to drop down a wire size to fully engage bracket	Educate patient: (1) Reasons for avoiding hard foods (2) To avoid pen chewing
Band loose	Band is too big for tooth	Select correct sized band for 'snug' fit and cement in place	
	Patient is eating sticky foods/sweets	Remove any remaining cement and re-cement band	Educate patient about reasons for avoiding sticky foods
		When one band of a quad/TPA becomes loose it is necessary to remove the quad/TPA and re-cement both bands	

Table 25.1 Fixed appliance (*Cont.*)

Lost elastic module or wire ligature		Replace If tooth has relapsed, may need to drop down to more flexible archwire to re-align	
Teeth feel loose	A slight increase in mobility is normal during tooth movement	Check mobility of affected tooth/teeth. Reassure patient	Warn patient in advance that this is likely to happen
	Tooth in traumatic occlusion with opposing arch	Check occlusion. Consider these options: (1) Fit a removable bite-plane appliance (2) Place an intrusion bend in wire in opposing arch (3) Take steps to reduce overbite	
	Root resorption	(1) Take radiographs to check how many teeth are affected and to what extent (2) Discuss with patient (3) If limited—rest for 3 months before recommencing active tooth movement (4) If marked—? discontinue treatment	
Tooth/teeth are painful	Some discomfort is normal after fitting and adjustment of FA	Reassure patient. Advise proprietary painkillers	Warn patient in advance that this is likely to happen especially for first few days after fitting/adjustment
	Tooth/teeth in traumatic occlusion	Check occlusion. Consider the following: (1) Fit a removable bite-plane appliance (2) Place an intrusion bend in wire in opposing arch (3) Take steps to reduce overbite	
	Periapical pathology	(1) Take careful history (2) Check vitality (3) Check response to percussion (4) Take periapical X-ray If diagnosis confirmed, remove attachment from tooth and refer patient to their dentist for further management. If practicable, defer further active tooth movement until radiographic signs of apical healing	
	Periodontal problem	(1) Take careful history (2) Probe affected tooth/teeth (3) Take periapical radiograph If diagnosis confirmed, remove attachment from tooth/teeth and refer patient to their dentist for further management	
Nance bulb or quad digging into palate		(1) Reassess need to continue with nance/quad (2) If need to continue, remove and adjust so that no longer digging into palate	Use gentle forces to minimize strain on anchorage (excessive forces can result in forward movement of molars to which nance is attached)
Sheath soldered to band on molar for attachment of palatal arch or quad has detached	Often occurs due to patient factors (e.g. eating hard/chewy foods)	Remove palatal arch/quad and band. Re-solder new sheath and replace band and palatal arch/quad	Advise patient to avoid hard/sticky foods or 'fiddling' with arch/quad
Patient hit in/around mouth		(1) Take periapical radiograph of affected tooth/teeth, if root fracture, splint affected tooth/teeth with heavy archwire (2) If brackets knocked off, replace if moisture control possible (if not, defer for 1 week) (3) If archwire distorted, remove arch-wire and place light flexible archwire (4) If teeth displaced, attempt re-positioning and place light flexible archwire (5) Monitor vitality (6) Warn of risks of delayed concussion	

25.2 Removable appliance

See Table 25.2 for further information about removable appliances.

Table 25.2 Removable appliance

Patient's presenting complaint	Possible causes	Management	Learning points
Mouth watering	Inevitable when appliance first fitted. If persists usually reflects insufficient wear	Reassure patient and advise that it will resolve as mouth adapts to strange plastic object	Warn patient at time of fitting
Problems with speech	Inevitable when appliance first fitted. If persists usually reflects insufficient wear	Reassure patient and advise that it will resolve once mouth adapts to strange plastic object	Warn patient at time of fitting
Appliance loose	Appliance unretentive due to poor design	Consider adding additional clasps and/or a labial bow. If not feasible then re-make appliance with improved design	
	Clasps not retentive. NB: if patient habitually clicks appliance in and out the clasps flex and become less retentive	Adjust clasps	It is advisable to warn patients when fitting appliance not to click appliance in and out
Clasp fractured	Can occur if patient habitually clicks appliance in and out	Replace clasp (if working model not available will need new impression) Will need to fit repair as often some adjustment is required at chair-side	
Acrylic fractured (including bite-plane, buccal capping)		Check whether fractured portion needs to be replaced or not. If not, smooth fractured edge. If repair required, take new impression if working model not available. Will need to fit repair as often some adjustment is required at chair-side	
Redness on roof of mouth	Candida	(1) OHI and dietary advice (2) If marked infection or does not respond to (1), prescribe antifungal to be applied to fitting surface of appliance	
	Trauma from appliance components	Adjust as required	
Sore cracks at side of mouth	Angular cheilitis	(1) OHI and dietary advice (2) If marked infection or does not respond to (1), prescribe antifungal	

25.3 Functional appliance

See Table 25.3 for further information about functional appliances.

Table 25.3 Functional appliance (see also problems related to removable appliances)

Patient's presenting complaint	Possible causes	Management	Learning points
Appliance comes out at night	Appliance not retentive due to poor design	Consider adding additional clasps and/or a labial bow. If not feasible then re-make appliance with improved design	
	Clasps not retentive. NB: if patient habitually clicks appliance in and out, the clasps flex and become less retentive	Adjust clasps	It is advisable to warn patients when fitting appliance not to click appliance in and out
	Insufficient wear of appliance during day	Ask patient to increase daytime wear	

Table 25.3 Functional appliance (see also problems related to removable appliances) (*Cont.*)

Teeth and jaws ache	Common occurrence during initial stages of treatment	Reassure patient	Warn patient at time of fitting that this may occur

25.4 Headgear

See Table 25.4 for further information about headgear.

Table 25.4 Headgear

Patient's presenting complaint	Possible causes	Management	Learning points
Face-bow comes out of tubes at night		Adjust inner arms of face-bow	Advise patients at the time of fitting that if this problem does occur they should stop wearing the headgear and contact their orthodontist
Face-bow tipping down anteriorly and impinging on lower lip	If the force vector is below the centre of resistance of the molars they will tip distally	Adjust outer arms up to raise moment of force above centre of resistance of molar to counteract tipping	Ensure movement of force acting through centre of resistance of teeth at time of fitting and check at each visit
Face-bow tipping up anteriorly and impinging on upper lip	If the force vector is above the centre of resistance of the molars they will tip mesially	Adjust outer arms down to lower moment of force below centre of resistance of molar to counteract tipping	Ensure movement of force acting through centre of resistance of teeth at time of fitting and check at each visit

25.5 Miscellaneous

See Table 25.5 for miscellaneous further information.
See Fig. 25.2 for additional information on first aid.

Table 25.5 Miscellaneous

Patient's presenting complaint	Possible causes	Management	Learning points
Dentist fractures tooth during extraction leaving root fragment		(1) Take X-ray to investigate size of fragment (2) If large and/or will interfere with planned tooth movements, refer patient for removal of fractured portion (3) If small and/or does not interfere with tooth movements, keep under radiographic observation	
Appliance component missing? Inhaled or ingested		(1) If airway obstructed, call ambulance and try to remove obstruction (2) If there is a risk that the component has been inhaled then refer the patient to hospital for a chest X-ray and subsequent management (give patient another similar component to aid radiologist when examining films) (3) If there is a danger that the component is >5 cm and has been swallowed then seek the advice of the local hospital. If >6 days previously, object has probably passed through patient's system (see also Fig. 25.2)	

Table 25.5 Miscellaneous (*Cont.*)

Bonded retainer detached		If retainer not distorted and teeth still well aligned: (1) Isolate, etch, wash, and dry (2) Re-bond retainer with composite
		If retainer distorted and teeth still well aligned, either bend up new retainer at chair-side using flexible multistrand wire or take impression for laboratory to bond up new retainer
		If teeth have relapsed, discuss with patient whether to monitor or retreat
Bonded retainer partially detached		If remainder not distorted then re-bond to remaining teeth If remainder distorted then remove and place new bonded retainer
(1) Vacuum formed retainer ill-fitting *(2) Lost vacuum-formed retainer*		If tooth alignment has not relapsed, take impression for replacement retainer If teeth have relapsed, discuss with patient whether or not to make new retainer and monitor, or retreat
Mouth ulcers	Irritation from an orthodontic appliance may precipitate recurrent aphthous ulceration in a susceptible patient	Chlorhexidine mouthwash may help to reduce the associated discomfort and duration of the ulcers
Patient/parent questions need to extract		(1) Ask why patient/parent concerned—if due to process of extraction, explain and reassure (2) If due to concerns regarding perceived disadvantages of extractions—discuss rationale for treatment plan (3) Reassess if alternative approach can be used

FA, fixed appliance; GI, glass ionomer; NT, nickel titanium; OHI, oral hygiene instruction; Quad, quadhelix; SS, stainless steel; TPA, transpalatal arch; X-ray, radiograph.

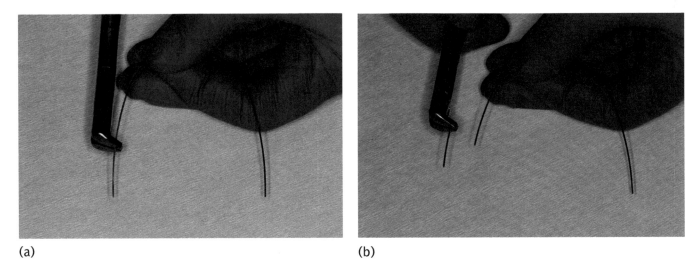

(a)   (b)

Fig. 25.1 The distal end cutting plier holds onto the cut end of wire to prevent injury. (a) Prior to cutting; (b) showing cut end held by cutter.

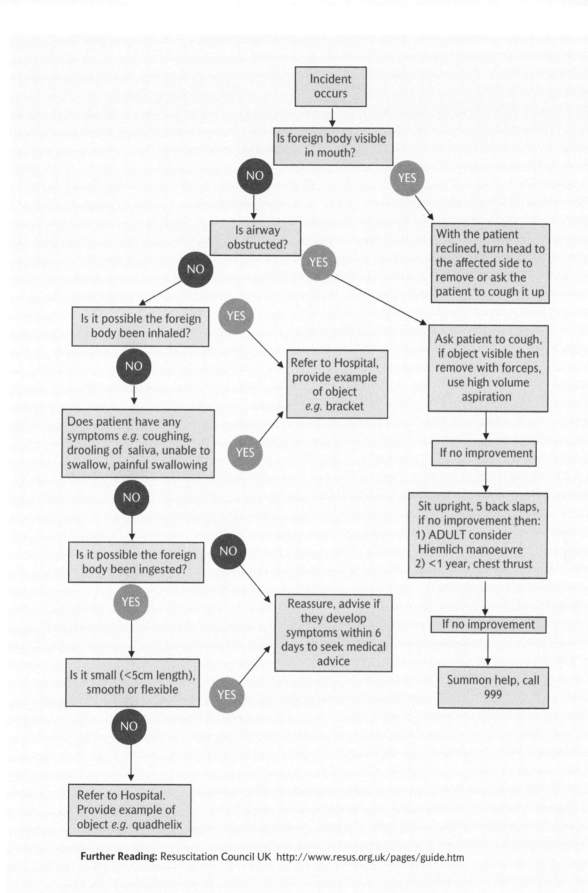

Further Reading: Resuscitation Council UK http://www.resus.org.uk/pages/guide.htm

Fig. 25.2 Flow diagram showing management of missing appliance component which may have been ingested or inhaled. Reproduced with the kind permission of the British Orthodontic Society.

Principal sources and further reading

Dowsing, P., Murray, A., and Sandler, P. J. (2015). Emergencies in orthodontics. Part 1: Management of general orthodontic problems as well as common problems with fixed appliances. *Dental Update* 2015, **42**, 131–40. [DOI: 10.12968/denu.2015.42.2.131] [PubMed: 26058226]

Dowsing, P., Sandler, P. J., and Murray, A. (2015). Emergencies in orthodontics. Part 2: Management of removable appliances, functional appliances and other adjuncts to orthodontic Treatment. *Dental Update* 2015, **42**, 221–8. [DOI: 10.12968/denu.2015.42.3.221] [PubMed: 26076540]
Two useful articles.

Definitions

Anchorage The resistance to unwanted tooth movement.

Angulation Degree of tip of a tooth in the mesiodistal plane.

Anterior open bite There is no vertical overlap of the incisors when the buccal segment teeth are in occlusion.

Balancing extraction Extraction of the same (or adjacent) tooth on the opposite side of the arch to preserve symmetry.

Bimaxillary dental proclination Both upper and lower incisors are proclined relative to their skeletal bases.

Bimaxillary dental retroclination Both upper and lower incisors are retroclined relative to their skeletal bases.

Bodily movement Equal movement of the root apex and crown of a tooth in the same direction.

Buccal crossbite The buccal cusps of the lower premolars and/or molars occlude buccally to the buccal cusps of the upper premolars and/or molars.

Centric occlusion Position of maximum interdigitation.

Centric relation The condyle is in its most superior anterior position in the glenoid fossa.

Cingulum plateau The convexity of the cervical third of the lingual/palatal aspect of the incisors and canines.

Clear aligner therapy Treatment provided by removable clear plastic appliances.

Compensating extraction Extraction of the same tooth in the opposing arch.

Competent lips Upper and lower lips contact without muscular activity at rest.

Complete overbite The lower incisors occlude with the upper incisors or palatal mucosa.

Crowding Where there is insufficient space to accommodate the teeth in perfect alignment in an arch, or segment of an arch.

Curve of Spee Curvature of the occlusal plane in the sagittal plane.

Dento-alveolar compensation The inclination of the teeth compensates for the underlying skeletal pattern, so that the occlusal relationship between the arches is less marked.

Ectopic tooth The tooth is in the incorrect position because it either developed in the wrong position or erupted into the wrong position.

Hypodontia This term is used when one or more permanent teeth (excluding third molars) are congenitally absent.

Ideal occlusion Anatomically perfect arrangement of the teeth. Rare.

Impaction Impeded tooth eruption, usually because of displacement of the tooth or mechanical obstruction (e.g. crowding or a supernumerary tooth).

Inclination Degree of tip of a tooth in the labiopalatal plane.

Incompetent lips Some muscular activity is required for the lips to meet together.

Incomplete overbite The lower incisors do not occlude with the opposing upper incisors or the palatal mucosa when the buccal segment teeth are in occlusion.

Intermaxillary Between the arches.

Intramaxillary Within the same arch.

Leeway space The difference in mesio-distal dimension between the deciduous canine, first molar, and second molar, and their permanent successors (canine, first premolar, and second premolar).

Lingual crossbite The buccal cusps of the lower premolars and/or molars occlude lingually to the lingual cusps of the upper premolars or molars. Sometimes referred to as a scissors bite.

Malocclusion Variation from ideal occlusion which might result in dental health and/or psychosocial implications for the individual. NB: the borderline between normal occlusion and malocclusion is contentious (see Chapter 1).

Mandibular deviation The path of closure of the mandible starts from a postured position.

Mandibular displacement When closing from the rest position, the mandible displaces (either laterally or anteriorly) to avoid a premature contact.

Midline diastema A space between the central incisors of >0.5 mm. Most common in the upper arch.

Migration Physiological (minor) movement of a tooth.

Normal occlusion Acceptable variation from ideal occlusion.

Overbite Vertical overlap of the upper and lower incisors when viewed anteriorly: one-third to one-half coverage of the lower incisors is normal; where the overbite is greater than one-half it is described as being increased; where the overbite is less than one-third it is described as being reduced.

Overjet Distance between the upper and lower incisors in the horizontal plane. Normal overjet is 2–4 mm.

Post-treatment changes Changes in tooth position after completion of orthodontic treatment as a result of relapse towards the original malocclusion and/or age changes.

Posterior open bite When the teeth are in occlusion, there is a space between the posterior teeth.

Relapse The return, following correction, of the features of the original malocclusion.

Reverse overjet The lower incisors lie anterior to the upper incisors. When only one or two incisors are involved, the term anterior crossbite is commonly used.

Rotation A tooth is rotated (twisted) around its long axis.

Settling Favourable changes in the occlusion after orthodontic appliances are removed at the end of treatment.

Spacing Where the teeth do not touch interproximally and there are gaps between adjacent teeth. Can be localized or generalized.

Tilting movement Movement of the root apex and crown of a tooth in opposite directions around a fulcrum.

Torque Movement of the root apex buccolingually, either with no or minimal movement of the crown in the same direction.

Traumatic overbite The occlusion of the incisors has caused ulceration to the mucosa in the opposing arch.

Uprighting Mesial or distal movement of the root apex so that the root and crown of the tooth are at an ideal angulation.

Orthodontic assessment form

Patient details	
Name	Referrer:
Address	
	Reason for referral
Tel Contact:	
Date of birth:	

History	
Patient's complaint	Habits
	Growth status
Motivation	Medical history
Dental history (including trauma and previous treatments)	
	Socio-behaviour factors

Extra-oral examination	
Anteroposterior	Smile aesthetics
Vertical	Soft tissues
Transverse	
	TMJ

Intra-oral examination		
Teeth present:	Lower arch	
Oral hygiene		
Periondontal health	Upper arch	
Tooth quality		
Teeth in occlusion		
Incisor relationship	*Molars* Right	Left
Overjet = mm	*Canines* Right	Left
Overbite	Crossbites	
Centrelines	Displacements	

Index